THE HORSE'S HEALTH FROM A TO Z

An Equine Veterinary Dictionary

Other books by Peter D. Rossdale
(not published by David & Charles)

Your Horse
The Horse from Conception to Maturity

THE
HORSE'S HEALTH
FROM A TO Z
An Equine Veterinary Dictionary

PETER D. ROSSDALE MA, FRCVS

AND

SUSAN M. WREFORD

ARCO PUBLISHING COMPANY, INC.
New York

Published by Arco Publishing Company, Inc.
219 Park Avenue South, New York, N.Y. 10003

Library of Congress Catalog Card Number 73-89678

ISBN 0 668 03414 9

Printed in Great Britain

CONTENTS

LIST OF ILLUSTRATIONS

PLATES

7

ACKNOWLEDGEMENTS

We would like to acknowledge many friends and colleagues who have helped with this book, in particular: Michael D. N. Hunt, MA, VetMB, MRCVS and Derek Thurlbourn for drawing the diagrams; Jenny Crossman and Elizabeth Wilson for help in preparing the manuscript; and Sidney W. Ricketts, BSc, BVSc, MRCVS for reading it in its final form.

We have also received much helpful advice from Raymond Hopes, BVMS, MRCVS, Colin K. Peace, MA, VetMB, MRCVS and Jack C. Sewell, BVSc, MRCVS (QDAH).

Figures 34 and 35 have been reproduced from *Lameness in Horses* by O. R. Adams, with the permission of the publishers Lea & Febiger, Philadelphia. Figures 5, 6, 7, 8, 13, 18, 19, 20, 29, 32, 36, 37 and 43 have been reproduced from Sisson & Grossman's *Anatomy of Domestic Animals* (W. B. Saunders & Co Ltd, Philadelphia) with the permission of Mrs L. C. Grossman.

INTRODUCTION
AND ETYMOLOGY

Veterinary language, especially that of the horse, is becoming increasingly difficult to understand. This is why we feel there is a need for an equine veterinary dictionary. We have tried to keep the book as simple as possible by defining diseases under their common names (though the medical ones are included for reference). In this way we hope the horse-owner will discover what his or her veterinarian means and the veterinary student will understand the terms used by horsemen, trainers and stud grooms.

Horsemen, for example, know about big leg; veterinarians call it lymphangitis; and to anyone in a trainer's yard it may be Monday morning leg.

Jargon in all walks of life causes barriers in communication. Professionals cannot converse freely with those who do not know the specialised terms they use; even within a profession groups of specialists can become isolated from one another. In compiling this book we aim to help reverse this trend as far as equine industries are concerned.

People are becoming more international in outlook. Whether they ride horses, train them, treat them or bet on them, they sometimes travel abroad to do so. It is not surprising then that there is a gradually emerging uniformity about words which can be spelt in more than one way.

In the dictionary we have taken a lead from America and in most cases have dropped diphthongs in the centre of words (eg anemia instead of traditional English anaemia). The policy extends to words such as hemorrhage (instead of haemorrhage), hemoglobin (for haemoglobin) and fetus for foetus.

However words in less common use, eg caecum, remain Anglicised. Traditional spelling is also retained when the choice of English or American occurs at the beginning of a word, eg oestrus not estrus. In any event, the reader will find English and American spellings cross-referenced, so should have little trouble finding the definition.

Although the book is intended primarily as a dictionary we have not resisted the temptation to expand on some entries. To save space for extra information we have eliminated many small words such as 'the' and are prepared for the style to be criticised as staccato. The following syllables should help the reader understand medical words:

a-/ab- or an-	negative or away from, as in abnormal
acou-	hear, as in acoustics
ad-	near, as in adrenal (near kidney)
adip-	fat, as in adipose tissue
-alg-	pain, as in analgesic (pain relieving) drug
anti-	against, as in anti-inflammatory
arthr-	joint, as in arthritis (joint inflammation)
articul-	joint, as in articulation
aur-	ear, as in auricle (flap of ear)
ba-	go, walk, as in abasia (faulty walking)
bacter-	small staff, rod, as in description of bacteria
bi-	two, as in bisexual
bi-/bio-	life, as in biochemistry
blast-	early stages of something growing, as in blastula
brachy-	short, as in brachydonty (having short teeth)
cardi-	heart, as in cardiologist (one who studies heart)
cav-	hollow, as in cavity
cephal-	head, as in encephalitis (inflamed brain or head)
cervic-	neck, as in cervical bones (vertebrae)
chondr-	cartilage, as in chondritis (inflamed cartilage)
-cid/e	kill, cut, as in bactericidal drug
contra-	against, as in contra-indicated drugs
crani-	skull, as in cranium
de-	down from, as in defecate
dent-	tooth, as in dentistry
derm-	skin, as in dermatitis (inflamed skin)
di-	two, as in diploid (having paired chromosomes)
dors-	back, as in dorsal vertebrae (bones of the back)
dys-	bad, as in dysfunction
ect-	outside, as in ectoderm (outer skin)
end-	inside, as in endometrium (uterus lining)
enter-	intestine, as in enteritis (inflamed intestine)
erythr-	red, as in erythrocyte (red blood cell)
extra-	outside, in addition to, as in extra-articular (outside a joint)
-facient	cause, as in abortifacient (agent causing abortion)
febr-	fever, as in febrile (characterised by fever)

gastr-	stomach, as in gastroenteritis (inflamed stomach)
glott-	tongue, as in epiglottis (cartilage at back of tongue)
helc-	ulcer, sore, as in helcoma (corneal ulcer)
hepat-	liver, as in hepatitis (inflammation of liver)
horm-	impulse, as in hormone
-itis	inflammation, as in carpitis (inflammation of knee)
lact-	milk, as in lactating mare
lapar-	flank, as in laparotomy (surgery into flank)
leuc-	white, as in leucocyte (white blood cell)
mal-	abnormal, as in malfunction
mening-	membrane, as in meningitis (inflamed membrane)
morph-	form, shape, as in amorphous (without shape, eg powdered drug)
ne-	young, as in neonate (foal)
neph-	kidney, as in nephritis (inflammation of kidneys)
neur-	nerve, as in neuron (nerve cell)
nutri-	nourish, as in nutrition
ophthalm-	eye, as in periodic ophthalmia (moon blindness)
or-	mouth, as in oral dose
-orchi-	testicle, as in cryptorchid (rig)
os-	bone, as in osteitis (inflamed bone)
pha-	say, speak, as in pharynx (voice box)
pharmac-	drug, as in pharmacology (science of drugs)
pharyn-	throat, as in pharynx
phleb-	vein, as in phlebitis (inflammation of vein)
pulmo-	lung, as in pulmonitis (inflammation of lungs)
ren-	kidneys, as in adrenal glands (glands near kidneys)
sarc-	flesh, as in sarcoid (a growth on skin)
thromb-	clot, lump, as in thrombus (blood clot in heart or blood vessel)
trache-	windpipe, as in tracheotomy (surgery through neck on windpipe)
vesic-	bladder or sac, as in vesicle (small blister on skin)

P.D.R. and S.M.W.

13

ABBREVIATIONS

Abbreviations most commonly used in the dictionary:

abbr.	abbreviation
approx.	approximately
C.	Centigrade
Ca	calcium
cf	compare
cm.	centimeter (100th of a meter) measure of distance
colloq.	colloquial/ly
cu. mm.	cubic millimeter
dim.	diminutive
E	East/ern
eg	for example
F.	Fahrenheit
Fr.	French
FSH	follicle stimulating hormone
gm./gms.	gram/s
gm./kg. body wt.	grams per kilogram body weight
Gr.	Greek
Hb	hemoglobin
Hg	mercury
ie	that is
IM	intramuscular/ly (by injection into muscle)
IU	international units
IV	intravenous/ly (by injection into vein)
L.	Latin
LH	luteinising hormone
μ (pronounced mew)	micron (measure of size)
ml.	millilitre (1,000th of a litre) measure of volume
mg.	milligram (1,000th of a gram) measure of weight
mμ	millimicron or micro μ (1,000th of a μ) measure of size
N	North/ern
neg.	negative
opp.	opposite
oz.	ounce
P	phosphorus
pl.	plural

Abbreviations

qv	which see
r.b.c.	red blood cell/s
S	South/ern
Sp.	Spanish
spp.	species
sub. cut.	subcutaneous/ly (by injection into skin)
syn./syns.	synonym/s
W	West/ern
wt.	weight

DICTIONARY

A

a-/an- Combining forms meaning negative.

ab- Combining form meaning away from.

abasia (a, neg.+Gr. basis, step) Inability to walk due to defect in co-ordination. **trembling a.** Quivering of legs. See neonatal maladjustment syndrome, cerebellar degeneration.

abdomen (belly, possibly from L. abdere, to hide) Body between chest and pelvis.

abdominal Of abdomen. **a. cavity** The area bounded by diaphragm in front, **a.** muscles below and at sides, spine and lumbar muscles above, pelvic outlet behind. Contains stomach and intestines (see alimentary canal), liver, kidneys, urinary bladder and sex organs. Enlarged in some colics, ascites, pregnancy. **a. sounds** See borborygmus.

abdominocentesis (abdomino + Gr. kentesis, puncture) Withdrawal of fluid through needle inserted into abdominal cavity.

abduct (ab- + L. ducere, to draw) Draw one part of body away from another, eg to **a.** a limb is to move it out of line as in some lamenesses.

aberrant (L. aberrans; ab, from + errare, to wander) Deviating from usual course, eg botfly larva's **a.** migration to equine brain (it usually stays in stomach).

ablate (L. ablatus, removed) Cut away or remove.

abort (L. aboriri, to miscarry) To expel fetus before it is viable. See abortion.

abortifacient (L. abortio + facere, to make) Substance which causes abortion, ie makes uterus contract.

abortion (L. abortio) Expulsion of fetus too underdeveloped to survive outside uterus; arbitrarily put at 300 days' pregnancy (after this usually termed premature birth). Signs of **a.** may be any or all of those at normal birth, although mammary development may be absent. A.

19

usually follows death of fetus but sometimes fetus may breathe and its heart begin to beat after delivery. **bacterial a.** Due to several types of bacteria, eg Streptococcus (most common in first 150 days), Escherichia coli (common at 150–300 days), Klebsiella, Salmonella abortus equi and, occasionally, Brucella abortus. **fungal a.** Due to fungus entering uterus through vagina when mare is in oestrus or after foaling. Fungus grows on placenta interfering with nourishment of fetus, causing **a.** usually at 200–300 days. Fungus may also enter fetal blood stream and cause lesions in liver and lungs. Diagnosis: on thickened placenta covered by brown exudate, white spots in lung and fungus in placenta. **physiological a.** That due to unknown cause, eg hormone deficiency in mare or fetus, chromosome abnormality resulting in faulty development, mare's poor diet, illness or excitement. **twin a.** That due to one twin dying and causing **a.** of the other. (Mare cannot easily carry twins to full term because uterus is not large enough for two placentae.) Mammary development with wax on teats and running of milk may start days or weeks before **a.**, probably on death of first twin. **viral a.** That due to virus, most commonly equine herpesvirus I (syn. rhinopneumonitis). The virus usually causes snotty nose in young horses but can cause **a.** without preliminary signs, singly or in epidemic form, from 6 months to full term. Diagnosis: on laboratory evidence of inclusion of bodies in nuclei of epithelial cells of liver and lungs. Virus can sometimes be grown in tissue culture. See plates 6 and 7.

abrasion (L. abrasio) Break in continuity of a body surface such as skin of mucous membrane. Usually caused by mechanical process, eg ill-fitting saddlery.

abscess (L. abscessus from ab-, away + cedere, to go) Cavity containing dead cells, bacteria and exudate (collectively called pus). May be acute, forming and bursting rapidly, or chronic, ie developing slowly and not bursting unless near body surface. Found in all tissues and organs. Causes: presence of foreign bodies, infection with bacteria or fungus, migrating parasitic larvae. See summer pneumonia, Corynebacterium, inflammation, sleepy foal disease, Staphylococcus, strangles, tuberculosis.

abscissa (L. ab, from + scindere, to cut) Horizontal line which, with ordinate (vertical line), is used as reference for recording data, as on a graph.

absorbefacient (L. absorbere, to absorb + facere, to make) Substance which promotes absorption. See dimethyl sulphoxide.

absorbent (L. absorbens from ab, away + sorbere, to suck) Medicine or dressing that promotes absorption, eg kaolin, cotton wool, gauze.

absorption (L. absorptio) Passage of fluid or substance into skin, mucous membranes, blood or lymph streams. See resorb.

acacia (Gr. akakia) Gummy exudate from stems and branches of Acacia senegal tree. Used as suspending agent or emollient in medicines, ointments.

acalcerosis Condition caused by lack of calcium in diet. See bones, diseases of.

acanthocyte (Gr. akankha, spiny + eidos, form) Abnormally-shaped red blood cell.

Acapron See quinuronium sulphate.

acariasis (Gr. akari, mite + iasis, a state of) Infestation with mites such as those causing mange, qv.

acataposis (a, neg. + Gr. kata, down + posis, drinking) Difficulty in swallowing. See grass sickness, choke.

accessory carpel bone One of 8 small bones of carpus (knee joint), placed behind and to outside of the other 7. In prominent position behind joint and may fracture, especially when jumping, causing lameness and pain. Diagnosis: on X-ray examination. Treat by screwing fractured part and resting for 6 months.

acclimatise To become used to new climate or management. Used in connection with horses travelling from one country to another.

acellular Not made up of cells, eg horn, hair.

acephalia See headlessness.

acepromazine maleate (trade name: Acetylpromazine) One of phenothiazine group of drugs. Used as tranquillisers before handling or anaesthesia.

acetabulum (in ancient Rome, cup to hold vinegar) Cup-shaped part of pelvis formed by ilium and ischium; receives head of femur to make hip joint.

acetic Of vinegar. Salt of **a.** acid is acetate.

acetonemia Rare condition of horses caused by acetone-like chemicals abnormally present in blood. (Common in cattle.)

acetylcholine Substance associated with transmitting nerve impulses; used to cause parasympathomimetic (qv) actions, eg stimulate alimentary canal in colic. See autonomic nervous system, carbachol.

Acetylpromazine Trade name. See acepromazine maleate.

acetylsalicylic acid (syn. aspirin) Colourless crystals or white granules. Odourless with slightly acid taste. Used to treat muscular pain, arthritis and reduce temperature, eg in setfast. May cause indigestion and hemorrhage if given repeatedly. Dose: 8–45gms.

Achromycin Trade name. See tetracycline hydrochloride.

acid (L. acidus from acere, to be sour) Sour, with properties the opposite of alkali. Compound that dissociates in aqueous solution to form hydrogen ions, turns litmus red and unites with bases to form salts. **a. base balance** Used in connection with buffering system of blood. Responsible for maintaining pH (qv) at about 7.40 units. **a. fast** Used in laboratory to denote that stained bacteria are colour fast in acid. **a. poisoning** See poisons.

acidemia (acid + Gr. haima, blood + –ia) Lowering of blood pH to below normal level of about 7.40 units.

acidosis Disturbance of acid base balance. **respiratory a.** Due to accumulation of carbon dioxide. **metabolic a.** Due to any acid other than carbon dioxide. See neonatal maladjustment syndrome.

acne (syns. contagious acne, Canadian pox, contagious pustular dermatitis, Staphylococcal dermatitis) Skin condition caused by infection with Corynebacterium pseudotuberculosis (Canadian pox) or Staphylococcus aureus. Small lumps develop in skin and form pimple, the top of which breaks, exuding pus. This mats with hairs and comes away as a scab, leaving moist, red area with small hole in centre. Staphylococcal infection tends to spread from central pustule and cause large raw areas. Often seen in yearlings when first saddled. Condition may be mistaken for ringworm, warble fly maggot or dermatophilus infection. (See separate headings.) Diagnosis: on finding organism in laboratory examination of pus and scabs. Treatment: apply antibiotic to sores and, in severe cases, also inject. Tack and grooming kit should be disinfected, especially girths and rubbers, horse should be isolated and not ridden.

aconite (L. aconitum, Gr. akoniton) Drug from dried root of Aconitum napellus (monkshood, wolfsbane, blue rocket). All parts of plant are poisonous and contain alkaloid aconitine. Previously used in liniments and for laminitis. **a. poisoning** Symptoms include colic, slowing of heart, muscular weakness, paralysis, dilated pupils, often resulting in death from asphyxia. No specific treatment.

acorn Fruit of oak tree. Can poison. See oak.

acou- Combining form meaning hear or of hearing.

acriflavine Orange-red crystalline odourless powder with acid taste. Used as antiseptic at 1 in 1,000 dilution.

ACTH See adreno-cortico-trophic hormone.

Acthar Trade name. See corticotrophin.

actino- (Gr. aktis, aktinos, a ray) Prefix meaning relation to a ray.

Actinobacillus Genus of micro-organisms of family Brucellaceae. Most common in horse is **A. equuli,** causal agent of sleepy foal disease.

active principle The substance responsible for effect of compound, eg morphine is **a.p.** of opium.

Actos Trade name. See corticotrophin.

acute (L. acutus, sharp) Sharp. In disease: having short, relatively severe course.

ad- (L. ad, to) Prefix meaning to, between, in addition to or near.

adaptation (L. adaptare, to fit) Adjustment to variations, eg newborn foal's **a.** to extra-uterine environment.

additive Something added, usually to diet, eg vitamin or mineral supplement.

adduct (L. adducere, to draw toward) To draw toward mid-line of a body or structure.

aden-/adeno- Combining form meaning gland.

adenitis Inflammation of a gland. See strangles, lymphangitis.

adenocarcinoma A tumour. See growth.

adenoma A tumour. See growth.

adenosarcoma A tumour. See growth.

adenovirus Virus causing upper respiratory tract disease. See virus.

adhesion (L. adhaesio, to stick to) Fibrous band abnormally joining two parts, eg between two loops of bowel following peritonitis (see colic); between tendon and tendon sheath; between iris and lens. See eye, diseases of: moon blindness. **a. healing** A scar.

adipo- (L. adeps, adipis, fat) Combining form meaning relationship to fat.

adipose (L. adiposus, fatty) Of fatty nature; fat.

adjustment Used in connection with newborn foals, eg normal or abnormal **a.** to extra-uterine environment. See neonatal maladjustment syndrome, behaviour.

adjuvant (L. adjuvans, aiding) Substance or drug which aids another. **Freund a.** (after Hungarian bacteriologist) Mixture of mineral oil and emulsifying agent used as vehicle for antigens of vaccine to increase immunising stimulus. Discontinued in horse influenza vaccine as it causes local reactions.

ad lib (abbr. L. ad libitum, at pleasure) Used in connection with feeding unlimited quantities.

administer To give drugs by various routes: through mouth (per os), through stomach, by injection (parenteral), under skin (subcutaneous), into muscle (intramuscular) or into vein (intravenous). See plate 25.

adrenal (L. ad, near + ren, kidney) In region of kidney. **a. glands** Two red-brown flattened organs about 10cm. long and 4cm. wide lying close to kidneys. They consist of capsule enclosing outer cortical layer and inner medulla. Glands are ductless and secrete hormones: outer layer, cortisol; inner layer, epinephrine (adrenaline).

Adrenalin Trade name. See adrenaline.

adrenaline (trade names: Adrenalin, Epinephrine) Substance secreted by medulla of adrenal gland. White or creamy-white crystalline odourless powder with slightly bitter taste. When injected causes rise in blood pressure (due to ability to constrict blood vessels and increase heart rate), dilation of pupils, inhibited movement of alimentary tract, formation of glucose from liver glycogen, sweating and fast breathing. Used locally to reduce bleeding by constricting blood vessel and, combined with local anaesthetics, to prevent rapid absorption from site of injection. Has no general action when given by mouth, so administered IV, 2–4ml. of 0.1% solution. See autonomic nervous system.

adreno- Prefix meaning relationship to adrenal gland.

adrenocortical Of cortex of adrenal gland.

adreno-cortico-trophic hormone (ACTH) Hormone secreted by anterior lobe of pituitary gland. It causes adrenal glands to produce cortisone. Synthetic ACTH injected to increase cortisone output for counteracting stress, shock, allergy, lymphangitis and oedema. Used in preference to cortisone which, if given repeatedly, may cause adrenal gland to cut its output.

adrenocorticotrophin See corticotrophin.

adult Mature or fully-grown horse, ie one over 5 years. See maturity, immaturity.

aerobic Describes bacteria able to grow only in oxygen. Cf anaerobic.

aerosol Solution of fine particles which can be atomised for sterilising, inhalation or spraying on to wounds, eg chlortetracycline hydrochloride.

afferent (L. ad, to + ferre, to carry) Conveying towards a centre, eg **a.** nerves convey impulses from periphery to central nervous system, ie brain and spinal cord. Cf efferent.

African horse sickness Acute or sub-acute virus infection endemic in Africa and present in Middle East and Asia since about 1960. It is spread by mosquitoes, not by direct contact. Horse family naturally affected (in horses mortality may reach 90%, donkeys are more resistant) but dogs, goats and other animals can be experimentally infected. There are 9 known strains of virus, which is present in blood tissues and internal organs; immunity against one strain will not necessarily protect against others. Strains can cause one of 4 types: horse sickness fever, pulmonary, cardiac and mixed. Each begins with fever reaching maybe 41°C. (105·8°F.). Horse sickness fever is mild, causing conjunctivitis, increased pulse rate and deep breathing, incubation 5–30 days. Pulmonary form characterised by acute oedema of lungs, fits of coughing and yellow discharge from nostrils. Breathing difficult and head and neck are distended. Finally animal chokes and appears to drown in its own secretions. Cardiac form incubates up to 3 weeks, fever develops slowly and persists longer than in pulmonary form. Swellings occur in head, neck and chest and small blood spots appear under tongue. There may be partial collapse, abdominal pain and restlessness. Recovery is more common than in pulmonary form. Mixed form common but often diagnosed only at post-mortem when heart and lung damage discovered. Often the result of double infection. Diagnosis: on symptoms and laboratory examination of blood. Immunity is produced by infection or vaccination, although vaccine must include all strains of virus to be effective. Control: vaccinate annually, kill mosquitoes, protect horses from being bitten. **A.h.s. vaccine, living** Mixture of several strains of virus weakened (attenuated) by repeated injection into mice. Used to protect against **A.h.s.** Injected in spring, 2–3 months before disease expected. Mares in advanced pregnancy should not be vaccinated and horses receiving first dose should be rested at least 3 weeks. Dose: 5ml. annually.

after-birth Fetal membranes consisting of placenta, amnion and cord (combined weight averages 15lb.). Normally expelled from uterus 10–140 minutes after foal has been delivered. Unlike cows, mares rarely eat **a.-b. a.-b., retention of** Fetal membranes retained longer than 10 hours after birth. May be serious (cause of infection). Treatment: palpation, prostaglandin. See birth. **a.-care** Special management and treatment of case following operation or illness. **a.-pains** Pain felt by mare following birth. Caused by contraction of uterus and expulsion of after-birth or birth hemorrhage, qv. Mare may roll violently and sweat.

agalactia (a, neg. + Gr. gala, milk + -ia) Failure of mammary glands to secrete milk. May affect mares who give birth to premature or stillborn foals. Cause unknown but probably related to hormonal disturbances. See mammary gland.

age Time lived. Measure of life dating from birth; best assessed by development and wear of teeth, qv. Some breeds take their official age from arbitrarily chosen registration date, eg Thoroughbred: 1 January (N hemisphere), 1 August (S hemisphere). In first year horse is called foal or weanling, second year a yearling, after seventh year it is termed aged. Life averages 20 years although 50 years has been recorded. See plates 27–9.

agglutination Reaction between bacteria and antibacterial substance (antibody) causing clumping of bacteria. Used in laboratory as test to identify bacteria. Also clumping together of any other cells, eg blood cells in the cross-matching of incompatible blood.

Agrazine Trade name. See phenothiazine.

air Colourless odourless gas of approx. 1 part oxygen, 4 parts nitrogen. Also contains ammonia, argon, carbon dioxide and organic matter.

alveolar a. That contained in air sacs of lungs. **a. passages** Tubes of head (nasal passages), larynx (voice box), trachea (windpipe), bronchi and small tubes of lung ending at air sacs (alveolae). **a. sac** See alveolus.

alae (pl. of ala) Cartilagenous plates which support entrance to nostrils. They consist of a broad lamina (qv) above and a narrow cornu (qv) below.

albinism (L. albus, white + -ism) Congenital absence of pigment in skin, hair and eyes. Complete **a.** rare in horses, usually confined to loss of pigment of iris so that dark area of pupil is surrounded by ring of white (wall-eyed). (See Albino, true.) Mating of albinos results in albino offspring but **a.** in only one parent produces coloured foal which, when inter-bred, has one-in-four chance of albino offspring. See Albino, coat colouring.

Albino Originally a colour, now developed to mean also a breed. **True A.** has pink iris to eye and entirely pink skin covered with white hair. Can be developed in almost any breed. Foundation sire of **A.** breed said to have been Old King, foaled in 1906 and believed to have been Arab-Morgan. Albinism may be aesthetically pleasing but must be suspect. Lack of pigment predisposes weakness, eg pink or blue eyes may have inferior vision. Pink skin, like white heels of coloured horses, tends to have low resistance to infection and is sunlight-sensitive. Popular as ceremonial and circus horse. Assn: American **A.** Assn, Inc, PO Box 79, Crabtree, Oregon (Zip no: 97335).

albumen See albumin.

albumin (L. albus, white) Protein found in animal and vegetable tissues; characterised by solubility in water and coagulation when heated; contains carbon, hydrogen, nitrogen, oxygen and sulphur. **A.** classed according to source of origin, eg egg **a.**, blood serum **a.**, milk **a.** As a food it is converted by digestion into suitable form for absorption into blood stream. **serum a.** That in blood. See blood tests.

albuminuria (albumin + Gr. ouron, urine) Albumin in urine. Sign of inflamed kidneys or damaged urinary tract, ie bladder, ureter, urethra. Affected horses usually lose condition. See cystitis, kidney disease.

alcohol (Arabic al-koh'l, something subtle) Colourless transparent volatile liquid. Used in laboratory to prepare and preserve anatomical and biological specimens, locally as antiseptic and astringent and sometimes given by mouth, as tonic, eg in beer/stout.

Alficetyn Trade name. See chloramphenicol.

alg- Combining form meaning pain.

algae (L. pl., seaweeds) Group of plants in which body is unicellular; includes seaweed and many fresh-water plants. Can be fed to horses, especially powdered seaweed, as source of iron and other minerals.

aliment (L. alimentum) Food or nutritive material.

alimentary canal/tract Colloq. guts, intestines or bowel. Tube extending length of body from lips to anus, in which digestion occurs. Various parts developed according to function and named in order—mouth, pharynx, gullet (oesophagus), stomach, small intestine, caecum, large colon, small colon, rectum. Last four parts (caecum, large and small colon, rectum) referred to as large intestine. Canal has three layers: an inner lining or mucous membrane containing digestive glands, middle muscular layer and outer peritoneal (qv) lining, except part from mouth to stomach and last part of rectum. Canal also receives products from salivary glands, liver, pancreas. It is suspended in abdomen by folds of peritoneum known as mesenteries, in which blood vessels pass to and from tube. Size and capacity of parts: gullet—1–2 meters; stomach— relatively small, 8–15 litres; small intestine—22 meters, 40–50 litres; caecum—1.25 meters, 25–30 litres; large colon—3–3.7 meters, 50–60 litres; small colon—3.5 meters; rectum—0.31 meters. See separate headings, colic.

alkali (Arabic al-qaliy, potash) Compound such as soda, potash, ammonia, which neutralises strong acids. Sodium bicarbonate used to treat bites, acid poisoning, diarrhoea and to counteract acidity of blood. **acid/a.** Measurement is written pH. See neonatal maladjustment syndrome. **a. disease** See selenium poisoning.

alkaloid (alkali + Gr. eidos, form) Substance found in plants. Usually has bitter taste and strong physiological action. Term also used for synthetic substances, eg procaine pethidine, which have actions similar to plant alkaloids. **A.**'s common in equine practice: arecoline, atropine, caffeine, cocaine, codeine, digitalin, digitoxin, ephedrine, ergometrine, heroin, hyoscine, hyoscyamine, morphine, physostigmine, pilocarpine, quinine, strychnine. See separate headings.

alkalosis Disturbance of acid base balance resulting in excess base or a deficit of acid or carbon dioxide. **metabolic a.** Excess base or deficit of any acid other than carbon dioxide. **respiratory a.** Increased breathing rate with too much loss of carbon dioxide.

allantoic fluid Brown or yellowish-brown waste fluid, formed partly by placenta and partly by fetal urine secreted by kidneys and passing through bladder and urachus; surrounds fetus but is separated from contact by amnion. Quantity at 45th day of pregnancy is 100ml.; at 100th day, 2,000ml.; at 300th day, 8,500ml. Contains flat rubber-like pad (hippomane, qv). Helps to protect fetus and lubricate birth canal at delivery. Escapes at beginning of 2nd stage labour when placenta ruptures. See birth: 2nd stage.

allantois (allanto, sausage + Gr. eidos, form) Outgrowth of hind gut of embryo which forms bladder, carries blood vessels in umbilical cord and later combines with chorion to form placenta. During development of foal, urine passes from fetal kidneys into bladder and then through urachus into sac formed by placenta. See allantoic fluid.

allele (Gr. allelon, of one another) One of two or more contrasting genes which determine inherited characters, eg size.

allergen (allergy + Gr. gennan, to produce) Substance which causes allergy; may be protein or non-protein. See antigen.

allergic Of allergy.

allergy Body's reaction to contact with, inhalation or ingestion of, antigen, qv. Form of sensitivity characterised by local reaction, eg rash or weals on skin. Horse injected with penicillin may suffer allergic reaction in form of filled legs and general malaise. Broken wind is allergic response to fungus which causes spasm of smooth muscle of small air passages (similar to asthma). Diseases caused by **a.** include hemolytic jaundice of newborn, purpura hemorrhagica, laminitis, nettle rash, photosensitisation, broken wind.

aloes Yellowish-brown or reddish-brown powder with nauseous bitter taste. Obtained from various species of aloe. Used as purgative, absorbed in small intestine and converted to anthraquinone derivatives which are carried in blood to large intestine where they increase gut movement (peristalsis) and intestinal secretions. Action usually limited to large intestine and may cause considerable griping. Takes 12–24 hours to produce effect which is helped by feeding bran mashes for 24–48 hours before dosing. Purging may last 3–24 hours. Dose: 10–15 gms. for horses up to 6 months; 15–20gms. up to a year; 20–25gms. up to 2 years; 25–30gms. 3 years and over. Drug now replaced by modern preparations such as danthron, qv.

alopecia Loss of hair. See bald.

alpha First letter of Gr. alphabet, written α. See globulin, prostaglandin, radiation. **a.-tocopherol** See tocopherol acetate.

Altan See danthron.

Alter Old Portuguese breed similar to Andalusian and probably developed from Minho.

alter Euphemism meaning to castrate.

alum (L. alumen; trade name: Stat) Colourless crystalline mass or white powder with sweetish taste. Used for astringent action in proprietary medicines for diarrhoea, in lotions with zinc sulphate to counter proud flesh and in toxoid preparations, eg tetanus toxoid. See lockjaw.

alveolae Pl. of alveolus.

alveolar Of an alveolus.

alveolus (L. dim. of alveus, hollow) Small sac-like cavity. **dental a.** Socket of teeth. **pulmonary a.** Minute air sac, many together form the inter-face between air and blood in lungs.

amaurosis (L. from Gr. amaurosis, darkening) Blindness without apparent lesion in eye, ie result of diseased optic nerve.

ambient (L. ambire, to surround) That which prevails. **a. temperature** That surrounding patient. See temperature, neonatal maladjustment syndrome.

amble See gait.

American Association of Equine Practitioners (AAEP) Route 5, 14 Hillcrest Circle, Golden, Colorado 80401. American equivalent of British Equine Veterinary Association, qv. **A. Quarter horse** Fast, strong breed with especially muscled-up hindquarters. Named **A.Q.h.** because first races in USA were over a quarter-mile. Descended mainly from English Thoroughbred stallion Janus, whose stock, mostly from Spanish mares, flourished in North Carolina and Virginia in the 1700s. A.Q.h. racing recently revived in States and type is popular for ranch work. Assns: **A.Q.h.** Assn, Amarillo, Texas; Western Horseman's Assn, c/o Mrs Hicks, Round Close, Yateley, Camberley, Surrey. **A. Saddle horse** Graceful breed, best examples being in USA. Now used primarily in show ring to display either 3 or 5 gaits, qv. Base of tail is vertical giving hair a fountain effect. This is achieved by nicking dock muscles and setting with a crupper (strap looped around base of tail and secured to saddle or roller). Breed influenced by English Thoroughbred, Morgan, Standardbred and, immediate forerunner, Kentucky Saddle horse. Assn: **A.S.h.** Breeders' Assn, 929 So. 4th Street, Louisville, Kentucky, USA (Zip no: 40203).

amino-acid Substance derived from digested protein.

ammonia (after Ammon, near whose temple in Libya it has been found) Pungent, water-soluble gas, NH_3. **a. solution** Clear colourless liquid with characteristic odour. Used to blister legs or, diluted, to relieve irritation from insect bites.

ammonium bicarbonate White crystals or fine powder with slight ammoniacal odour. Used to treat spasmodic or flatulent colic. Dose: 3–15gms. **a. carbonate** Drug with stimulant effect. **a chloride** White odourless powder with cool salty taste. Given by mouth to increase acidity of urine or as mild expectorant, qv. Dose: 3–15gms.

amnion Shiny transparent membrane surrounding fetus and containing amniotic fluid, qv. See plates 7, 11 and 12.

amnionitis Inflamation of amnion producing thickened membrane due to fungal or bacterial infection; may be associated with brown staining due to premature passing of meconium, qv.

amniotic fluid Clear colourless fluid surrounding fetus and containing acids, salts, cells and mucus; formed by fetal urine and secretion of amnion, volume increases from 120ml. to 3,600ml. during last 8 months of pregnancy.

amoeboid action Moving or eating like an amoeba, ie absorbing food by surrounding it, eg white blood cell.

amonium See ammonium.

amorphous (a, neg. + Gr. morphe, form) Having no definite form or shape; in pharmacy: not crystallised.

amphetamine (trade name: Benzedrine) Synthetic powder which stimulates nervous system. Occasionally used to increase respiration during anaesthesia. Can be used dishonestly as stimulant drug. See veterinary rules.

amphi- (Gr. amphi, on both sides) Prefix meaning on both sides; double.

amphiarthrosis (amphi- + Gr. arthrosis, joint) Form of articulation allowing little movement, the surfaces being connected by fibro-cartilage, eg vertebrae united by inter-vertebral fibro-cartilages (discs). See vertebra.

ampicillin (trade name: Penbritin) White micro-crystalline odourless powder with bitter taste. Synthetic penicillin particularly active against gram-positive and gram-negative bacteria. Given by mouth or injection. Dose: 10mg./kg. body wt. twice daily.

ampule (Fr. ampoule) Small glass container, usually used to store fluid drugs and sealed to preserve contents in sterile condition.

ampulla (L. a jug, pl. ampullae) Flask-like enlargement. **a. ductus deferentis** Enlargement in vas deferens, duct which extends from tail of epididymis to pelvic part of urethra; it is 6–8 ins. (15–20cm.) long and 1in. (2cm.) in diameter. There is no increase in lumen of tube but a

H.H.—C

thickening of wall due to numerous branched tubular glands. **a. of semi-circular canals** Enlargement at one end of the three semicircular canals in inner ear. **a. recti** Terminal part of rectum which is not surrounded by peritoneum.

amyloid (amylo-, starch + Gr. eidos, form) Abnormal material of complex nature, probably a glycoprotein, qv. May accumulate in abnormal quantities in various organs of body—particularly liver—causing amyloidosis disease. Can be a complication of wasting diseases such as glanders, strangles, tuberculosis.

ana- (Gr.) Prefix meaning upward, backward or repetition.

anabolism (Gr. anabole, a throwing up) The cells' conversion of simple substances into complex ones, eg food into protoplasm; building of muscle and generally putting on condition. Can be increased by injecting drugs. See steroids, anabolic. Cf catabolism, metabolism.

anabolite Product of anabolism.

anaemia See anemia.

anaerobe (an, neg. + Gr. aer, air + bios, life) Micro-organism that lives only in absence of oxygen. **facultative a.** Micro-organism able to live under either anaerobic or aerobic conditions. **obligate a.** Lives only in complete absence of oxygen, eg Clostridium tetani. See lockjaw.

anaerobic Growing only without oxygen.

anaesthesia Loss of sensation. **epidural a.** Injection of 5–15ml. of procaine or other local anaesthetic into epidural space, usually between 1st and 2nd tail (coccygeal) vertebrae. This blocks spinal nerves as they emerge from cord. Used for surgery of tail, vulva, anus, vagina, rectum, perineum; to repair recto-vaginal fistula and in difficult birth to eliminate excessive straining. **general a.** Where consciousness is lost. Used in major operations. A quick-acting barbiturate is given intravenously to cast horse into recumbency. Endotracheal tube (see volatile a. below) is inserted into windpipe and a. can be maintained for several hours, depending on time needed by surgeon. **local a.** Where effect is confined to a small area. Includes procaine injection into skin causing loss of sensation in that area. Used for stitching wounds, removing growths and simple operations, eg castration, Caslick (see separate headings). Can also be injected over nerve. See nerve block. **volatile a.** Gases such as chloroform, halothane, ether. Administered through mask or through closed circuit apparatus of tube in windpipe (endotracheal tube). A cuff around tube is inflated, sealing windpipe so that gas can be introduced into horse's air supply. See plate 25.

anaesthetic Agent which produces anaesthesia, qv.

anal (L. analis) Of the anus.

analeptic (Gr. analepsis, a repairing) Drug which stimulates central nervous system, eg amphetamine, caffeine. See veterinary rules.

analgesic (an, neg. + Gr. algesis, pain) Drug which relieves pain without causing unconsciousness. Pain from parts such as skin, muscles, bones, joints, responds to **a.**'s such as aspirin, phenylbutazone, oxyphenbutazone; pain from abdomen and alimentary tract, to pethidine and morphine derivates. Used in conditions such as setfast, pulled muscles, sprain, arthritis, colic.

analysis (ana- + Gr. lysis, dissolution) Determination of exact composition of substance or material. **qualitative a.** Nature of constituents. **quantitive a.** Proportion of constituent. See dope test.

anamnesis (Gr. anamnesis, a recalling) Collected medical history, ie previous abnormality or disease, date of appearance, duration.

anaphrodisia (an, neg. + Gr. Aphrodite, Venus + ia) Absence or loss of sexual desire.

anaphrodisiac Suppressing sexual desire; drug or treatment capable of this. See antiandrogen.

anaphylaxis (ana- + Gr. phylaxis, protection) State of shock produced experimentally or unintentionally, eg horse given foreign protein in transfusion of blood plasma may be sensitised by first administration and suffer **a.** on receiving second.

anasarca Accumulation of fluid in tissues below skin, particularly on wall of abdomen and chest. Caused by heart failure, allergy, malnutrition and septicemia.

35

anastomose To communicate, as in arrangement of arteries and veins which allows blood to flow past an obstruction, eg if one artery supplying foot is severed, other arteries **a.** so that blood flow to area is not restricted; in surgery portion of intestine can be removed (eg to correct a twist) and ends of gut anastomosed so that continuity is re-established. See twist.

anatomist One concerned with, or skilled in, anatomy. See conformation.

anatomy (ana- + Gr. temnein, to cut) Science of body structure and relationship of its parts. Knowledge of **a.** is based on dissection of body. **comparative a.** Comparison of different species. **morbid a.** That of diseased organs and tissues. **veterinary a.** That of domestic animals.

Andalusian Breed named after district of Spain. Influenced many breeds, including Criollo, Frederiksborg, Lipizzaner, Neapolitan and Friesian. Generally noble-looking with thick mane, although in Portugal a slighter type is used in bullfighting to jump away from bull. **A. Carthusian** Descended from those **A.** horses bred by monks in Carthusian monasteries in Jerez and Seville. **A. Thoroughbred** Fine-looking riding horse, usually grey. **A. Zapatero** Descended from **A.** horses bred by Zapata family, now bred privately and at military stud in Cordova. Usually grey.

andr-/andro- (Gr. aner or andros, man) Combining form meaning relationship to male.

androgen (andro- + Gr. gennan, to produce) Any male hormone. Produces masculine characteristics, eg testosterone. Cf antiandrogen. See sex hormones, male.

androsterone An androgen in urine of both sexes which carries male characteristics. Can be injected to help restore libido of gelding.

anemia (Gr. an, negative + haima, blood) Deficiency of red blood cells (erythrocytes) and hemoglobin per unit of blood. Normal r.b.c. count is 7–8 million per cu.mm. and Hb 14gms. per 100ml. Figures indicating **a.** would be 3–6 million r.b.c. per cu.mm. and 8–12gms. per 100ml. Signs might be pale mucous membranes and increased rate and force of heart beat. **A.** is due to: (1) loss of blood as a result of rupture of a vessel, external or internal bleeding (see hemorrhage); (2) increased destruction of r.b.c. (hemolytic **a.**) due to infection with bacteria, virus (see swamp fever), protozoa (see biliary fever), poisoning, immunological reaction (see hemolytic jaundice); (3) nutritional deficiency—bone marrow may cut output of r.b.c. and/or Hb due to deficiency of iron, copper cobalt or folic acid, or as a result of a generalised infection with toxin-producing bacteria such as Streptococci, E. coli. **A.** classed as normocytic, microcytic or macrocytic according to size of red cells; or normo-, hypo- and hyperchromic according to concentration of hemoglobin in each cell.

aneurine/a. hydrochloride (syns. thiamine hydrochloride, vitamin B_1) White crystalline powder with meat-like odour and bitter taste. Made synthetically, from rice polishings or yeast. Forms part of enzyme system essential for metabolism of carbohydrate. Deficiency causes acids to accumulate in tissues and a reduced absorption of glucose from gut. (Deficiency is rare as **a.h.** widely distributed in foodstuffs.) Used to treat bracken poisoning and said to have quietening effect in high doses. Dose: 100mg. daily by mouth or injection; as antidote: 50–100mg. sub. cut.

aneurysm Collapse of artery wall due to weakness caused by disease. **parasitic or verminous a.** That caused by migrating redworm larvae. Occurs in artery supplying intestines (anterior mesenteric). It may set up inflammation of artery (arteritis), causing blood to clot and stick to lining of vessel (thrombus), resulting in death; or blood clot may break into small parts which get carried in blood stream (see embolus) until they lodge in a vessel, blocking blood supply to part of gut. Peritonitis and colic (verminous colic) follow. Treatment: workers are trying to (1) perfect drug that will disperse blood clots, (2) find way of pinpointing clots, so they can be surgically removed. Prevention lies in controlling the parasite. See redworm. Cf ulcerative enteritis.

angina Feeling of suffocation and acute stabbing pain in humans, caused by lack of oxygen to heart muscle, also known as **a. pectoris.** Not known if horses feel it.

angioma (Gr. angeion, vessel + -oma) Tumour formed of blood vessels. See growth.

angle (L. angulus) Point of intersection of two borders or surfaces. **a of**

37

jaw Junction of horizontal and vertical of maxilla or lower jaw. See Arab.

angleberry Wart-like growth on skin. See growth.

Anglo-Arab Recognised cross of Thoroughbred/Arab. Popular as hack and hunter and to cross with pony breeds for children. To qualify for A.A. stud book, horse must be (1) produce of horse in Arab stud book or General Stud Book (Arabian Section) and horse in GSB (not Arabian section); (2) direct descendant of horses eligible as in (1); (3) bred abroad, entered in the country's stud book and accepted by Arab Horse Society, body controlling breed in England. Breed flourishes in France through Arab and Thoroughbred stallions of National Stud in Normandy (Le Haras du Pin, Orne). They lead premium (qv) lives, serving a few hundred mares in SW France. Assn: Arab Horse Soc. See Arab.

Anglo-Norman Three main types: draught, cavalry, trotter. Hybrid of latter two now being developed especially around Caen, Orne, for show-jumping. Originally developed in Normandy, France as powerful war horse. William the Conqueror said to have imported many into England. Breed deteriorated when haphazardly crossed with Mecklenburg and Danish cart horses. Later Arab, Thoroughbred and Norfolk trotter blood introduced, resulting in **A.N.** trotter, hardy type who tended to pull loads at the trot. Draught type, usually grey, developed with Percheron and Boulonnais strains and formerly used to pull mail carts. Cavalry type used by army and for sport.

anhidrosis (an, neg. + Gr. hidros, sweat + -osis) Lack of sweat. See dry coat.

anhydrase Enzyme concerned in removing water from a compound. **carbonic a.** Helps decompose carbonic acid into carbon dioxide and water, aiding transfer of carbon dioxide from tissues to blood and alveolar air.

animal nursing auxiliary Lay assistant who has passed examination set by Royal College of Veterinary Surgeons; diploma designated RANA.

Animycetin Trade name. See chloramphenicol.

aniso- (Gr. anisos, unequal, uneven) Combining form meaning unequal or dissimilar.

anisocytosis (aniso- + Gr. kytos, hollow vessel + -osis) Having red blood cells (erythrocytes) of unequal size.

ankylosis Abnormal fusion of joint surfaces. See arthritis.

anode (Gr. ana, up + hodos, way) Positive pole of galvanic battery or electric source. Cf cathode.

anodyne (an, neg. + Gr. odine, pain) Drug or medicament that relieves pain, eg atropine, codeine, hyoscine, morphine, pethidine. See colic.

anoestrus Sexual inactivity, usually in mares during winter. See oestrous cycle.

anophthalmia (an, neg. + Gr. ophthalmos, eye) Absence of both eyes. Rare cogenital fault requiring destruction on humane grounds. In some cases minute vestiges of eyeball are present (microphthamia).

anorchid (an, neg. + Gr. orchis, testis) Male without either testis in scrotum. See rig.

anorexia Complete absence of appetite. See appetite, lack of.

anorgasmy (an, neg. + orgasm) Failure to ejaculate. See behaviour, male sexual.

anovular Not accompanied by discharge of an ovum, eg occasionally, mare's oestrous period. See oestrous cycle.

Anovulin Trade name. See hydroxymethylprogesterone.

anoxemia (an, neg. + oxygen + Gr. haima, blood) No oxygen in blood.

anoxia Absence of oxygen.

antacid Drug which corrects excessive acidity of gut, eg bicarbonate.

antagonism (Gr. antagonism, struggle) Opposing, as between muscles, medicines, eg groups of muscles such as flexors and extensors of limb said to be antagonistic to one another; one type of antibiotic may be antagonistic to another, each reducing the other's capacity to kill bacteria, eg penicillin and Chloromycetin.

ante- (L., before) Prefix meaning before in time or place, eg **a.**-natal, before birth.

Antepar Trade name. See piperazine salts.

anterior A position which is forward, in front of or towards the head end of body, eg shin is anterior aspect of cannon bone. Descriptions of markings use **a.**, eg bay with white off-pastern extending to **a.** aspect of fetlock. Cf posterior.

antero-posterior From front to back, eg. X-ray beam said to be **a.p.** when machine is in front of, and photographic plate behind, limb.

anthelmintic (ant- + Gr. helmins, worms; syns. worm powders, vermicide, vermifuge) Drug or substance which kills intestinal parasites (worms). Usually given in feed or by stomach tube. Acts only on those parasites in alimentary canal, not on larval forms which migrate through organs and blood vessels. In common use in horses: piperazine salts (seatworm and whiteworm), levamisole hydrochloride (lungworm), dichlorvos, phenothiazine, pyrantel tartrate, thiabendazole (redworm).

anthrax (Gr. anthrax, coal, carbuncle) Infectious notifiable disease (see veterinary rules, Ministry of Agriculture). Rare in horse and man, caused by anthrax bacillus. More common in cattle and sheep.

anthropo- (Gr. anthropos, man) Combining form meaning relationship to humans.

anthropozoonosis Disease transmitted between man and animal; in the horse: glanders, encephalomyelitis.

anti- Combining form meaning against, eg in antidote.

antiabortifacient Drug given to prevent abortion, eg progesterone, luteinising hormone.

antiandrogen Any hormone which reduces effect of an androgen, ie decreases masculinity.

antibacterial Killing bacteria; drug or substance which does so, eg antibiotics, sulphonomides.

antibiotic (anti- + Gr. bios, life) Substance or drug which kills or inhibits multiplication of bacteria. **bacteriocidal a.** One which kills bacteria, eg neomycin, penicillin. **bacteriostatic a.** One which reduces growth and reproduction of bacteria, eg chloramphenicol (Chloromycetin), chlorotetracycline hydrochloride (Aureomycin), oxytetracycline (Terramycin), tetracycline (Achromycin). **A.** may have both -cidal and -static powers, eg Streptomycin. **broad spectrum a.** Effective against wide range of bacteria, eg neomycin, Chloromycetin. **fungicidal a.** Effective against fungal organisms, such as those causing ringworm and uterine infections, eg nystatin. Any **a.** may cause side-effects such as allergy, filling of legs, loss of appetite, persistent diarrhoea.

antibody Substance produced by body as a result of an antigen, and which reacts specifically with that antigen. **A.** is classed according to its action, ie anti-enzyme, antitoxin, bacteriolysin, hemolysin, agglutinin, blood group **a.**

anticoagulant Substance which prevents clotting of blood, eg sodium acid citrate. 120ml. of solution containing 2% sodium acid citrate and 2.5% dextrose prevents clotting of 400ml. of blood (such as when collected for transfusion).

anticonvulsant Substance or drug which stops or relieves convulsions. Used to treat newborn foals. See Mysoline, Epanutin and neonatal maladjustment syndrome.

antidiarrhoeal Drug or substance that combats diarrhoea.

antidiuretic hormone Hormone secreted by posterior pituitary. Reduces amount of urine formed by acting on kidney tubules, causing them to resorb greater quantities of water. Hormone release is reduced by cold, pain, changes in fluid balance of blood, chemical agents.

antidote (L. antidotum, from Gr. anti, against + didonai, to give) Substance used to combat effect of poison. See poisons.

antifungal Substance which kills or suppresses reproduction and growth of fungus. See antibiotic, ringworm, fungus.

antigen Substance, usually a protein, which stimulates body's production of antibodies (immune bodies). Can be bacteria, virus, blood corpuscles, serum or toxin.

antigen/antibody reaction Result when antigenic material contacts antibody in tissues or in laboratory experiment. Includes agglutination, precipitation, hemagglutination, complement fixation, neutralisation.

antigenicity Potency of an antigen, qv.

antihemorrhagic Stopping hemorrhage; drug that prevents or stops it. See coagulation, bleeding.

antihistamine Drug that counteracts action of histamine, eg promethazine hydrochloride, corticosteroids.

anti-inflammatory Reducing inflammation (qv); drug, substance or process which reduces or suppresses it. Those in common use in equine practice: Butazolidin (phenylbutazone), Tanderil (oxyphenbutazone), corticosteroids, cold water, ice packs.

antipruritic Drug which allays itching and local irritation.

antipyretic Temperature-reducing; drug with this action, eg pethidine hydrochloride, salicylate (aspirin), quinine (rarely used in equine medicine). Acts by reducing production of heat or increasing its loss.

antisepsis (anti- + Gr. sepsis, putrefaction) Prevention of sepsis or putrefaction by inhibiting or destroying a micro-organism. See antiseptic.

antiseptic Preventing decay; drug or substance which does so by controlling, not necessarily killing, micro-organism. Cf disinfectant. (See benzalkonium chloride solution.) **a. poisoning** Result of contaminated water or accidental administration. Symptoms include convulsions, coma, shock. Treatment: give soothing substances (demulcents), saline (intravenously) and corticosteroids.

antiserum Serum that contains antibodies. Prepared by injecting horse or other animal with specific antigen so that large quantities of antibodies circulate in blood. This is then purified in laboratory to concentrate the antibody required. See tetanus toxoid, antigen, antibody.

antispasmodic Preventing spasms, eg of painful, overactive gut. Drug that does so.

antitetanic Preventing tetanus; drug that does so. See lockjaw, tetanus toxoid.

antitoxin (anti- + Gr. toxicon, poison) Counteracting the action of toxin; substance (antibody) that does so.

antiviral Drug or substance which destroys viruses or suppresses their growth. Not available for use on horses. See interferon. Cf vaccine.

Antoban Trade name. See piperazine salts.

Antostab Trade name. See serum gonadotrophin.

Antrycide sulphate Trade name. See quinapyramine sulphate.

Antuitrin S Trade name. See chorionic gonadotrophin.

anuria (an, neg. + Gr. ouron, urine) Little or no excretion of urine. Caused by lack of kidney secretion due to low fluid intake, excess sweating, obstructed urinary passage (see stone) or ruptured bladder. See bladder, rupture of.

anus Terminal part of alimentary tract. Sphincter muscle which keeps feces in rectum. Is normally tense, but may become relaxed in diarrhoea. Is sometimes torn by forelegs of foal (see rectovaginal fistula). Should be noted for signs of parasite infestation (see seatworm).

aorta Trunk of main artery beginning at base of left ventricle. It passes upwards and forwards, then curves sharply backwards to reach spine at 8th or 9th thoracic vertebra; passes backwards underneath spine, lying first between the lungs, then passing through diaphragm to enter abdomen, where it divides, under the 5th or 6th lumbar vertebra, into two common iliac arteries. May rupture causing fatal hemorrhage if its walls are weakened by redworm larvae or long-standing nutritional disturbance. See plate 36.

aortic Of the aorta. **a. arch** See arteries, table of. **a. semilunar valve** Three semilunar cusps, each with a nodule on the free edge. Valve opens during contraction of heart, allowing blood to pass from left ventricle into aorta. It closes as heart relaxes, preventing blood from returning. Closure of valve forms part of 2nd heart sound. May be infected by bacteria or redworm larvae (see endocarditis). Inefficiency of action is termed incompetence, and hardening of cusps (with consequent narrowing of the opening), stenosis. See plate 36.

apathy Loss of interest in surroundings. Sympton of many illnesses especially those involving fever and pain.

apex Pointed extremity or top of an organ or part, eg **a.** of heart.

aphonia (a, neg. + Gr. phone, voice) Loss of voice, as caused by Hobday (qv) operation. Rarely congenital.

aphtha Small ulcer. See stomatitis.

apices (L.) Pl. of apex.

apnoea (a, neg. + Gr. pnoia, breath) Cessation of breathing, eg in asphyxiated newborn, during anaesthesia or in disease, when it may follow periods of rapid breathing. **terminal a.** State where heart beats but breathing stops. Horse will die in minutes without emergency measures. See neonatal maladjustment syndrome.

apo-, ap- (Gr. apo, from) Prefix meaning separation or derivation.

apocrine (Gr. apokrinestha, to be secreted) Glandular secretion which is concentrated at one end of secreting cell then thrown off, eg milk from mammary gland. Cf holocrine and merocrine.

apoplexy (Gr. apoplexia) Condition associated with acute vascular lesions of brain, ie hemorrhage, thrombosis or embolism; marked by coma and paralysis. Rare in horses although similar signs found in newborn foals or adults with head injuries. See cerebellar degeneration.

apothecary (Gr. apotheke, storehouse) One who prepares and dispenses drugs.

Appaloosa (spotted horse) Probably exported from Near East or Spain to Mexico about 1600 and named from breed developed by Indians of Palouse area of Washington State, N America. Now found in most parts of world, popular as circus, drum and saddle horse. Body pink-skinned with predominantly white hair, spotted black or brown, the pattern often strikingly regular over quarters. Whatever the coat's appearance, **A.** strain easy to identify by feeling raised skin patches and noting patterned hoofs, possibly with vertical stripes. Some Arab blood present. Assns: **A.** Horse Soc., c/o Col V. D. S. Williams, East Burnham Park, Farnham Royal, Buckinghamshire; British Spotted Horse Soc.; **A.** Horse Club (America).

appetite (L. appetere, to desire) Conditioned reflex depending on past associations (hunger describes sensation from stomach movements caused by lack of food). **A.** decreases in dehydration, fluid imbalance, overwork, nervous tension, fever. Can be increased by drugs such as anabolic steroids and possibly tonics, most of which contain vitamins A, B_1 and B_{12} and minerals including iron, copper, cobalt, manganese and strychnine. **depraved a.** (pica) Desire for substance not classed as food, eg tree bark, soil, dung, after-birth. May be result of mineral or other deficiency, of boredom or of physiological upset, eg if horse is given antibiotic it may nibble feces to replace intestine's natural flora. (Fresh dung can be mixed with water and given by stomach tube.) **lack of a.** (anorexia) Occurs in colic and severe illness and is usually a sign of ill-health.

aprosopia See facelessness.

Aqua Mephyton Trade name. See concentrated vitamin K solution.

Arab/Arabian Breed thought to be the oldest (it was bred in Asia, more than 5,000 years ago). Later developed as it is today by jealously guarded breeding in Arabian desert, where there were 5 strains of Asil or pure-bred **A.**, most widespread being Kuhaylan. (Word comes from kuhl, a paint women used around their eyes, the connection being that **A.** has dark, kuhl-coloured skin—though the coat may be almost any colour.) **A.** has great beauty, high spirits, proud carriage, long mane and tail, wide, deep-angled jaw and dished profile with

45

large, low-set eyes. Darley A. (imported 1704 and bred by Anazeh tribe on fringe of Syrian desert) is ancestor of majority of Thorough-breds. Breed seems to be only one which suffers cerebellar degeneration. Assns: **A.** Horse Soc., 32 St James's Place, London SW1; Secretary: Lt.-Col J. A. Denney, Sackville Lodge, Lye Green, Crowborough, Sussex (Crowborough 5448). **A.** Horse Club Registry of America, 332 So. Michigan Ave, Chicago, Illinois (Zip no: 60604).

Arachnida Class of Arthropoda which includes marine kingcrabs, scorpions, spiders, parasitic ticks, mites and all their relatives. Those important in equine veterinary medicine: sub-class Euarachnida, order Acarina, sub-order Ixodides, family Ixodidae (see ticks), sub-order Trombidiformes, genus Demodex (see mange) and genus Trombicula (see harvest mite), sub-order Sarcoptiformes, family Oribatidae (see oribatid mite and tapeworm), family Sarcoptidae, genus Sarcoptes (see mange), family Psoroptidae, genus Psoroptes (see mange) and genus Chorioptes (see mange).

arc (L. arcus, bow) Part of circumference of a circle. **reflex a.** Term describing route of nervous impulse reflex, eg from skin to central nervous system and returning to muscle, as in reaction to pin-prick.

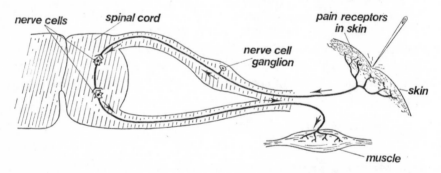

1 Reflex arc (or nervous pathway); impulse is transmitted from skin to spinal cord and back to muscle, causing it to contract

arch (L. arcus, bow) Anatomical term, eg aortic **a.**, part of aorta from heart to beneath spine.

ARCS Abbr. Associate of the Royal College of Science.

Ardennes Breed originally from **A.** mountains and area spanning French/Belgian border. Old-established, hardy type used by Napoleon's cavalry and in World War I. Crossing with Brabancon breed has produced some draught families, while other strains are 14–15 hands. Especially popular in Sweden, where they make up more than half the horse population.

arecoline hydrobromide White crystalline odourless powder with bitter taste. Alkaloid obtained from seeds of Areca catechu. Contracts involuntary muscle, eg in alimentary tract, uterus and air passages; contracts pupils, slows heart rate and stimulates salivary glands. Action reversed by atropine. Dose: 15–60mg. by injection as a purgative to treat impacted colic. See colic.

areola (L. dim. of area, space) Minute space in tissue. **a. tissue** Special cells which fill spaces between muscles or under skin.

arrhythmia (a, neg. + Gr. rhythmos, rhythm) Irregular heart beat or rhythm, eg dropped beat. Diagnosed by electrocardiogram but can be heard with a stethoscope. **sinus a.** Disturbed SA (sino-atrial) node. See electrocardiogram.

arsenic Medicinal forms include Fowler's and Donovan's solutions, now rarely used. A. tends to accumulate in liver and is slowly released to other tissues. Toxicity varies with solubility but in massive doses it causes rapid death. Symptons include abdominal pain, staggering, collapse and paralysis; in less acute cases: salivation, thirst, diarrhoea (sometimes bloodstained), exhaustion, loss of appetite, trembling and subnormal temperature. At post-mortem: acutely inflamed alimentary tract; swollen mucous membranes which come away when rubbed. Diagnosis: symptons confirmed by urine analysis; at post-mortem liver is most useful material for chemical analysis. Treatment: saline purgative followed by kaolin. Sodium thiosulphate 10gms. in 100ml. water IV and 30gms. in about 300ml. of water by mouth.

arteritis See equine viral arteritis.

arterial Of an artery.

arteriole (L. arteriola) Minute artery leading from larger artery to capillary, qv.

arteriosclerosis Hardening of artery walls.

artery (L. and Gr. arteria, from aer, air + terein, to keep, because **a.**'s were once thought to hold air) Tube forming part of system which conveys blood to all parts of body. Has thick walls of elastic tissue and muscle formed of outer coat (adventitia), middle coat (media) and inner coat (intima). It carries bright red blood (due to high oxygen content) at high pressure, in contrast to vein or capillary. Most **a.**'s divide and branch until they end in arterioles. For main ones see **a.** table.

TABLE OF MAJOR ARTERIES

Part	Artery	Origin	Area of supply or continuing artery
chest	coronary (right & left)	aorta	heart muscle
chest	pulmonary	right ventricle	lungs
chest/ abdomen	aorta	left ventricle	all parts of body other than lungs
chest	common brachiocephalic	branch of aorta	forelegs, head and neck
chest	brachiocephalic	brachiocephalic trunk	head, neck and right foreleg
head & neck	occipital	common carotid	brain and spinal cord
head & neck	internal carotid	common carotid	brain
head & neck	external carotid	common carotid	upper jaw, pharynx, tongue, lips, face, eyes and ears
head & neck	internal maxillary	external carotid	lower jaw, meninges, eyelids, nasal passage and palate
right foreleg	brachial—right	brachiocephalic	right foreleg
left foreleg	brachial—left	common brachiocephalic trunk	left foreleg
forelegs	brachial	brachiocephalic and common brachiocephalic	shoulders and forelegs
forelegs	median	brachial	forelegs below elbow

Part	Artery	Origin	Area of supply or continuing artery
forelegs	common digital	median	medial and lateral digital
forelegs	medial and lateral	common digital	forelegs below fetlock
hindlegs	femoral	external iliac	popliteal **a.**, belly muscle, udder, penis, stifle region, muscles of hindquarters
hindlegs	popliteal	femoral	stifle joint, muscles at bases of 2nd thigh, hock, cannon bone and lower part of leg
hindlegs	common plantar	popliteal	medial and lateral plantar **a.**
hindlegs	medial and lateral **plantar**	common plantar	hindlegs below fetlock
chest	thoracic aorta	ascending aorta	oesophagus, intercostal muscles, substance of lungs
abdomen	abdominal aorta	thoracic **aorta**	contents of abdominal cavity
abdomen	anterior mesenteric	abdominal aorta	small intestine, caecum, part of large colon
abdomen	renal (left & right)	abdominal aorta	kidneys
abdomen	posterior mesenteric	abdominal aorta	colon and rectum
genital organs	internal spermatic (male) (left & right)	abdominal aorta	spermatic cord and testes
genital organs	utero-ovarian (left & right)	abdominal aorta	ovaries and uterus
back	lumbar	abdominal **aorta**	skin and muscles of back

Part	Artery	Origin	Area of supply or continuing artery
hindquarters	internal iliac	abdominal aorta	contents of pelvic cavity, perineum, penis, clitoris, tail, muscles of hindquarters
abdomen	umbilical	internal iliac	placenta in fetal life, round ligament of bladder (adult)
abdomen	external iliac	abdominal aorta	femoral a., uterus, muscles of back (psoas)

arthr- Combining form meaning joint.

arthritic Of, or affected with, arthritis.

arthritis (Gr. arthron, joint + -itis) Joint inflammation, caused by trauma, infection or stress. Any joint affected but most common are knee (carpus), fetlock and inter-vertebral joints. **infective a.** See joint-ill. **osteo-a.** Ulceration of joint surface and rarification of bone below with growth of new bone (oesteophyte). See joint mice. **rheumatoid a.** Chronic disease not known in horses. **serous a.** Inflammation of joint membrane producing increased joint oil (synovia) and swelling. See windgall, bog spavin. If prolonged, leads to osteo-**a. ankylosing a.** Destruction of joint surface following infection or injury. Results in fusion of underlying bones, eliminating movement.

arthro- Combining form meaning relationship to a joint.

arthrocele (arthro- + Gr. kele, tumour). Swollen joint. See windgall, joint.

arthrocentesis Punctures of a joint to draw off fluid. See synovial fluid.

arthrochondritis Inflamed joint cartilage. See joint.

Arthropod parasites (Arthropoda) (Gr. arthro-, joint + pous, foot) Phylum of animal kingdom of which Arachnida (qv) and Insecta (qv) are main classes. Members have hard exoskeleton and paired, jointed legs. Some are important in human and veterinary medicine, because they suck blood and act as vectors, qv. See tick.

articular (L. articularis) Of a joint.

articulation Junction between two or more bones. See joints.

artifact (L. ars, art + factum, made) Artificial structure or feature, eg mark on X-ray photograph which may resemble fracture or bone damage.

artificial Unnatural; by mechanical process. **a. insemination** (AI) Putting stallion semen into mare's uterus. Fresh semen can fertilise egg after **a.i.** and even frozen equine semen is now successful. (Freezing is more difficult than when using cattle semen.) Breeding authorities have yet to sanction use of **a.i. a. respiration** Breathing with help of eg oxygen mask (may be necessary in treating shock, respiratory stress). **a. vagina** (AV) Apparatus used to collect semen for laboratory examination. Usually rubber sheath surrounded by warm water inside flask-like cylinder. When stallion has mounted mare, penis is directed into **a.v.** See also condom.

Artiodactyla (Gr. artios, even + daktylos, finger) Order of ungulates with an even number of toes; includes ruminants, pigs, deer, antelope. Cf Perissodactyla, order to which horses belong.

arytenoid (Gr. arytaina, ladle + eidos, form) Jug-shaped. **a. cartilage** See wind.

Ascaris (pl. ascarides) Genus of nematode parasite. See whiteworm.

ascending Having an upward course. **a. aorta** That part of large artery which passes from base of heart to beneath spine.

Aschheim-Zondek test (after German gynecologists, Selmar **A.** and Bernhardt **Z.**) Pregnancy test in humans; female's urine is injected into mouse. Similar test adopted in horses, using blood instead of urine. See pregnancy tests.

ascites Collection of fluid in abdomen. Caused by toxins in blood (septicemia) or obstructed blood flow to liver. Usually accompanied by oedema in other parts of body. Fluid consists of blood plasma without some of larger protein molecules. (Urine may collect in abdomen in cases of ruptured bladder.)

ascitic Of, or characterised by, ascites.

ascorbic acid (syn. vitamin C) Odourless colourless crystals or white crystalline powder with acid taste. Essential to all animals, but horses unlikely to suffer deficiency. Dose: 0.5–1gm. IV, to help treat anemia or chronic hemorrhage. See bleeder.

asepsis (a, neg. + Gr. sepesthai, to decay) Absence of septic matter or freedom from organisms. See antiseptic, disinfectant.

aspect (L. aspectus from aspicere, to look toward) That part of a surface viewed from a particular direction, eg dorsal **a.,** from above.

Aspergillus (L. aspergere, to scatter) Genus of fungi, including several common moulds. **A. maydis** Cause of type of paralysis and inco-ord-ination (May stalk disease) in S Africa. See fungi.

asphxia (a, neg. + Gr. sphyxis, pulse) Suffocation; condition of decreased oxygen and increased carbon dioxide content of blood and tissues. **a. neonatorum** Faulty breathing in the foal. Birth subjects foal to a degree of **a.** from which it rapidly recovers, in normal situations, as breathing starts. See breath.

aspirator Apparatus for sucking fluids and matter from a cavity; used in surgery.

aspirin See acetylsalicylic acid.

ass Member of Equidae similar to donkey and probably its ancestor. Two sub-species, Onager (the wild **a.** of Bible) and Kiang. Types include **Nubian wild a.** (Equus asinus africanus); **Somali wild a.** (Equus asinus somalicus); **Indian wild a.** (Equus hemionus khur). Usually about 12 hands; grey or dun with pale belly; dark dorsal stripe between short, dark mane and dark, tufted tail; long ears and boxy hoofs. Makes braying noise instead of whinny (see equine sounds). Has 62 chromosomes, qv.

Association of the British Pharmaceutical Industry 162 Regent Street, London W1R 6DD (01 734 9061). See also British Veterinary Codex. **A. of Veterinary Anaesthetists** c/o B. Mitchell, Dept of Experimental Surgery, 408 Gilmerton Road, Edinburgh 9 (031 664 3262).

asthma (Gr. asthma, panting) Disease characterised by difficult breathing (dyspnoea) and accompanied by wheezing due to spasmodic contraction of bronchi, qv. Usually caused by allergy and complicated by bronchitis. See broken wind.

astringent Drug or chemical which causes contraction of blood vessels and stops discharge. **a. lotion** Often mixture of copper and sulphate and used to check growth of proud flesh.

astrocyte (astro- + Gr. kytos, hollow vessel) Star-shaped cell; as found in nervous tissue, eg brain.

Astryl Trade name. See sodium glycarsamate.

asymptomatic Not showing or causing symptoms or signs.

asynchronism Disturbed co-ordination. See neonatal maladjustment syndrome, wobbler.

atavism (L. atavus, grandfather) Remote inheritance rather than from immediate ancestors, due to chance combining of genes.

ataxia (Gr. ataxia, lack of order) Failure in muscle co-ordination. See wobbler, cerebellar degeneration.

atelectasis (Gr. ateles, imperfect + ektasis, expansion) Incomplete expansion at birth, or subsequent collapse, of air sacs in lungs. See broken wind, neonatal maladjustment syndrome.

atelectatic Of atelectasis.

atheroma (Gr. athere, gruel + -oma) Lesion of arteries characterised by degenerative changes.

atherosclerosis Lesion of arteries in which deposits occur in inner lining resulting in yellowish plaques containing cholesterol and other fatty material. May occur in aorta of horses and cause heart murmurs or rupture of artery.

atlas First cervical vertebra articulating with skull.

atresia (a, neg. + Gr. tresia, a hole + -ia) Absence or closure of normal body opening. May be congenital as in absence of part of rectum and small colon. See meconium retention.

atrial fibrillation Condition in which heart beats irregularly (arrhythmia) due to rapid and ineffectual contractions (flutter) of first chambers. Causes reduced performance and, months or years later, enlarged heart and death. Diagnosis: on ECG recordings. Treatment: digitalis and quinidine sulphate can sometimes revert heart beat to normal rhythm.

atrio-ventricular valves Those guarding opening between first and second chamber (atrium and ventricle) on left and right sides of heart. See mitral and tricuspid valves.

atrium (L., Gr. atrion, hall) A chamber; anatomical term, eg either of first chambers of heart, qv.

atrophy (L. and Gr. atrophia) Wasting or diminution in size of cell, tissue, organ or part. **muscle a.** Wasting of muscle due to lack of use, in lameness or paralysis.

atropine Alkaloid contained in plants of the family Solanaceae (deadly nightshade), dwale (blanewort), henbane and thornapple. **a. poisoning** Symptoms: dry mouth, increased pulse and respiratory rate, extreme dilation of pupils, blindness, restlessness, muscular trembling followed by fall in temperature, convulsions, paralysis and death. Diagnosis: place a drop of horse's urine into eye of a healthy animal, eg cat, and observe the dilation of pupil in bright light half an hour later. Treatment is largely ineffectual. **a. sulphate** Colourless odourless alkaloid crystals, synthetic or extracted from Hyoscyamus muticus. Antagonises effects of arecoline and diminishes secretions from salivary, bronchial and alimentary glands. Causes increased heart rate, dilated pupils. Used before operations or with purgative to reduce pain caused by excessive stimulation of alimentary tract. Given by injection, by mouth or in eye drops, ointments. Dose: by injection 15–30mg. See purgatives; eye, diseases of.

attenuation (L., attenuation from add to + tenuis, thin) Altered virulence of a micro-organism by passage through host species or by repeated growth on laboratory media; process used to prepare vaccine, qv.

54

atypical (a, neg. + Gr. types, type or model) Not conforming to typical pattern; of unusual type, eg signs of disease may be **a.** of a particular syndrome. **a. behaviour** See vices.

audiovisual Relating to senses of sound and sight.

aur- Combining form meaning ear.

Aureomycin Trade name. See chlortetracycline hydrochloride.

aureomycin hydrochloride See chlortetracycline hydrochloride.

auricle (L. auricula, a little ear) The external ear, ie pinna or flap of ear. Also atrium or first chamber of heart. See ear, heart.

auscultate To listen to body's internal sounds, ie those from heart, lungs or alimentary canal. See stethoscope, heart sounds, murmur, borborygmus.

Australian (Waler) Breed developed in New South Wales. No other type recognised as national breed, but draught horses (developed from Shire, Suffolk Punch and Clydesdale), ponies (from Timor stock), polo ponies and Thoroughbreds bred in most states. **A. Veterinary Association** See Australian Veterinary Journal. **A. Veterinary Journal** Monthly journal of **A.** Veterinary Association, 76 Paramatta Road, Camperdown, New South Wales, Australia 2050.

aut-/auto- (Gr. autos, self) Prefix meaning relationship to self.

autoclave (auto- + L. clavis, key) Apparatus used for sterilising instruments, swabs etc. Relies on heat produced by steam under pressure.

autointoxicant Toxin produced in body.

autointoxication Effect of toxin generated by micro-organisms normally present in body, eg those in gut can, in certain conditions, produce a harmful toxin causing diarrhoea or colic.

autolysis (auto- + Gr. lysis, dissolution) Disintegration of cells and tissues by their own enzymes; process of dissolution after death.

autonomic nervous system Arrangement of nerves regulating actions not under conscious (voluntary) control. Composed of sympathetic (or accelerator) and parasympathetic systems and characterised by a junction (synapse) between spinal cord and nerve-ending in organ or tissue. (Place of junction known as a ganglion.) Action of the 2 systems is usually antagonistic, eg pupil of eye, dilated by sympathetic, constricted by parasympathetic; heart rate increased by sympathetic, slowed by parasympathetic; gut movement, decreased by sympathetic, increased by parasympathetic; secretion of glands in lungs and alimentary canal, decreased by sympathetic, increased by parasympathetic; blood pressure, increased by sympathetic, lowered by parasympathetic. Drug which mimics action of sympathetic nerves (energy) is adrenaline. Drug which mimics action of parasympathetic nerves (rest) is acetylcholine.

autopsy (auto- + Gr. opsis, view) See post-mortem.

AV Abbr. artificial vagina, qv.

Avelignese Small Italian draught and pack horse, virtually same as Haflinger, qv.

avitaminosis Deficiency of vitamins in diet. See appetite.

axilla Area between shoulder and chest through which vital nerves and arteries travel. See brachial plexus.

axis (L., Gr. axon, axle) (1) Imaginary line dividing body or part of it symmetrically. (2) Second cervical vertebra. See vertebra.

azoturia See setfast.

B

Babesan Trade name. See quinuronium sulphate.

Babesia Genus of protozoan parasites. See biliary fever.

babesiasis/babesiosis Infected with Babesia. See biliary fever.

Bacillus (L., little rod) Genus of micro-organism of family Bacillaceae, order Eubacteriales, includes gram-positive, aerobic, spore-forming bacteria; some cause disease (pathogenic). **B. anthracis** (syn. anthrax bacillus) Causal organism of anthrax.

bacillus (pl. bacilli) Any rod-shaped bacterium belonging to order Eubacteriales, eg Escherichia coli, found in feces and sometimes mare's genital tract, Klebsiella pneumonia, causes venereal disease, Mycobacterium tuberculosis (T.b.), Clostridium tetani (lockjaw). Cf coccus.

bacitracin Substance produced by gram-positive organism Bacillus subtilis. Used as antibiotic against gram-positive bacteria.

back Part of horse's body from withers to tail. **broken b.** Fracture of one or more vertebrae, may result in severed or pinched spinal cord causing paralysed hindlegs. **dipped or hollow b.** Depressed vertebral column behind withers giving sunken look. See muscles, spine, vertebra.

backbone Vertebral column or spine. Series of bones (vertebrae) which form column extending length of body; acts as support for legs and ribs and forms bony canal for main nerve trunk (spinal cord). See spine, spinal cord.

backflow Flow of fluid in an abnormal direction, eg **b.** of blood from second to first chamber of heart, due to faulty valve action. See heart, vulvular stenosis.

back-raking Removal of feces from rectum, eg before rectal examination of colic case.

bacteremia Bacteria in blood.

bacteria (pl. of bacterium) Extremely small chlorophyll-free unicellular organisms, which multiply by simple division. (Also called germs, microbes, micro-organisms. Cf fungi, which are multicellular with sexual reproduction, and viruses, minute particles invisible with ordinary microscope, which reproduce only in living cells.) **B.** classified by (1) reaction to stains (dye): eg gram-negative, gram-positive, acid fast; (2) shape: eg coccus—round, bacillus—cylindrical rods, vibrio—comma shaped, actinomyces—with branching filaments, spirochaete—long and flexible, twisted around long axis; (3) size: eg average diameter of a coccus is about 1/25,000th of an inch; (4) arrangement: eg strings—streptococci (distinguishable from staphylococci which have grape arrangement), capsules—around some **b.** and can be demonstrated by staining, eg Klebsiella; (5) spore formation: oval or round bodies in framework and in cell membrane of **b.**, eg Clostridium tetani; (6) flagella: long, delicate threads on motile **b.**, eg Escherichia coli. **b., cultivation of** In laboratory **b.** should be grown on/in special substances known as media, eg fluid media containing meat extract, broth or peptone; solid media made of gelatine (albumin from tendons and cartilage) or agar (dried seaweed); selective media, those favouring growth of certain **b.**, eg which are coloured by dye.

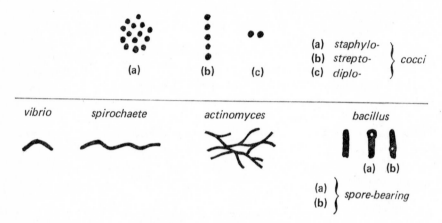

2   Different types of bacteria

Material containing the **b.** is placed on/in sterile media and incubated overnight at 38°C. Colonies grow on solid media and a sediment of **b.** accumulates in liquid media. Sediment or colony can then be examined under microscope and tested further. **b., identification of B.** are classified by how they grow in fluid and solid media, their biochemical activity, eg side reactions during growth as in Klebsiella, which split urea, Streptococci which ferment carbohydrate.

bacterial Of bacteria. **b. abortion** See abortion. **b. diseases**

Specific disease	Causal organism
acne	Staphylococcus aureus
	Corynebacterium pyogenes
anthrax	Bacillus anthracis
botulism	Clostridium botulinum
brucellosis	Brucella abortus
glanders	Loefflerella mallei (syns. Pfeifferella mallei, Malleomyces mallei)
leptospirosis	Leptospira pomona
lockjaw	Clostridium tetani
malignant oedema	Clostridium septicum

salmonellosis

Salmonella typhimurium
Salmonella abortus equi
Salmonella enteritidis

sleepy foal disease — Actinobacillus equuli
strangles — Streptococcus equi
summer pneumonia — Corynebacterium equi
tuberculosis — Mycobacterium tuberculosis
ulcerative lymphangitis — Corynebacterium
pseudotuberculosis

Non-specific disease

abcess (1,2)
diarrhoea (3)

joint-ill (1,2,3,4)
lymphangitis (1,2)
meningitis (1,2,3)
uterine infection (metritis)
(1,2,3,4,5)
pneumonia (1,2,3)
snotty nose (1,2,6,7)

Bacteria

1 Staphylococcus aureus
2 Streptococcus pyogenes var.
   equi (S. zooepidemicus)
3 Escherichia coli
4 Klebsiella pneumoniae
5 Pseudomonas pyocyanea
6 Hemophilus influenzae
7 Bordetella species

Figures in brackets indicate most common causal bacteria.

bactericidal (bacterium + L. caedere, to kill) Drug or substance which destroys bacteria, eg penicillin. See antibiotic.

bacterin Bacterial vaccine.

bacteriolysis (bacteria + Gr. lysis, dissolution) Breaking up of bacteria.

bacteriophage (bacteria + Gr. phagein, to eat) Virus which kills bacteria.

bacteriostasis (bacteria + Gr. stasis, stoppage) The inhibiting of bacterial growth by drugs or other substances.

bacteriostatic Drug or substance which inhibits growth or multiplication of bacteria, eg sulphonamide. See antibiotic.

Bacterium Genus of micro-organisms known as Coli-typhoid group. Cause infections especially of intestines, urinary and genital (urogenital) tracts. (Gram-negative, non-sporing bacteria, some motile, others non-motile.) See Escherichia coli, Salmonella enteritides, S. abortivo equina, S. typhimurium, Actinobacillus equuli, Klebsiella pneumoniae.

bacterium (L., Gr. bakerior, little rod; pl. bacteria) See bacteria.

bag Colloq. for mamary glands, qv.

balance (L. bilanx) Term used in physiological states. **fluid b.** Proportions of fluids in body parts such as tissue spaces, cells, blood.

balanic Of glans penis or glans clitoridis.

balanitis Inflamed glans penis.

balano- (Gr. balanos, an acorn) Combining form meaning relationship to glans penis or glans clitoridis.

balanoposthitis (balano + Gr. posthe, prepuce) Inflamed glans penis and prepuce.

bald Without hair. B. patches may be due to horse rubbing coat, destruction of hair follicles after injury, radiation or diseases of skin, eg ringworm. See skin, diseases of.

Balearic Distinct ancient breed of Majorca, in B. group of islands. Has delicate roman-nosed head which it carries bent against neck at fast paces. Mane is short, indicating B. may be descendant of ancient Greek type thought to have been naturally hogged and brought to islands during Greek occupation.

baleri Form of trypanosomiasis of horses, sheep, goats and cattle in French Sudan; caused by Trypanosoma pecaudi. Marked by fever, body swellings and emaciation.

ball Spherical mass; bolus; powdered drug mixed with syrup or treacle to form a mass and usually given with balling gun. Once popular but superseded by liquid drugs given through stomach tube.

ballottement See pregnancy tests.

bar (1) Part of upper gum between front teeth (incisors) and either tusks (absent in mare) or premolars. Area bears no teeth and takes bit of bridle. (2) Continuation of wall of foot; turns inward at heel to run parallel with frog. Forms part of weight-bearing surface. See foot.

Barb Native breed of Morocco, Algeria and W Africa around Lake Tchad. Delicate-looking, with particularly low-set tail. Can thrive on poor food, like Arab, but is less spirited than its more popular neighbour. Virtually extinct outside natural home due to extensive crossing, particularly with Arab. **B.** and Arab are ancestors of English Thoroughbred.

Barbary horse Old name for Barb, qv.

barbiturate Class of drug used as anaesthetic (or, dishonestly, as stopper dope; see veterinary rules). Symptoms of **b.** poisoning: shallow breathing, lethargy, coma, absence of normal reflexes, dilated pupils. Can cause death from respiratory failure (due to depression of nerve centres). Treatment: give stimulant drugs, eg nikethamide, leptazol, picrotoxin.

barker See neonatal maladjustment syndrome.

barley Annual grasses of Hordeum species. Cereal grain often fed to horses. **b. straw** Used for bedding but considered inferior to wheat straw because horses tend to eat it. See food.

baroreceptor Sensory nerve-ending stimulated by changes in pressure. See nerve-ending.

barren Sterile; infertile. **b. mare** One that is not pregnant; also barrener. See infertility.

barrier Obstruction. **blood-brain b.** Division between blood and central nervous system. Term means substances and drugs in blood cannot necessarily pass into nervous system. **placental b.** Placental membrane between maternal and fetal blood. It is selective, allowing only certain substances to pass to fetus.

base (L., Gr. basis) Foundation or lowest part; a substance which takes up hydrogen ions and thereby makes a solution more alkaline. **b. deficit** Lack of base (alkaline salts) in blood, resulting in acidity. Present in diarrhoea, convulsions. See blood tests, biochemical (7). **b.-narrow** Term of conformation: describes forelegs set close together on brisket, or hindlegs on quarters. Legs often splay wide at hooves (toe-wide). **b.-wide** Limbs set wide apart on body and often closer together at hooves (toe-narrow).

basophil (Gr. basis, base + philein, to love) Histological term denoting structure or cell easily stained with basic dyes.

bastard strangles See strangles.

Basuto/Basuto pony One of most sure-footed breeds. Developed in S Africa from Cape horse, Arab, Barb and, later, English Thoroughbred. Used for polo and general riding in S Africa, where it is still crossed with Arab.

Batak (or Deli) Pony of hills of Sumatra. Takes name either from island's B. inhabitants or port of Deli, where many are shipped to Singapore. Usually brown or skewbald with crested neck and delicate head due to Arab influence.

bay See coat colouring.

bear's foot (syn. Helleborus viridis) Plant containing drug similar to digitalis. Causes diarrhoea and heart reaction.

beat A pulsation of heart or artery. See pulse. **dropped b.** An irregular b. **ectopic b.** Heart beat originating at some point other than sino-atrial node. See electrocardiogram.

Beberbeck Breed resembling heavy Thoroughbred, usually over 16 hands and chestnut or bay. Developed in Beber-bach region of E Germany from local mares, Arab and Thoroughbred stallions. Rule of B. breeding was that Thoroughbred-sired fillies were covered by only B. stallions. B. stud sold to Polish government after World War I.

beer Alcoholic drink from barley and hops. Given as conditioner.

Beetewk Draught breed developed from mares around **B.** river, Veronej province, Russia, and Dutch stallions, with progeny being bred to Orlov trotters, qv.

behaviour Demeanour. Most horses' natural **b.** is inhibited by domestication but patterns do exist. Those described are typical of a normal, healthy horse—deviation may indicate ill-health. **atypical b.** See vices. **eating b.** The horse is now a continuous feeder, a grazer (see evolution) and seldom takes more than a mouthful or two before moving a step. When stabled it should be fed little and often, because stomach is small for horse's size (see food). It sometimes nibbles tree bark or dung (see appetite, depraved) but does not usually graze where it defecates. Foal nibbles solid food at about 8 days old. **foal b.** Foal is born with head unsteady, eyes open, ears back and tail tucked down. It quickly rights itself on to brisket and paws with forelegs, moving away from mare, causing umbilical cord to break (see birth). Mare nuzzles and licks foal and when, a quarter of an hour after birth, it tries to stand, she nickers (see equine sounds). After repeated efforts it finally stands, maybe three-quarters of an hour after birth. At about an hour old, foal's lips make sucking movements as it searches for mare's udder. It sniffs and licks any object and eventually finds way along mare's flank to stifle, which it may suck vigorously before finding teats. After about 2 hours it walks easily, gets up and down, nurses and, if humans approach, seeks mare's side. If mare appears in pain (qv), foal shows distress by whinnying and circling round her. Sleep and awareness of danger steadily increase, though foals carefully handled in first few hours show less fear and are more tractable later. (**abnormal foal b.** See neonatal maladjustment syndrome.) **general b.** (temperament) Probably inherited (see gene) and affected by training. Some claim sire is more likely than dam to pass on temperament and that energetic **b.** is more easily transmitted than passive **b.** White, palomino and grey horses are thought more tractable and tend to be cautious (because they are conspicuous to enemies) while chestnuts are less tractable. Few judges now claim aggressive nature for certain points of conformation, eg small ears, small eyes. Fighting, by kicking and biting, is usual between a stallion and any other entire male or gelding who tries to oust him as herd leader. **herd b.** In the wild, a herd roams little at night. As most foals are born during darkness, herd is unlikely to move before new foals can travel. Herd leader is usually a stallion who, especially during spring and summer, stays near whichever mare is in season. Herd leader (can also be old or large horse) can be identified by watching feeding order. Grey horses often act as look-outs. (See general **b.**) **male sexual b.** Colt may show erection and mounting at 6–8 months, but is unlikely to mate before 10–12 months. Penis is comparable to human penis (vascular-muscular type) therefore entry into mare (intromission) depends on full erection. Stallion shows three phases: (1) courtship, (2) erection and mounting, (3) intromission and ejaculation. In courtship stallion neighs on seeing receptive mare, arches neck and curls upper lip (flehmen posture), nudges mare, smells vulva and bites skin of her rump. Erection is gradual until, when complete, penis is 12–20ins. long. (In captivity, experienced stallion may achieve erection when taken to covering yard, before seeing mare.) Immature stallion may try to mount mare sideways and might mount 1–4 times before intromission. Ejaculation, on average, is 13 seconds later and recognised by flagging of tail. Some stud grooms, to be certain it has occurred, hold base of stallion's penis to feel flow of semen. Sexual drive (libido) is keenest in spring, which coincides with mare's natural breeding season. (See plates 1–5.) (**abnormal male b.** includes savaging mare, sometimes instead of ejaculating, and masturbation, qv.) **mare b.** Mare's bond with foal develops as she licks and sniffs it soon after birth. When she stands, maybe 30 minutes later, she will shelter it from intruders. Attachment increases until she weans foal, about 10 months later (in wild state), by being unco-operative when it wants to suck (see weaning). Occasionally mare lets another foal suck, but usually accepts only her own (see fostering). (**abnormal mare b.** Some mares are hostile towards foal and may savage it. Occasionally mares show lesbian **b.** by mounting one another.) **b. during pain.** See birth, colic, setfast; plates 8–10. **resting b.** Horse sleeps intermittently for about 7 hours of the 24, mostly in hottest part of day, though habits vary according to breed. Most horses sleep standing up and rest by lying down to expose body to sun. Horse may paw ground before lying down, lowering first shoulders, then quarters. It rests on one side, with legs outstretched, or on side of chest with a forelimb and a hindlimb flexed under body. (It cannot rest, dog-like, on sternum, as bone forms a sharp ridge.) On rising, forelegs stretch ahead and chest rises as hocks take weight. **social b.** When horses first meet they show 4 stages of acceptance: (1) they circle, watching one another, (2) touch nostrils, (3) investigate the other's body and tail with tip of muzzle, (4) if mutual tolerance is agreed, nibble one another's necks. Horses prefer particular herd-mates, usually of the same social rank

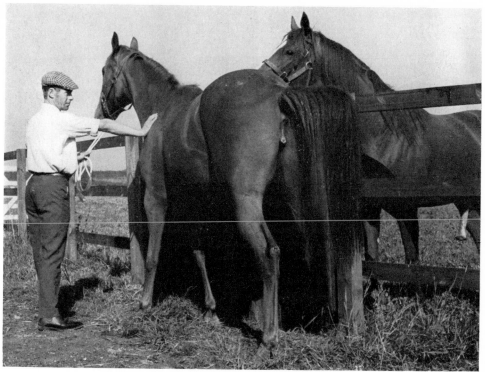

1 Teasing a mare. The teaser, with penis erect, smells and bites the mare. She shows by accepting this behaviour and winking her vulva that she is sexually receptive

2 Covering boots are put on to minimise any injury if the mare kicks the stallion

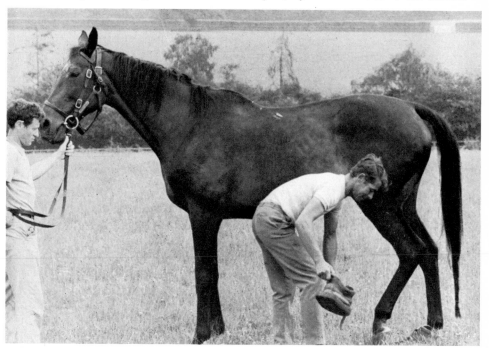

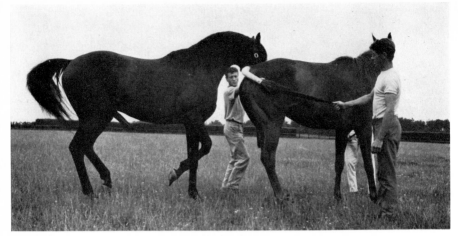

3 The stallion is held behind the mare . . .

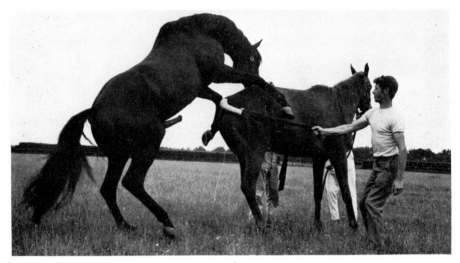

4 . . . mounts her . . .

5 . . . and achieves intromission. When covering is supervised by handlers (instead of the stallion running with his mares), it is often in a closed covering yard

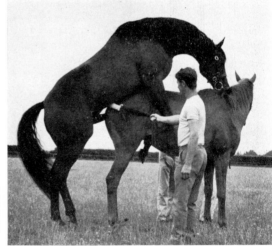

(see also equine sounds). **voiding b.** Adult defecates 5–12 times a day and urinates 7–11 times, though figures depend on breed, climate, diet and amount of work. Horse does not defecate where it grazes, but will walk to particular area. Entire horse tends to back into area, but mare faces patch, so that field of mares soon becomes horse-sick. A gelded animal may change habit from that of stallion to that of mare. Entire horse (but not mare) smells ground before and after defecating. He also sniffs ground after urinating. The sexes adopt similar stance to urinate—hind legs pushed back and apart. The stallion walks away, lashing tail and flexing penile muscles. Mare may wink vulva, as if in season. (If she has foal at foot she will defecate and urinate more carefully to avoid contaminating udder.) See Ethological Society.

belching Expulsion of gas via mouth. Uncommon in horses due to strong sphincter muscle at gullet's entrance to stomach.

belladonna (syn. deadly nightshade) (1) Plant poisonous to horses. See nightshade poisoning. (2) Fine green powder with slight odour and bitter taste. Prepared from leaves of Atropa belladonna. Similar action to atropine sulphate, qv. Dose 1–3gms.

belly (1) Abdomen, qv. (2) Fleshy part of muscle.

bemegride sodium (trade name: Megimide sodium) Fine white odourless powder. Stimulates central nervous system and used to lighten barbiturate anaesthesia after operations. Dose: 20 mg./kg. body wt. IV.

Benadryl Trade name for antihistamine (qv) drug.

benign Non-malignant, eg growth which does not recur when removed. See metastasis, growth.

benzalkonium chloride solution (trade names: Drapolene, Marinol, PRQ Antiseptic, Roccal, Zephiran) Clear colourless liquid with aromatic odour and bitter taste. Used 1 part to 50 parts water or 1 in 500 with alcohol for pre-operative sterilisation of hands and arms. Instruments, but not rubber, may be stored in 1 in 2,000 dilution.

benzamine penicillin (trade names: Dibencil, Penidural) White odourless tasteless powder. Antibacterial action which when given by intramuscular injection is released slowly over several days.

Benzedrine Trade name. See amphetamine.

benzene hexachloride See gamma.

benzoin Balsamic resin obtained from Styrax benzoin. Used as inhalant, qv.

benzyl benzoate (trade name: Spasmodin) Colourless crystalline or oily liquid with faint aroma and sharp burning taste. Used to treat sarcoptic mange. See mange.

benzylpenicillin (syn. penicillin; trade names: Crystapen, Falapen, Penavlon, Solupen) Fine white crystalline powder obtained by growing Penicillium notatum in suitable culture medium. Bacteriostatic drug and, in high dosage, bactericidal against gram-positive bacteria, eg Clostridium, Corynebacterium, Leptospira, Streptococci. Relatively inactive against gram-negative bacteria. Dose: 3–6mg./kg. body wt. IM. See infection, strangles, joint-ill, pneumonia, uterus (infection of).

Berkfurin-E Trade name. See nitrofurantoin.

beta Second letter of Gr. alphabet. See globulin, radiation. **b. hemolysis** Clear zone round growth of Streptococcus on blood agar media; due to break down of blood (hemolysis) by toxins produced by germ. See Streptococcus pyogenes.

betamethasone sodium phosphate (trade names: Betsolan, Betnesol) Absorbent crystalline powder with slight odour. Potent anti-inflammatory steroid. For uses and side effects see cortisone acetate. Dose: 10–30mg. IM or 2–10mg. injected into joint.

Betnesol See betamethasone sodium phosphate.

Betsolan/B. eye and ear drops Trade names. Drops contain betamethasone sodium phosphate, qv.

BEVA See British Equine Veterinary Association.

Bhutia Native pony of India, particularly Nepal. Sure-footed and hardy. Usually grey and about 13 hands (slightly larger than other native of India, the Spiti).

bi- (L. bi, two) Combining form meaning two or twice.

bicarbonate Salt with two equivalents of carbonic acid to one base, eg **sodium b.**, counteracts acidity in stomach and blood, makes urine more alkaline and used to treat excess staling. Dose: 15–60gms. by mouth. In severe diarrhoea: 10ml. of a 5% solution per kg. body wt. IV.

biceps (bi- + caput, head) Muscle having two heads. See muscles, table of.

bicipital Relating to biceps muscle, eg **b.** groove on front of humerus bone. **b. bursitis** Inflamed bursa between biceps brachi muscle and **b.** groove. Symptoms are those of shoulder lameness, including shortened stride and stumbling. Diagnosis: on signs, swelling at point of shoulder, pain when joint is manipulated. Treatment: inject bursa with corticosteroids.

bicornuate (bi- + L. cornutus, horned) Having two horns, eg uterus.

bicuspid (bi- + L. cuspis, point) Having two cusps, eg molar teeth or **b.** valve of heart.

b.i.d. Abbr. for L. bis in die, twice a day. Used on prescriptions to advise frequency of dose.

big head (syns. osteodystrophia fibrosa, miller's disease) Disease of horses on unbalanced diets, high in phosphorus (P) and low in calcium (Ca) such as cereal, hays and bran. Usually affects horses 2–7 years old. Can be produced by diets with a ratio of Ca to P of 1:3 or greater, irrespective of total Ca intake. Low Ca intake (2–3gms. per day) and a Ca/P ratio of 1:13 causes symptoms within 5 months. A Ca intake of 26gms. per day and a Ca/P ratio of 1:5 produces signs in a year. Normal Ca/P ratio in a diet should be 1.3:1. Soft fibrous tissue forms in bones and first symptoms are lameness, arching of back and creaking joints. Erosions of joint cartilage develop and, in advanced cases, bones may break and tendons become sprained. If not treated, condition results in swollen lower jaw and enlarged face. Treatment: give diet with Ca/P ratio of 2:1. Cereal hay should be supplemented with alfalfa, or clover and limestone (20–40gms. daily).

big leg (syns. lymphangitis, Monday morning leg) Non-contagious disease characterized by fever, lymphangitis and swelling of one or both hindlegs. Usually starts abruptly with a temperature around 41°C., shivering, pain, rapid pulse and respiration. Limb is hot and swollen with beading of lymphatics on the inside. Horse loses appetite, may sweat and become constipated. Acute stage lasts 2 days, swelling persists much longer and occasionally abscesses develop and serum oozes from affected limb. Condition is associated with superficial wounds and infection of lymphatic system. Treatment: give antibiotics (eg penicillin), pethidine, corticosteroids and exercise. Once a limb has been affected, recurrence is common, the subcutaneous tissue may become fibrous and the limb permanently thickened and enlarged. See plate 39, also lymphangitis.

Bigourdan/B. ameliore (improved **B.**) Extinct branch of Tarbenian family developed to add height to Tarbenian and since lost in that breed, which is virtually Anglo-Arab.

bilateral (bi- + L. latus, side) Having or affecting two sides, eg **b.** cataract affecting both eyes. See also rig.

bile Brown or greenish-yellow fluid secreted by liver and carried in bile duct to intestines. It aids emulsification and absorption of fats and contains acids, pigments, carbonate, cholesterol and mucin. It is constantly secreted by the horse which, unlike other species, does not have a gall-bladder in which to store it. See bilirubin, biliverdin.

bili- (L. bilis, bile) Combining form meaning relationship to bile.

biliary fever Serious condition caused by Babesia (parasites which live in red blood cells and are transferred from host to host by blood-sucking insects). After a bite, parasite incubates 5–21 days. Symptoms: depression, thirst, watery eyes with swollen lids, intense jaundice (turning all tissues deep yellow) and minute hemorrhages on mucosal surfaces. These signs are followed by constipation or diarrhoea and in some cases oedema of limbs, head and abdomen. The urine is red due to presence of hemoglobin and there is severe anemia. Bad cases become emaciated and inco-ordinated and die in about 12 days. Recovery and convalescence takes weeks or months. Diagnosis: by examination of blood smears for presence of parasites. These begin to disappear from circulation soon after day of bite so smears should be made as early as possible. Treatment: diminazene aceturate (dose: 3.5mg./kg. body wt. IM); phenamidine isethionate (0.03ml. of 40% solution sub. cut.); quinuronium sulphate (0.6mg. sub. cut.).

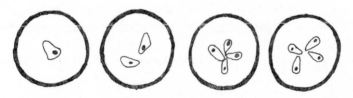

3 Various stages of Babesia reproduction in red blood cells; the organism causes biliary fever

bilirubin (L. bili + L. ruber, red) Bile pigment formed from hemo-globin when red blood cells are destroyed by special cells. Liver normally changes **b.** into biliverdin (qv) but it may be found in urine and tissues in cases of jaundice. See blood (biochemical tests: 4), hemo-globin, red blood cells, jaundice.

bilirubinemia (bilirubin + Gr. haima, blood) Abnormal amount of bilirubin in blood stream.

bilirubinuria Abnormal amount of bilirubin in urine.

biliverdin (bili- + L. viridis, green) Green pigment which liver forms from bilirubin, before it passes to intestines.

bimastic Having 2 mammary glands, eg mare.

biniodide An iodide with 2 atoms of iodine in each molecule, eg **b.** of mercury, used as blister, qv. See red mercuric oxide.

bio- (Gr. bios, life) Combining form meaning relationship to life.

bio-assay Method of estimating strength of drug by noting its effect on animals, compared with that of a standard preparation.

biologicals Medicines prepared from living organisms, eg serums, vaccines, antigens, antitoxins.

biometry (bio- + Gr. metron, measure) Science of statistics applied to biological facts; mathematical expression of biological data.

biopsy (bio + Gr. opsis, vision) Removal of a minute portion of tissue to study in laboratory, eg portion of growth, uterus, bone or liver. A **b.** punch or needle is used, depending on site and tissue involved, eg liver **b.** is performed through flank, uterine **b.** through vagina.

birdsville disease Condition found in Australia if horses graze Indigofera dominii plant. Symptoms: wandering in circles, pushing head against objects. Treatment: recent work suggests certain types of protein, eg peanut meal, gelatin, may help counteract toxicity of the plant.

birth (syns. labour, parturition, confinement, foaling) Act of expelling foal and its membranes from uterus, through **b.** canal. Occurs between 7 p.m. and 7. a.m. in 90%of mares. Relatively fast and completed in 3 stages. **1st stage b.** (hotting up) Surface veins stand out and mare may run milk. Uterus contracts causing signs of pain (unease—pawing ground, looking round at flanks, flehmen posture, lifting hindleg, raising tail, hindquarter cringing, see plates 8–10). Signs appear in increasingly intense phases, between which mare may rest or eat. Muscles in uterus wall bear down on contents in waves passing towards cervix, which dilates. Fetal head and limbs are propelled into **b.** canal. This stage may last minutes to several hours. May occur hours, days or weeks before foaling and be repeated several times. Mare said to hot up and cool off. Finally, placenta ruptures. **2nd stage b.** Starts when mare 'breaks water' (placenta ruptures, allowing escape of yellowish (allantoic) fluid). Mare shows most of signs of 1st stage plus straining. Many mares get up and down several times but 95% complete delivery when down. Mare may half roll, apparently to alter foal's position for easier delivery, or lie with back against wall. Abdominal muscles contract to supplement action of uterus by reducing size of abdomen. Foal is forced along **b.** canal until only hindlegs are left in vagina. 2nd stage lasts 5–60 minutes and averages 20 minutes (see plates 11–14). **3rd stage b.** Foal paws with forefeet, dragging hindfeet clear of vagina. Mare usually stays down for up to 40 minutes. She usually delivers fetal membranes (after-birth) about an hour after foal, but it may be 5 minutes–10 hours. Mare may roll and show other signs of pain as uterus returns to non-pregnant size (involution) and placenta separates from uterine wall. **b. canal** Fetus's route from uterus to outside: cervix, vagina and vulva, encased in pelvis. **b., hazards of** Include trauma and **b.** hemorrhage. See also dystocia; recto-vaginal fistula; uterus, prolapse of; vaginal bruising; after-birth, retention of. **b. hemorrhage** (syn. parturient hemorrhage) Bleeding during or immediately after delivery of foal. Two types— internal and external. Internal is result of ruptured artery in membrane (broad ligament) supporting uterus. At birth this is enlarged to accommodate extra blood flow necessary for pregnant uterus. Rupture allows blood to escape but it may be contained oy peritoneum and surrounding tissues. However if blood breaks through peritoneum, so it can flow into abdominal cavity, mare **bleeds to death.** External bleeding is from lining of uterus after separation of after-birth. Some blood may be from placenta. Condition is not usually fatal but causes pain and can lead to uterine infection. Symptoms: pain, sweating, rolling, curling upper lip, pawing ground, rapid breathing and pulse, pale mucous membranes which become chalk-white in fatal cases. Swelling may appear to one side of vulva. Initially mare may be reluctant to proceed with 2nd stage labour, may roll during delivery and if she survives, may be jaundiced (best seen on sclera of eyes and lining of gums) after 24 or 48 hours. Treatment: quiet handling, rest, pain relieving drugs, tranquillisers, blood coagulating agents, transfusion of whole blood—but this is ineffective unless plenty is available, eg over 10 litres. Prevention: no specific measures though copper deficiency may be associated with fatal hemorrhage. Avoid using twitch for at least 24 hours after foaling as its use may start hemorrhage. Cf vaginal bruising. **b. management** As far as possible mares should be allowed to foal without interference but should be watched for signs of abnormality. Many breeds foal outdoors but Thoroughbreds nearly always in a loose box; this should be at least 12ft. by 12ft. with good ventilation and clean bedding, which should not be shaken as this can contaminate atmosphere with dust. Mare should be watched at a distance and breaking of water recognised. Within 5–10 minutes of this the shiny amniotic membrane should appear at vulval lips. After thoroughly washing hands attendant should feel in vagina for foal's muzzle and forelegs and if mare's vulva has been stitched (Caslick operation) it should be cut with straight scissors. Further action unnecessary unless 2nd stage is delayed, ie straining does not occur or is not associated with a progressive appearance of foal. After complete delivery the umbilical cord should be left to rupture when mare gets to her feet or foal struggles. Mare should not be disturbed or made to get up prematurely. During final stages of delivery amnion can be removed from foal's head. This is unnecessary for normal healthy foal but may prevent an unhealthy one suffocating. Amnion can be tied to cord after it has ruptured, to provide a weight which helps delivery of after-birth. **pre-b. position** For about 4 months before **b.** fetus lies on back with head and limbs flexed. In 1st and early 2nd stage labour body rotates and forelegs extend. Foal passes into **b.** canal with forelegs stretched out, one slightly ahead of the other. See dystocia, presentation, position, posture.

bisexual (bi- + L. sexus, sex) Having gonads of both sexes. See intersex.

bishop (after a Mr **B.** who originated deceitful practice of marking teeth) To make grooves in table surface of front teeth (incisors) so animal appears younger than it is.

bis in die (L., twice a day) See b.i.d.

bismuth (trade name: Forgastrin) Tasteless, odourless creamy-white powder. Given internally to sooth stomach and intestine or applied externally as protective ointment, lotion or powder. Dose: foals 2–4gms., adults 15–30gms.

bite To grip with teeth. See behaviour, general.

black See coat colouring. **b. leg** An acute infectious disease caused by Clostridium chauvoei, characterised by toxic degeneration of muscles. Common in cattle but rare in horses.

bladder (L. cystis) Any membranous sac, but usually means urinary **b.** Hollow muscular organ roughly pear-shaped and capable of holding up to a gallon of urine. **b., rupture of** (syn. patent **b.**) Colloq. for condition of newborn foal in which hole or tear in **b.** wall causes continual escape of urine into abdomen. May be result of faulty development or injury during birth. Signs appear 2–4 days after birth and include failure to pass normal stream of urine, crouching and straining (must be distinguished from more common condition of meconium retention, qv). Abdomen becomes distended with fluid which can be drawn off. See paracentesis. Treated by operation under general anaesthesia to close tear. Most cases survive if diagnosed early, otherwise foal dies from pressure of diaphragm on lungs, causing suffocation.

blasto- (Gr blastos, germ) Combining form meaning relationship to bud; particularly used in connection with embryo.

blastocoele (blasto- + Gr. koilos, hollow) See blastula.

blastoderm (blasto- + Gr. derma, skin) See blastula.

blastomycosis See epizootic lymphangitis.

blastula Cell mass (blastoderm) and fluid-filled cavity (blastocoele) formed from division of fertilised ovum. See embryology.

blaze White marking (qv) over forehead and bridge of nose.

bleb Fluid sac or vesicle beneath skin, eg **b.** of local anaesthetic injected beneath skin.

bleeder Horse which suffers from nosebleeds (epistaxis) or tendency to break blood vessels. Source of hemorrhage may be mucous membrane of nasal passages, throat, guttural pouch or lungs; may occur at rest, at exercise, or when horse lowers head after coming in from exercise. Frequently fatal; no reliable cure, though coagulant drugs, vitamin C and antibiotics may help if cause is infection. Rest is essential to allow lesion time to heal.

blepharitis Inflammation of eyelids. Caused by injury, flies, infection with bacteria.

blepharo- (Gr. blepharon, eyelid) Combining form meaning relationship to eyelid or eyelash.

blepharospasm (blepharo- + Gr. spasmos, spasm) Spasm of eyelid muscles, occurs in painful conditions of eyeball, especially when subjected to light.

blind Unable to see. May be result of damage or disease of eyeball, optic nerve or brain. Horse **b.** in only one eye is not severely handicapped. Newborn foal may be temporaily **b.** following convulsions. See eye, diseases of: moon blindness; neonatal maladjustment syndrome; anophthalmia.

blister (L. vesicular) (1) Collection of fluid that causes horny upper layer of skin to rise, separating it from parts below. May be filled with blood. See blood **b.** (2) Colloq. for fluids and ointments that cause counter-irritation and are used to treat tendon injuries or inflamed joints. **B.** may be cantharides (Spanish fly), red mercuric iodide or ammonia compound (which all cause small **b.**'s) or mustard or turpentine, which make skin peel.

bloat See colic.

block Obstruction or stoppage. Used in connection with impulse through heart muscle, local anaesthesia (nerve **b.**) or colloq. for stoppage in alimentary tract. See colic, heart, nerve **b.**

blood Red fluid circulating in arteries, capillaries and veins and driven by pumping action of heart. Consists of about 40% cells and 60% fluid (plasma). Cells are mainly red (erythrocytes)—8,000,000 per cu.mm. Rest are white (leucocytes)—7–8,000 per cu.mm., or platelets (200,000 per cu.mm.). Plasma contains water, proteins, salt, sugars, enzymes, vitamins and minerals. **B.** takes nourishment and oxygen to body cells, carries waste material and gas (carbon dioxide) to organs of excretion, ie lungs, gut, kidneys, and transports hormones. It is one of 3 vehicles for body water, the others being intracellular and interstitial fluids (see fluid balance). **b. blister** (syn. hematoma) Collection of b.-stained fluid in muscle. It lifts skin, area often becoming gradually larger until it needs lancing and washing out with antibiotics. Common sites: brisket and hindquarters, resulting from kick or other injury. **clotted b.** See coagulation. **cord b.** That in umbilical arteries and veins. **b. diseases** Changes in composition of **b.** may be due to: (1) Condition in part of body, eg diarrhoea causes loss of body fluid (see dehydration) and therefore **b.** becomes more concentrated (hemoconcentration). Liver disease may alter protein and enzyme levels (see liver disease). (2) Infection with parasites (see biliary fever), bacteria or virus (see swamp fever). (3) Hemolytic diseases (see hemolytic jaundice). (4) Primary conditions (see anemia, leukemia). **b. in feces** Sign of enteritis due to bacterial/parasitic infection. **B.** is dark if bleeding is some distance from rectum and bright if it is close to anus. **b. groups/types** Various inherited systems are present in red **b.** cells (erythrocytes). Red cell groups are designated A, C, D, K, P, Q, U and X and further divided into factors. The serum protein can be divided into systems: albumin (AL), transferrin (TF), esterase (ES), PR, 6 PGD and PGM. These systems are further divided into factors.

RED CELL GROUPS

SYSTEMS	A	C	D	K	P	Q	U	X
FACTORS	$A_1,A,H,-$	$C,-$	D_1,E_1,E_2,J_2,E'	$K,-$	$P_1,P,-$	Q,R,S	$U,-$	$X,-$

PROTEIN POLYMORPHISM GROUPS

SYSTEM	ALBUMIN (AL)	TRANSFERRIN (TF)	ESTERASE (ES)	PR	6PGD	PGM
FACTORS	F,S	D,F_1,F_2,G,H,M,O,R	F,G,H,I,S	L,N,S	F,S	F,S

Systems and factors can help establish parentage of a foal and record of **b.** type will one day be necessary to qualify for General Stud Book (Thoroughbreds). (Reference: Scott, Michael, BSc, ARCS.) **occult b.** That present in such small quantities that it can be detected only by laboratory tests. **peripheral b.** That circulating in, or close to, skin. **placental b.** That in placenta. **b. plasma** That part of whole blood in which red and white cells are suspended. If anticoagulated **b.** is allowed to stand plasma is seen as clear fluid above sediment of cells; contains water, proteins and salts. **b. pressure** Pressure in arteries (high) and in capillaries and veins (low). During contraction (systole) of heart, pressure is about 120mm.Hg in arteries, but during relaxation (diastole) it falls to about 80mm.Hg. In veins pressure may be as low as 5mm.Hg and close to heart there may be small negative pressure when **b.** is sucked into chambers. Estimating arterial pressure is impracticable in the horse, although it has been tried using a cuff around tail or limbs.

Pressure can be gauged by inserting catheter into artery and connecting it to measuring apparatus, but this is usually done only in experiments. **b. serum** Clear fluid which separates when **b.** clots. Similar to plasma but does not contain fibrinogen. **b. tests** Examination of **b.** samples in laboratory to aid diagnosis of disease. Hematology is examination of cellular content; biochemical tests determine levels of minerals, salts, enzymes, proteins; serological tests show **b.** groups and the presence of antibodies. Hematology: (1) Red **b.** cell count—the number of red cells (erythrocytes) per cu.mm. Normal range 7–10 million per cu.mm. depending on age and state of fitness. (2) Hemoglobin content—measured in gms. per 100ml., normal 12–17gms./100ml. (3) Packed cell volume (hematocrit or PCV)—proportion of cells to plasma expressed as a percentage. Normal range, depending on age and fitness, 33–45%. (4) White **b.** cell count—number of white cells per cu.mm. of **b.** Normal range 5–10,000 per cu.mm. (5) Differential white **b.** cell count, polymorphs 50%, lymphocytes 45%, monocytes 2%, eosinophils 1%, basophils 2% of total white cell count. (6) Platelet count, normal 2–300,000/cu.mm. (7) Erythrocyte sedimentation rate (ESR)—rate at which red **b.** cells (erythrocytes) separate from plasma if sample of **b.** is left to stand. Sample usually left at room temperature and measured in millimetres per hour. Normal range 10–50. Not usually significant in horses. For all these tests **b.** is collected into bottles containing an anti-coagulant to prevent clotting. Red cell count, hemoglobin and packed cell volume can show anemia, qv. White cell count can indicate infection; see infection, diagnosis of. Platelets help clotting. Biochemical tests: (1) Total serum protein (TSP)—amount of protein per 100ml. of serum. Normal range 5–7gms. per 100ml. (2) Albumin and globulin—albumin/globulin ratio of TSP. Normal ratio about 1:0.7 (that is 3gms. per 100ml. albumin and about 2.1gms. per 100ml. globulin). TSP increases in disturbed fluid balance and decreases in chronic conditions. Albumin/globulin ratio is reversed (eg 0.5:1.0) in infectious disease and albumin levels may fall below 2gms. per 100ml. in liver disease. (3) Serum enzymes—serum glutamic oxaloacetic transaminase (SGOT), creatinine phosphokinase (CPK) and serum alkaline phosphatase (SAP). Levels are measures of liver and muscle activity. They rise in disease of tissues (see setfast; heart, diseases of; liver, diseases of; bone, diseases of). Normal levels: SGOT—80–200 international units (IU); SAP—50–150 IU depending on age, higher in young animals; CPK—30–60 IU. (4) Bilirubin—bile pigment. Normal: less than 4mg./100ml. Tests can distinguish between bilirubin (bile pigment) which has entered **b.** before passing through liver from that which entered afterwards (see jaundice). (5) Calcium and phosphorus levels—normal range: calcium 10–14gms. per 100ml. of serum. Calcium/phosphorus ratio in young animals is normally about 4:2.5 and in 3-year-olds and over, 4:1. Changes occur in bone disease, rickets and dietary deficiency or excess of either mineral (see calcium/phosphorus ratio). Most biochemical tests are performed on serum. **B.** is collected into clean bottle and left at room temperature, so that it clots, leaving serum separate. Plasma is used to measure (6) hormone levels—progesterone, oestrogen, cortisol. Blood is collected into an anticoagulant (eg heparin) and centifuged to separate cells from plasma. (7) **B.** gases (oxygen and carbon dioxide) and acidity (pH) can be measured in **b.** collected from a vein but arterial samples are necessary to study lung function. These tests are not routine but help diagnose acid states of **b.** (as a result of metabolic or respiratory dysfunction), foal conditions, diarrhoea, broken wind and other diseases of lungs and liver. **B.** can form basis of function tests, eg using dye, such as bromosulpthalein (qv), to measure its rate of disappearance from **b.** (This shows liver function.) **B.** can also be examined for unnatural substances, such as dope (barbiturates, minerals, toxins, see dope test). Serological tests: Levels of antibody can be measured in serum and expressed in titre, ie the lowest dilution of serum at which antigen/antibody reaction occurs in test tube, eg in brucellosis 1 in 10 titre is negative and 1 in 40 positive. These tests are used to diagnose virus infections. Initially (acute phase) the body has not reacted to infection and level of antibodies in **b.** has not been affected. A sample at this stage can be compared with one taken 2 or 3 weeks later (convalescent phase) when titre is higher. This is evidence of an infection of the antibody used in test, eg a horse with fever and cough is tested for levels of influenza virus antibodies in acute phase (result 1 in 100). In convalescent stage, serum level is 1 in 640— definite evidence of infection with influenza. See also pregnancy tests, cross-matching. **b. transfusion** Giving **b.** of one horse to another. The donor **b.** is collected into bottle containing anticoagulant and transfused with apparatus attached to a needle or catheter inserted into recipient's vein, usually the jugular. Before transfusion it is usual to cross-match to ensure compatibility. See cross-matching. **b. in urine** Sign of setfast, infection or stone (calculi) in bladder or urethra. Stallion may bleed from the urethra after repeated attempts at service due to rupture of small vessel at distal end of penis. Giving phenothiazine can cause red-coloured urine. **b. vessels** Arteries, capillaries and veins. The system of tubes carrying **b.** from heart to body tissues and organs and returning it to heart to complete circulation. **whole b.** That which contains all its elements. See anemia, plasma, red cells, white cells.

blue Colour of dye, eg methylene **b.** used as antiseptic and in laboratory for staining. **b. bottle** See Calliphora. **b. roan** See coat colouring.

body (L. corpus, Gr. soma) Whole of horse, or main part. **inclusion b.** Particle in cell infected with virus.

bog spavin Swollen hock joint due to increased synovial fluid. Caused by faulty conformation, injury, nutritional deficiency, anemia, allergy and infection with bacteria or virus. Symptoms: fluctuating swelling over front inside of hock and two smaller swellings on outside of joint about hand's breadth below point of hock. Treatment: identify cause, treat accordingly and possibly inject corticosteroids into joint and apply deep heat. See also spavin, plate 38.

boil External abscess. Treatment: apply warm poultice until ripe; lance or allow to burst, use antibiotics if necessary. **blind b.** Abscess which does not form a core and may not burst. Affects especially saddle area. Cf warble fly, acne.

bolus (L., Gr. bolos, lump) (1) Mass of food. Hay or other nutrient is ground between molars and mixed with saliva to form **b.** which is swallowed. (2) Rounded mass larger than a pill. See ball, choke.

bone Hard substance making up body's skeleton, on which soft tissues hang. Consists of 35% living and 65% non-living material. Half weight of **b.** is non-living calcium phosphate which, with fluid of **b.**, is constantly changing; entire calcium content of skeleton is replaced about every 200 days. Covered by membrane (periosteum) and if, as in a long **b.**, it has a hollow (marrow) this is lined with membrane (endosteum). Consists mainly of a ground substance or matrix arranged around living cells in concentric rings. These rings form cylinders (lamellae) through which fine (Haversian) canals travel along axis of **b.** These canals contain small arteries and veins to supply **b.** cells. Cells immediately round Haversian canals are osteoblasts, which secrete matrix of **b. B.** varies according to place in skeleton and may be compact, spongy, or a mixture, eg hind cannon (metatarsal) has a compact shaft with a spongy inside which helps to give lightness and strength. Long **b.**'s grow at either end from cartilage in which calcium is laid down, so changing calcium into **b.** Life of molecule of calcium can be examined by making it radio-active and following it with a geiger counter. Typically, a molecule of calcium might stay in **b.** for 10 days, then travel in blood stream. Equine blood contains 4 parts calcium (12mg. per 100ml.) to 1 part phosphorus (4mg. per 100ml.). **b., diseases of** Can affect structure, outer lining (periosteum), growth plate (epiphysis) or cavity and marrow. Conditions are caries, rickets, osteoarthritis (see arthritis), epiphysitis, osteitis, periostitis, osteoarthropathy, exostosis, osteodystrophy, fracture. **b. flour/b. meal** Source of calcium and phosphorus; included in some compound feeds. See calcium/phosphorus ratio. **b.'s of foreleg** Shoulder blade (scapula), arm (humerus), forearm (radius and ulna), knee (carpus, containing 8 small **b.'s**), cannon **b.** (metacarpus, equivalent of **b.'s** between human wrist and knuckles), digits (1st, 2nd and 3rd phalanx **b.'s**, equivalent to human finger). **b.'s of hind leg** Hip (pelvic girdle or os coxae), which joins its fellow on opposite side at symphysis and articulates above with sacrum—hip is composed of ileum, ischium and pubis; thigh (femur) which articulates with pelvis at top end and with tibia and patella below; second thigh (tibia and fibula), hock (tarsus, containing 6 small **b.'s**, equivalent to human ankle), cannon (metatarsal); digits similar to those of foreleg. See skeleton, cartilage.

booster Colloq. 2nd or subsequent dose of vaccine to enhance protection against eg influenza, lockjaw. See vaccinate.

boot Leather and metal cover for part of limb, eg hock **b.**, ankle **b.**, foot **b.** Used to protect when travelling, racing etc or to hold dressing in place.

borate Salt of boric acid, qv.

borborygmus (pl. borborygmi) Sound from food, fluid and gas passing through intestines by movement of alimentary tract. Can be heard with naked ear or stethoscope. Loud in diarrhoea and spasmodic colic; decreased in cases of blocked alimentary tract. See colic, peristalsis, twist.

boric acid White shining scales, crystals or powder; odourless, non-irritant, with slightly bitter taste. Applied to wounds, ulcers, mucous membranes and as mouthwash or eye lotion.

borna disease An infectious viral disease affecting brain. Causes fever, paralysis, muscular tremors and hypersensitivity with death 1–3 weeks later. Recorded only in Germany and similar to encephalomyelitis, qv.

bot Botfly larva which lives in horse's stomach. Belongs to order Diptera, family Oestridae. 5 species of genus Gasterophilus, 3 of which live in Britain—G. intestinalis, G. nasalis and G. hemorrhoidalis. (Others are G. pecorum and G. inermis.) Fly is about ½in. long (13mm.), resembles bee but cannot suck, bite or feed because its mouth parts are degenerate. Life cycle: adult fly is active in early summer and September, making humming sound as it flies. On warm days it hovers close to horse, with egg ready at rear (ovipositor) and lays up to 300 eggs an hour. Each hatches in 9–12 days but first larva cannot develop until it is licked into a horse's mouth. The larvae of G. inermis and G. hemorrhoidalis can pierce cheek to enter mouth. In mouth, larva penetrates mucosa and burrows down wall of gullet. G. intestinalis wanders in tongue 20–30 days. The 2nd and 3rd larvae (**b.** maggots) live in stomach, although those of G. inermis and G. pecorum are also found in pharynx and gullet. Maggot is

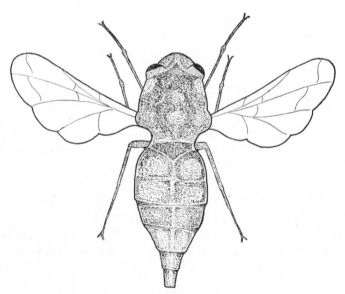

4 Botfly (Gasterophilus intestinalis)—female

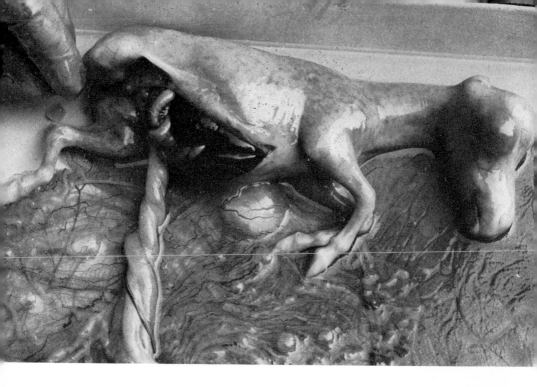

6 160-day fetus lying on the placenta. The abdomen has been opened to show the liver and intestines. Note umbilical cord (lower left) and unformed eyes. See *cord, fetus, embryology*

7 Amnion opened to show 205-day fetus. See *fetus, embryology*

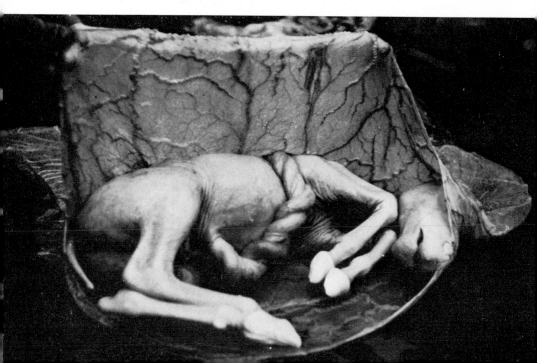

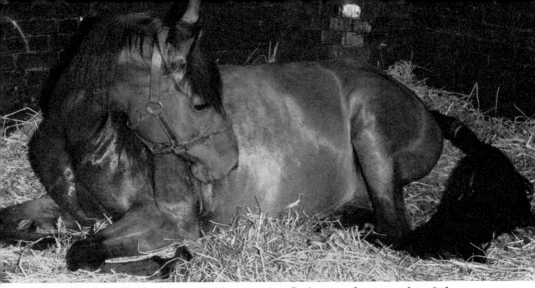

8 Signs of pain—looking round at flanks, sweating on neck and chest

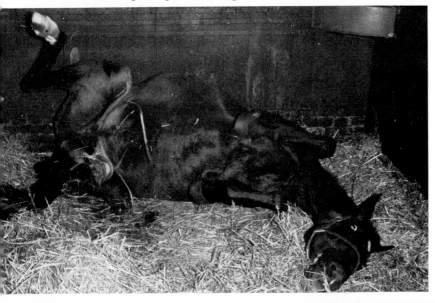

9 Rolling

10 Pawing the ground.
See *birth, colic*

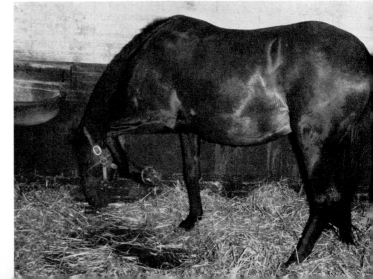

thought to live on host's food for about 10 months. It drops off stomach wall and either attaches to rectum or passes straight out. On the ground it wriggles to a crevice to pupate. The pupal stage lasts about 3 weeks, then adult fly emerges and cycle is complete. Adult flies can cause horses to panic and gallop into each other or into fences; maggots cause inflamed stomach or other parts of digestive tract and disrupt digestion. Treatment: see dicophane, carbon disulphide, haloxon, metriphonate. See plate 26.

botulism Rare fatal disease caused by taking in toxin of Clostridium botulinum. Symptoms appear 3–7 days later and include paralysis of limbs, jaw, throat and tongue, which hangs from mouth. Horse cannot swallow, collapses and dies. Cf lockjaw.

bouillon Broth or soup used in laboratory to grow and identify bacteria. See laboratory tests.

Boulonnais Strong, fast draught horse named after a breeding area in Pas-de-Calais dept of France, around Boulogne, Two types: Abbeville, medium size and Dunkirk, larger and heavier. Used for driving and farm work and improved by Arab and Barb stallions brought home by French crusaders. Generally strawberry or blue roan, dapple grey or black; resembles Percheron, qv.

bowed tendon Colloq. for inflamed deep and superficial flexor tendons and their sheaths (tendinitis/tendonitis) of forelimb. Shows as bulge in normally straight line behind cannon bone. Treatment: (1) physiotherapy, hot and cold applications, ie poultice or deep heat by shortwave plus cold water from hose or iced bandages; (2) massage and supporting bandage; (3) surgery by stabbing, splitting, transplant; (4) blistering or firing (now dying out on humane grounds, see plate 17); (5) injections of corticosteroids IM or into tendon sheath. Requires 3–24 months' rest depending on severity. See plate 19.

box shrub (Buxus sempervirens) Ornamental shrub containing alkaloids. If eaten by horse can cause pain, convulsions, dysentery or death from asphyxia.

Boyle's law (after British physicist Robert B.) At a constant temperature volume of gas is inversely proportional to pressure on gas, ie the greater the pressure, the smaller the volume (conversely the less the pressure the more the gas expands).

BP Abbr. British Pharmacopoeia, qv.

Brabancon Belgian draught horse probably named after Brabant province. Many were crossed with Rhenish and Ardennes. Also bred in Russia in Gorki (Gorky/Gorkiy) province.

brachial Of the foreleg. **b. plexus** See nerves, table of.

brachy- (Gr. brachys, short) Combining form meaning short.

brachycardia See bradycardia.

brachydonty Having short teeth. Used in study of horse's evolution, length of teeth helping determine age of fossil. **B.** abnormal in present-day horse and may indicate crib-biting. Opp. hyposodonty. See evolution, teeth.

bracken poisoning Caused by eating young bracken. It contains an enzyme which inactivates thiamine, causing deficiency. Symptoms: inco-ordination, staggering and unnatural stance, eg feet well spread and back arched. Severe muscular tremors develop, death is preceded by chronic spasms and drawing back of head (opisthotonus). Treatment: 50–100ml. thiamine (aneurine hydrochloride, BPC) sub. cut.

brady- (Gr. bradys, slow) Combining form meaning slow.

bradycardia (brady-+Gr. kardia, heart) Abnormally slow heart rate.

brain (L. encephalon, Gr. enkephalos) Part of central nervous system occupying skull (cranium). Weighs about 23 oz. (650gms.) and forms about 0.7% of body weight in medium-sized horse. It consists of 3 main segments: cerebrum (or cerebral hemispheres), cerebellum and medulla. These are divided into secondary segments and derivatives: medulla oblongata, pons cerebellum, anterior cerebella peduncles, anterior medullary velum, corpora guadrigemina, cerebral peduncles, optic thalami, hypothalamic tegmenta, pineal body, pituitary body, optic nerves and retinae, cerebral hemispheres, olfactory tracts and bulb. All segments contain nerve cells (grey matter) and nerve fibres (white matter) and parts are specialised to control certain functions, eg cerebellum, movement; medulla oblongata, breathing. B. also contains cavities: 4th ventricle, cerebral aqueduct, back and front parts of 3rd ventricle, lateral ventricles and olfactory continuations. **b. cortex** External layer of any part of **b. b., diseases of** Include abscess and growth. Both are rare. Abscess causes drowsiness and inco-ordination (similar to encephalomyelitis, qv) and may be due to Streptococcus equi infection. Growth (syns. neoplasm, tumour) is usually a slowly developing abscess which causes chronic changes in **b.** See also cerebellar degeneration. **b. hemorrhage** Bleeding into **b.** Result of kick, knock etc or, in foals, of difficult birth. See neonatal maladjustment syndrome. **b., injury of** Most common after collision or rearing over backwards. Symptoms which vary with extent and site of injury, include semi- or complete unconsciousness, convulsions, inco-ordination, failure of eye pupils to contract in bright light, blindness, bleeding from nostrils and/ or ears. Any of these may continue to some degree after initial recovery. **b. parasites** Botfly or redworm larvae occasionally wander to **b.,** damaging tissue.

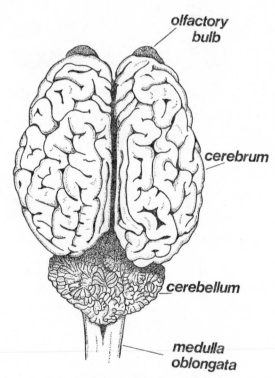

5 Brain from above

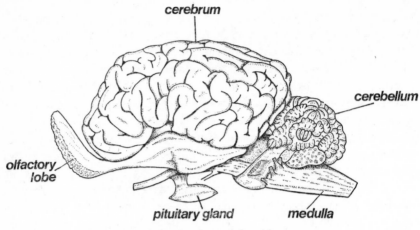

cerebrum

cerebellum

olfactory
lobe

pituitary gland

medulla

6 Brain from left side

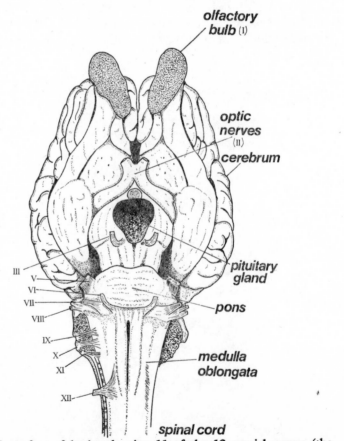

olfactory
bulb (I)

optic
nerves
(II)

cerebrum

pituitary
gland

III
V
VI
VII
VIII

pons

IX
X
XI

medulla
oblongata

XII

spinal cord

7 Undersurface of brain, showing 11 of the 12 cranial nerves (the
emergence of the fourth or trochlear nerve is not visible)

bran Food obtained from outer coat of cereal grain, usually wheat. See food.

branch Division or offshoot; anatomically: distribution of blood vessels, lymphatics, nerves, air tubes.

break See fracture, wound.

breaking of water Colloq. for escape of fluid from vagina at start of 2nd stage labour. See allantoic fluid, birth.

breast Front part of chest, usually pectoral region, ie in front of fore-legs. Cf brisket. **b. bone** (syn. sternum) Bone in centre of chest. Keel-shaped in horse.

breath (L. spiritus, halitus) That air taken into lungs due to expansion of chest (inspiration) and expelled by contraction of chest (expiration). **bad b.** Sign of constipation, colic, decayed teeth, sinusitis, some forms of pneumonia. **first b.** That taken by foal when born as it struggles to break amnion; may be series of gasps followed by rhythm. Cf asphyxia neonatorum.

breathing Alternate inspiration and expiration of air. **b. rate** (respiration) Adult: 12–20 breaths per minute at rest. The younger the horse, faster the rate. Increased in exertion, fever, pneumonia, acidity of blood (acidemia), anemia. See also broken wind, wind.

breech See dystocia.

breed (1) To reproduce. See behaviour, oestrous cycle, embryology, Society for the Study of Animal Breeding. (2) A division within species Equus caballus. See names of various breeds.

Breton horse Bred in Brittany, France. Three types: **B.** heavy draught, usually grey or bay with light 'feathers', bred near coast, about 16 hands; **B.** mountain draught, up to 14/15 hands; **B.** draught post, lighter type.

brevi- (L. brevis, short) Combining form meaning short.

Brevidil Trade name. See suxamethonium.

Brevital Trade name. Type of short-acting anaesthetic.

bridle Harness for horse's head, usually leather straps attached to metal piece (bit) in mouth. Used by veterinarians to control horse being examined when twitch (qv) would be unnecessarily severe or dangerous. See birth hemorrhage.

Brietal sodium Trade name. See methohexitone sodium.

brisket Area of body over sternum bone. Horses said to lie **on b.** when head, neck and withers are off ground, forelegs slightly flexed and one hindleg is beneath body. More common position of rest than lying flat on one side of body. See behaviour.

British Equine Veterinary Association (BEVA) Founded in 1960 as division of British Veterinary Association. Publishers of Equine Veterinary Journal, 7 Mansfield Street, London W1M 0AT (01 636 6541) **B. Horse Society** Body which governs light and heavy horse societies, sets standards in the show-ring and examines riding instructors. National Equestrian Centre, Kenilworth, Warwickshire CV8 2LR (Coventry 27192) or c/o 35 Belgrave Square, London SW1 (01 235 6431). **B. Pharmacopoeia** (BP) Book listing drugs, their actions, uses, etc. Published by direction of General Medical Council by Pharmaceutical Press. See **B.** Veterinary Codex. **B. Show Jumping Association** A division of **B.** Horse Society, qv. **B. Veterinary Association** See Veterinary Record. **B. Veterinary Codex** Book containing actions, usage and dosage of drugs, vaccines, etc. Published for the Pharmaceutical Soc. of Gt Britain by the Pharmaceutical Press, 17 Bloomsbury Square, London WC1, in 1953, and since then in a new edition and supplements. **B. Veterinary Hospital Association** (BVHA) Formed in 1972; c/o H. Andrew, 39, Hawkshead Road, Paisley, Scotland (Paisley 3464). See veterinary hospital. **B. Veterinary Journal** Independent magazine founded as Veterinary Journal in 1875 by George Fleming, MRCVS. Published every two months by Bailliere Tindall Ltd, 7 Henrietta Street, London WC2 (01 836 3386). **B. Veterinary Radiological Association** c/o S. W. Douglas, School of Veterinary Medicine, Madingley Road, Cambridge, CB3 0ES.

broken wind (syns. heaves, atelectasis, chronic pulmonary emphysema) Condition affecting 4-year-olds and over, characterised by difficult breathing. Occurs in most countries but commonly where horses are stabled and fed mouldy hay. Thought to be caused by allergy to fungus, particularly moulds containing Aspergillus species, Alternaria species and Hormodendrum species. Antibody reaction induces spasm of muscles in wall of small air ducts and bronchioles so that air is trapped in air sacs (alveoli). These may eventually rupture so that 2 or more fuse (emphysema). Condition often accompanied by infected and inflamed air passages (bronchitis). The acute form occurs suddenly with difficult breathing (dyspnoea) and is similar to acute human asthma. Attack may coincide with change of environment, eg from field to stable. Attacks more common during hot, humid weather. Signs include heaving belly, flared nostrils, rhythmic movement of anus and surrounding area (perineum) coinciding with breathing, restlessness, profuse or patchy sweating and tendency to resent handling, deep, nonproductive cough and loud wheezing. Attacks are not fatal but may last several minutes and occur daily if management is unaltered. Case then progresses into chronic form. This may have history of mild respiratory fault. Horse may cough when walked from warm air into cold and breathing becomes faster with double expiration. Bronchitis usually develops, with more coughing and slight nasal discharge. Condition may have functional or structural basis. In functional form, air sacs are enlarged and their walls undamaged, so horse may become normal. In structural form air sacs have been damaged. It usually takes months or years to develop and is irreversible. Diagnosis: on symptoms, sounds from the lungs and positive skin reaction to test doses of common moulds. Treatment: fresh, dust-free air. Stabled horses should be placed on peat moss and fed good-quality hay. Antihistamine drugs and antibiotics may help if bronchitis is present.

bromosulpthalein (syn. BSP) Dye used to measure activity of liver. It is injected into vein and catheter placed in jugular vein to collect blood samples for laboratory examination at intervals up to 20 minutes. Mature horses should remove at least 20% of BSP per minute.

bronchi Pl. of bronchus.

bronchial (L. bronchialis) Of bronchi, bronchiol, bronchioli, bronchiolus, bronchus.

bronchiolitis Inflamed bronchioles when tubes become full of exudate (cells and fluid). Associated with viral and bacterial infection, eg herpesvirus, Streptococci, Staphylococci. See bronchitis, catarrh, cough, snotty nose.

bronchitis Inflammation of larger bronchial tubes of lungs due to infection or irritation by foreign material, eg dust. Usually accompanies broken wind (emphysema) and follows infection with a virus, eg one belonging to herpes group. See bronchiolitis; broken wind; snotty nose; abortion, viral.

bronchopneumonia Bacterial, viral or fungal infection of small air tubes and air sacs of lungs.

bronchus (syn. bronchiolus; L., Gr. bronchos; pl. bronchi) A large air passage in lungs. Stems from windpipe (trachea) and divides into bronchioles.

broth Liquid used in laboratory for cultivating micro-organisms.

Brucella abortus (after Sir David Bruce) Abortion caused by Brucella genus of bacteria. Rare in horses but can occur if mares graze near infected cattle. See abortion, brucellosis.

brucellosis Condition caused by bacteria of family Brucellaceae, order Eubacteriales. Characterised by stiffness, due to abscesses or infection in joints. Can be spread by draining fistulous withers. Diagnosis: on blood tests. See blood (serological tests).

bruise Injury to superficial structure of body, eg skin.

bruised Structure containing bruise, eg **b.** sole (syn. stone bruise). See foot.

bruit Abnormal sound in heart beat. See heart sounds.

brush When inside of one limb strikes inside of another, cf speedy cutting. See gait.

buccal (L. buccalis from bucca, cheek) Of the cheek, qv.

bucked knee (syn. knee sprung) Deformity of knee (carpal) joint resulting in permanently flexed joint. Usually seen in foals; condition improves by 6 months. **b. shin,** (syns. sore shin, metacarpal periostitis) Inflamed lining of cannon bone, most common in Thoroughbred 2-year-olds. Usually in one or both forelegs. Caused by galloping on firm ground. The membrane (periosteum) lining bone becomes detached and new bone is formed. Symptoms include pain, swelling and lameness. Treatment: rest, cooling lotions, cold applications, corticosteroids and DMSO. See stress fracture, plate 20.

Budyonovsky Russian breed popular for eventing and first in Britain found to harbour Parafilaria multipapillosa, qv.

buffer Substance in fluid which lessens change in acidity or alkalinity when acids or alkalis are added.

bulbo-urethral Two glands about 4cm. (2ins.) long and 2.5cm. (1in.) wide near urethra. They open into urethra via 6–8 ducts and their secretion (seminal plasma) nourishes and transports spermatozoa.

bulbs of heel Back part of foot formed by digital cushion, part of periopic corium (qv) and lateral cartilages (qv). Subject to bruising by over-reach.

bulla Large blister filled with serous fluid. See blister.

bull nosed foot Hoof rasped in front so that toe is cut short.

bundle Anatomical term for collection of fibres, eg **b.** branches. See heart impulse.

Burmese (syn. Shan) Strong but slow pony, bred by hill tribes of Shan state in central Burma. Similar to Mongolian and the faster Manipur.

burn Lesion resulting from contact with hot liquid or fire. **chemical b.** One due to corrosive substance. See blister.

bursa (L., Gr. a wine skin; pl. bursae) Sac or cavity filled with fluid (synovial) at places where friction is likely to occur, eg in joints.

bursatti See stomach worm.

bursitis Inflamed bursa caused by injury or infection, eg brucellosis. Common sites include bursa at point of elbow (syns. shoe boil, capped elbow), at hock (syn. capped hock), at hip (trochanteric **b.**, syn. whorlbone). See whorlbone lameness, hygroma, bicipital **b.** Treatment:

drain fluid with needle and inject corticosteroids.

Buscopan Trade name. Antispasmodic (qv) drug used to treat some colics and obstructed gullet.

Buta-Leucotropin Trade name. See phenylbutazone.

Butazolidin (syn. bute) Trade name. See phenylbutazone.

button Anatomical term for knob-like structure, eg lower end of second and fourth metacarpal and metatarsal bones. See splint.

buttress foot (syns. pyramaditis, pyramidal disease) Bone enlargement at front of pedal bone, causing swelling on front of foot at coronary band. May be result of fracture of bone, or arthritis. Diagnosis: on lameness, pain and swelling.

BVMS/BVM&S Abbrs. Bachelor of Veterinary Medicine and Surgery.

BVSc Abbr. Bachelor of Veterinary Science.

C

Ca Abbr. for calcium.

cachexia (cac- + Gr. hexis, habit) Wasting and malnutrition. See metabolism, wasting.

cadaver (L. from cadere, to fall, perish; syn. carcass) Corpse, dead body. See carcass, rigor mortis.

cadmium Toxic metal. **c. poisoning** Rare condition of horses grazing near zinc smelters. Main symptom: acute diarrhoea.

caecum (L., blind gut) Large comma-shaped sac between small intestine and colon; about 1.25m. (4ft.) long with capacity of about 25 litres (7 gallons) in adult horse. Consists of base, body and apex and occupies central lower abdomen. See alimentary canal.

caesarean section Surgical removal of fetus, performed under general anaesthesia. The flank or abdomen is opened (laparotomy), uterus exposed and fetus extracted. **C.s.** necessary if fetus cannot pass through birth canal because part or parts are lodged against mare's pelvis. (Attempts should first be made to correct malalignment by manipulation, see dystocia.) **C.s.** has replaced embryotomy (cutting fetus into pieces with a special instrument—embryotome—so it can be delivered through birth canal).

caffeine White powder or silky glistening odourless particles with bitter taste. From dried leaves of Camellia sinensis. Stimulates central nervous system and helps muscle efficiency, increases breathing rate and acts as diuretic. Considered a stimulant dope in racehorses. See veterinary rules.

calcareous (L. calcarius) Of lime or calcium. **c. deposits** May form in ligaments after chronic inflammation.

calciferol White or colourless crystalline powder, odourless and tasteless. Has action and uses of vitamin D. See concentrated vitamin D solution.

calcification (calcium + L. facere, to make) The depositing of calcium salts, eg **c.** of cartilage at growing ends of bones. See growth plate.

calcium (L. calx, lime; abbr. Ca) Yellow metal or basic element; atomic weight 40.08; present in body tissues and important in coagulation of blood. C. and phosphorus are main minerals in bone. **c. borogluconate** White odourless powder or transparent scales. Given as 10–40% solution to treat poisoning by chloroform, carbon tetrachloride or lead; also in rare cases of mares showing signs like milk fever after foaling, ie unsteadiness, twitching of superficial muscles, lying down for long periods. **c. carbonate** See chalk. **C. Disodium Verserate** Trade name. See sodium calcium edetate. **c. hydrogen phosphate** White crystalline odourless slightly salty-tasting powder. Given as source of calcium and phosphorus. Dose 4–8gms. See bone flour. **c. and phosphorus** (abbrs. Ca, P) Minerals required for bone and teeth formation; they account for more than 70% of mineral content of body. Too little of either limits usefulness of the other. Adequate quantities in a proportion of Ca to P of 1.3:1.0 and adequate vitamin D are essential for proper utilisation in body. Mature horse of 1,000lb. needs about 15gms. per day of Ca and P. Young horse of 400lb., about 10gms. of Ca and 8gms. of P. **c./phosphorus ratio** Proportion of Ca to P in diet. **c sulphate** See plaster of Paris.

calculus See stone.

calf See gaskin.

Calliphore (Gr. Kallos, beauty + phoros, bearing) Genus of scavenging fly which lays eggs in decaying matter or on wounds. **C. vomitoria** Common blowfly or bluebottle.

callus A formation of new bone in soft, fibrous tissues between ends of broken bone; may project from beneath skin as hard lump, as in fracture of splint bone. See splint.

calor Heat; one of main signs of inflammation, qv.

calorie Unit of heat **large c.** (written kilocalorie or C.). Heat required to raise temperature of 1kg. of water 1 degree centigrade. Used in study of metabolism. **small c.** Amount of heat needed to raise temperature of 1gm. of water 1 degree centigrade.

calorific (L. calor, heat + facere, to make) Heat-producing.

calorimeter (L. calor, heat + Gr. metron, measure) Instrument that measures heat exchange.

Camargue Pony of marshy C. district of France, S of Arles. Usually grey or white (but not albino, qv). Some still roam and breed in feral herds of about 15 mares per stallion. Renowned for their looks—they have particularly long manes and tails—stamina and ability to sprint. Used to round up C. bulls. Many geldings and barren mares ridden by tourists in summer and turned loose with stallions, mares and foals to spend bitter winter on marshes. Country of origin doubtful, possibly N Africa, Tibet or China. Julius Caesar said to have created stud farms before C. pony reverted to its feral life. See plate 23.

camped Fault of conformation in which forelegs (c. in front) or hindlegs (c. behind) are extended too far from body.

Canadian pox See acne.

canal Narrow tube or channel in body, eg alimentary c., qv, birth c., qv.

cancellous Spongy. Used in connection with bone tissues.

cancer (L., crab) Growth which is malignant, ie forms secondary growths. Relatively rare in horses. See growth.

Candida (L. candidus, glowing white) Genus of yeast-like fungus. **C. albicans** May infect uterus and genital tract or foal's tongue, causing greyish-white coating; infection may follow antibiotic treatment.

canine (L. caninus) Of dog, eg **c.** tooth. See teeth.

canker See thrush. **c. of ear** Infection of ear by Staphylococcus or mites. Uncommon in horses.

cannon Bone between knee and fetlock. See metacarpal.

cannula (L. canna, reed) Tube inserted into body for transfusing or drawing off fluid. **trocar and c.** Metal instrument for cannulating organ or part inflated with gas, pus or fluid. Cf catheter.

cannulate To insert tube.

cantharadin Glistening colourless crystals obtained from cantharides, qv. Irritates skin, causing redness, burning and blistering. Used to blister legs. Blistering liquid: mix colophony (1.2gms.) and cantharadin (0.4gm.) in castor oil (2.5ml.) and add acetone to make up to 100ml. See blister.

cantharides Dried Spanish fly, Cantharis (blister bug) or dried beetle.

canthus Inner and outer angle of eye, qv.

capacity (L. capacitas from capere, to take) Expression of measurement. **cranial c.** Amount of space in skull. **vital c.** Amount of air that can be forcefully expelled from lung after full inhalation. C. measured metrically in cubic centimetres (cc); 1cc=1ml. (millilitre).

Cape horse Extinct ancestor of Basuto pony bred from first horses imported into S Africa—4 Arab/Barb types— in 1650s. Highly prized for looks and stamina in Boer War but breed later deteriorated. Used in 1820s in Basutoland by the invading Zulus, then developed into today's Basuto.

capillary (L. capillaris, hair-like) Minute tube; smallest type of blood vessel connecting arteries with veins. Has extremely thin wall, which allows exchange of gases, nutritive and waste materials between blood and tissues through which it passes. Lymph vessels also have **c.** system.

capped elbow Swollen point of elbow (over olecranon) due to inflamed bursa and/or bruising of skin and underlying tissues. Often caused by hindfoot when getting up. **c. hock** See hock.

capsule (L. capsula, a little box) Structure which encloses organ or part, eg fibrous **c.** surrounding kidney or ovary; joint **c.**, membrane enclosing cavity of joint, qv.

capsulitis Inflamed joint capsule. See arthritis.

Carbachol Trade name. See carbachol.

carbachol Small colourless crystals or white powder with faint fishy odour. Stimulates movement of alimentary canal and bladder, also smooth muscle of pregnant uterus. Used to treat colic due to mild stoppage. Given in a 1 in 1,000 solution sub. cut. or IM. Antidote: atropine.

carbohydrate (syn. sugar) Food substance found in vegetable and animal tissue, viz., starch, glucose, lactose and fructose. In plants starch and fructose are built up from carbon dioxide under influence of light; in animals glucose derived from breakdown of **c.** in food and built up into glycogen (qv) and glucose. Lactose is produced in mammary glands from glucose and secreted in milk.

carbon bisulphide/disulphide Clear colourless highly refractive liquid with characteristic odour. Used as anthelmintic (qv) against botfly larvae. Given through stomach tube. Dose: foals 4–8ml., adults 8–16ml. (Horses should be fasted before treatment.) Highly toxic drug requiring great care. Signs of poisoning include excitement, colic and, in extreme cases, convulsions and death.

carbon tetrachloride (a tetrachloromethane) Clear colourless liquid with burning taste. Used as anthelmintic; largely replaced by piperazine salts, qv. **c.t. poisoning** Death may occur 3–4 days after administration. Symptoms: spasm and coma. Antidote: calcium borogluconate IV.

carbuncle (L. carbunculus, little coat) Type of abscess involving skin and subcutaneous tissue, usually has multiple drainage points and caused by staphylococcal germ. See abscess.

carcass (Fr. carcasse; syn. cadaver) Dead body. Parts of equine **c.** can be utilised—hooves to make glue, flesh to feed dogs. Meat has sweet taste.

carcinogen Substance or virus which induces formation of growth, eg wart. See growth.

carcinoma (Gr. karkinoma from karkinos, crab, cancer) Type of malignant growth composed of epithelial cells. See growth.

cardiac (L. cardicus from Gr. kardiakos, heart) Of the heart. **c. output** Amount of blood pumped from heart during each beat (stroke volume), or amount pumped per unit time. Falls in heart disease such as atrial fibrillation. See heart rate.

cardiogram (cardio- + Gr. gramma, a writing) Tracing made by machine known as cardiograph, as in electrocardiogram, qv.

cardiograph (cardio- + Gr. graphein, to write) Instrument which records a cardiogram.

cardiologist Person with particular knowledge of diagnosing and treating heart disease.

caries (L., rottenness) Decay or death of bone. See bone, diseases of.

Caritrol Trade name. See diethylcarbamazine citrate.

carotid (Gr. karotis from karos, deep sleep) Main artery of neck. See arteries, table of. **c. body** Collection of special cells sensitive to alterations of oxygen and carbon dioxide concentrations in blood. Able to affect breathing by nervous reflex to help keep concentrations within normal limits. **c. sinus** Part of **c.** artery sensitive to alterations in blood pressure and able to exert nervous control of heart rate and blood pressure.

carpal (L. carpalis) Of the carpus (knee). **c. bones, fracture of**

Any of 8 may be broken, but radial, third **c.** bone and accessory most likely. Trauma is most common cause. Symptoms: similar to those of carpitis, ie heat, pain, swelling and lameness. Diagnosis: by careful X-ray examination from several different angles, because number of bones involved may mask fracture in one. See slab fracture. **c. joint** Formed by 8 bones in 2 rows: proximal and distal. Proximal: radial, intermediate, ulnar and accessory (pisiform). Distal: first, second, third and fourth **c.** bones. Radial is largest bone of proximal row and its front edge is usually where arthritis develops. **c. joints** The 3 small joints which make up knee joint: (1) between radius and proximal row of **c.** bones; (2) intercarpal joint, between the two rows of **c.** bones; (3) carpo-metacarpal joint, between distal row of **c.** bones and upper end of metacarpal (cannon and splint bones). The joint capsule is common to all 3 joints. Synovial membrane is arranged so that second 2 compartments communicate, but first is separate.

carpitis (syn. popped knee) Inflamed carpal (knee) joint causing distended capsule and soft enlargements, resistance to flexion and pain on movement or pressure (see arthritis). Severe cases may be caused by broken carpal bones. See plate 40.

carpus (L., Gr. karpos) Joint between forearm and cannon, commonly called knee; equivalent to human wrist.

carrier Individual harbouring micro-organisms capable of causing disease but without producing signs; a distributor of infection, eg individual carrying strangles germ in glands may cause outbreak of disease when in contact with susceptible horses. C.'s help spread encephalo-myelitis, swamp fever, etc.

cartilage (L. cartilago; colloq. gristle) Specialised tissue of cells surrounded by ground substance. Provides embryo's skeleton, most of which gradually hardens into bone. **articular c.** Caps bones forming joint to provide surface for movement. **costal c.** That at ends of ribs where they join sternum. **cricoid c.** That forming a ring. **elastic c.** Pliable, occurs where muscles and membranes need support, eg voice box, windpipe and between nostrils (nasal septum). **fibro c.** Fibrous **c.** in, eg, skull. **growth (epiphyseal) c.** That at ends of long bones and which forms new bone. See growth plate.

caseation (L. caseus, cheese) Abscess of decaying tissue and cells resembling cheese. See Corynebacterium equi.

casein (L. caseus, cheese) Main protein of milk.

Caslick (after American veterinarian E. A. C.; syn stitching) Operation performed under local anaesthesia in which lips forming upper part of vulva are stitched together to prevent air entering vagina. Necessary in mares that have poor conformation (ie vulva sloping from normal vertical position). Mare that has had C. should be cut, with straight scissors, immediately before foaling and re-stitched afterwards.

Caspian pony Rediscovered in 1965 around C. Sea. Some run wild, others are used as pack ponies. Usually 9–11 hands. May be ancestor of Arab and direct descendant of horse which roamed Zagros Mountains on Persia/Iraq border in prehistoric times.

cassette (Fr., a little box) X-ray film container which prevents exposure to light but through which X-rays can pass; may contain an intensifying screen. See radiation.

cast See anaesthesia, plaster of Paris.

castor oil Colourless or pale yellow liquid from seeds of Ricinus communis. Has slight odour and nauseating taste. Sometimes used in foals up to 12 hours old to help passage of meconium (qv). Dose: 60–90ml., in a drink. Also used with zinc in soothing ointment for sores etc. **c.o. plant (Ricinus communis) poisoning** Symptoms, several days after ingestion: inco-ordination, sweating, diarrhoea, muscle spasms and heart tremor. May cause death. At post-mortem gut lining is inflamed, lymph glands swollen and gut, liver, kidney and possibly windpipe and lungs are fluid-filled. Treatment: specific antiserum, but this is unlikely to be available, so use anti-shock measures. See shock.

castrate (syns. alter, cut, emasculate) To remove gonads, rendering individual sterile.

castration (L. castratio) Surgical removal of testes; either under sedation and local anaesthesia with horse standing or under general anaesthesia. (C. in Britain illegal without an anaesthetic.) Usually performed at 1 or 2 years; sometimes at 3 months. Castrated male (colloq. gelding) does not develop stallion's physique, eg thick, slightly crested neck or, often excitable, temperament and rarely shows any sexual interest in females. Cf vasectomy. See emasculator.

cata- (Gr. kata, down) Prefix meaning down.

catabiosis (Gr. katabiosis, a passing life) Normal ageing of cells.

catabolic Of catabolism.

catabolism (Gr. katabole, a throwing down) Breaking down of protein and loss of muscle. One of 2 types of metabolism (cf. anabolism). Rate of **c.** (catabolic rate) usually increases with age.

catabolite Product of catabolism.

cataplasm (L. cataplasma, Gr. kataplasma) Poultice, qv.

cataract See eye, diseases of.

catarrh (L. catarrhus from Gr. katarrhein, to flow down) Purulent or semi-purulent discharge produced by an inflamed mucous membrane. May be in nose or alimentary canal. See snotty nose, colic.

catecholamine Compound with action that mimics that of sympathetic nervous system (see autonomic nervous system), eg adrenaline.

catechu Pale-brown odourless powder with bitter taste. Powerful astringent, used to treat persistent diarrhoea. Dose: 4–12gms.

catgut Material prepared from sheep's intestine and used to stitch wounds. **chromic c.** That sterilised and impregnated with chromium trioxide. See suture.

cathartic See purgative.

catheter (Gr. katheter; syn. cannula) Surgical instrument, usually made of nylon or plastic, for drawing fluids from, or introducing them into, any cavity of body. **uterine c.** One used to infuse infected uterus with, eg antibiotic solution. **indwelling c.** One left in place for a long time, eg in vein or uterus. Cf cannula.

catheterisation Act of passing a catheter.

cathode (Gr. kata, down + hodos, way) Negative electrode or pole of galvanic circuit.

cauda Tail or tail-like appendage, eg **c.** epididymis, tail of epididymis, qv.

caudal Of tail or inferior end.

cause (L. causa) Process which brings about condition or disease. **exciting c.** That which leads directly to specific condition, eg Streptococcus equi causes strangles. **predisposing c.** Something which renders horse more liable to specific condition without actually producing it, eg poor conformation of leg leading to sprain of tendon.

caustic (L. causticus, Gr. kaustikos) Corrosive: destructive to living tissue, eg silver nitrate, qv.

cautery (L. cauterium, Gr. kauterion) Application of caustic substance, hot iron or electric current. See firing, diathermy.

cava (pl. of cavum) See vein.

cavity (L. cavitas) Space or potential space in body, eg abdominal **c.,** qv.

cavum (L., pl. cava) Anatomical cavity or space.

Cayuse Pony of Red Indians of America. Descended from Mustang by careless cross-breeding.

Ceform Trade name. See cephaloridine.

cell (L. cella, compartment) Minute unit of protoplasm, singular in such organisms as bacteria or certain protozoa, eg amoeba; or organised into complex systems forming tissues of body. Differs widely in size, structure and function but usually consists of protoplasm divided into cytoplasm and nucleus; although nucleus absent in bacteria and red blood cells. Main types: **adipose c.** See fat. **blood c.** See red and white blood **c. bone c.** qv. **cancerous c.** See growth. **cartilage c.** qv. **connective tissue c.** qv. **egg c.** See gamete, ovum and embryology. **endothelium c.** qv. **follicle c.** qv. **germ c.** Sex **c.** or gamete. **granulosa c.** qv. **hepatic c.** See liver. **nerve c.** qv. **muscle c.** qv. **phagocytic c.** See phagocyte. **sensory c.** See nerve. **spermatazoon c.** qv. See also embryology, gamete.

cement (L. cementum) See teeth.

centesis (Gr. kentesis) See abdominocentesis, paracentesis.

centigrade (L. centum, hundred + gradus, a step) Scale of heat measurement with freezing point of water at zero and boiling point at 100 degrees. See temperature, weights and measures.

centigram One hundredth part of a gram. Abbr. cgm. See weights and measures.

centimetre Linear measurement of metric system; one hundredth part of a metre; approx. 0.394 inch. Abbr. cm. **cubic c.** Unit of mass or cube, each side of which measures one **c.** Abbr. cu.cm. or cc.

Central Veterinary Society One of oldest veterinary societies, c/o M. Findlay, 6 Woodthorpe Road, London SW15 6UQ (01 788 8224).

centre (Gr. kentron, L. centrum) Collection of nerve cells concerned with particular function, eg breathing **c.** controls respiration. See brain.

centrifuge (centre + L. fugere, to flee) Machine which spins, exerting a centrifugal force; used in laboratory for separating, eg cells from plasma in blood (see hematocrit, blood tests), sediment from water in urine.

centrosome (centro- + Gr. soma, body) Area of cell cytoplasm important in mitosis, qv.

centrum (L., Gr. kentron) Anatomical term for a central structure, eg **c.** of vertebra.

cephalic (L. cephalicus, Gr. kephalikos) Of head or head-end of body, eg **c.** vein.

cephaloridine (trade names: Ceforn, Ceporin) Antibiotic with wide range of activity against gram-positive and gram-negative bacteria. Particularly useful in kidney, bladder and lung infections.

Ceporin Trade name. See cephaloridine.

cereal (L. cerealis) Edible grain such as barley, oats. See food.

cerebellar Of the cerebellum (part of brain, qv). **c. degeneration/hypo-plasia** Rare disease of cerebellum which causes muscle inco-ordination (ataxia), head tremor and faulty blink response. Usually appears in first few months and worsens until foal dies or has to be destroyed. May be hereditary. Arab seems to be only breed affected, though similar disease reported in Gotland and Oldenburg breeds.

cerebellum (from L. cerebrum, brain) Part of brain controlling co-ordination. See brain.

cerebrospinal Of the brain and spinal cord. **c. fluid** (CSF) Fluid which bathes spinal cord and brain stem; contains salts, minerals, sugar, small amounts of protein, a few cells. Can be withdrawn for lab. examination by inserting needle into cisterna magna at base of skull (see occiput) or into space above spinal cord in back (lumbar puncture). Protein and cell content increase in inflammatory conditions.

cerumen (L. from cera, wax) Earwax.

cervical (L. cervicalis from cervix, neck) Of the neck (eg **c.** vertebra) or cervix (eg **c.** swab).

cervicitis Inflamed cervix. May be due to infection or to injury (eg during foaling).

cervix (pl. cervices) Muscular neck of uterus, can be seen through speculum inserted into vagina; changes in tone, colour and moistness in various states of oestrous cycle and pregnancy. See oestrous cycle.

cesarian See caesarian section.

Cestoda See tapeworm.

chalk (calcium carbonate) Fine white or off-white odourless tasteless powder. Absorbent and antacid, used in mixtures to treat diarrhoea. Dose: 30–120gms.

chamber (L. camera, Gr. kamara) Enclosed space. **anterior c. of eye.** Space between cornea and lens. **c.'s of heart** Atrium (auricle) and ventricle, also known as first and second **c.'s**. See eye, heart.

channel (L. canalis, a water pipe) Groove through which fluid flows, eg blood **c.**, lymph **c.**

character Nature of object or organism. **acquired c.** Modification as result of environment, such as some behaviour or stunted growth. **mendelian c.'s** Used in genetics (Mendel's law) for distinct characteristics dependent on inherited material (genes); may be recessive or dominant. **sex c.'s** Those of reproduction and differences between male and female. **sex-linked c.** One transmitted to only one sex, the genes for which are carried on sex chromosome. See Mendel's law, chromosome.

Charolais French breed of 15–16 hands, developed from English Thoroughbred.

check apparatus System of ligaments forming part of stay apparatus, qv. Foreleg: superior and inferior check ligaments, superficial and deep flexor tendons; hindleg: tarsal (inferior) check ligament and deep digital flexor tendon. Structures help support lower part of leg and prevent overextension.

cheek Skin either side of face. Inner side (buccal membrane) may be ulcerated by rough caps on teeth, penetrating wounds or injury from bit.

chemistry (Gr. chemeia) Science of elements and compounds of elements. **analytical c.** That of analysis. **forensic c.** That applied to solution of legal problems (see veterinary rules). **organic c.** That of compounds containing carbon, ie those associated with organic as opposed to inorganic substances. **physical c.** That of relationship of chemical and physical properties.

chemoreceptor Nerve cell sensitive to chemical substances, eg those of smell and taste; or to chemical changes in blood stream, eg reduced oxygen or increased carbon dioxide tension. See nerve cell.

chemotherapy Treatment of disease by chemicals which affect causative germ but do not harm patient. See antibiotic.

chest (syns. thorax, thoracic cavity) Part of body bounded by rib cage and diaphragm. Contains heart, an important artery (aorta), a main vein (vena cava), lungs, gullet, (oesophagus), thymus and lymph glands.

chestnut (1) Horny growth just above inside of each knee (carpal)

106

joint and 3 inches below inside of each hock. May be vestige of hoof of 2- or 3-toed horse (see evolution) and probably as individual as human fingerprint. Photographed to use in racehorses' identity papers in some states of America. Cf. ergot. See donkey, plate 40. (2) See coat colouring, also for liver **c**.

chewing Movement of lower jaw from side to side by which food is ground between upper and lower molars. **c. disease** Incessant, abnormal **c.** after eating yellow star plant. **nervous c.** Symptom of brain damage suffered by newborn foal (see neonatal maladjustment syndrome).

cheyne-stokes respiration Gradual increase and decrease in depth of breathing. Occurs in heart failure, during anaesthesia or after brain injury.

chigger See flea.

chill Attack of involuntary muscular contractions accompanied by sense of cold. Term used by horsemen for undiagnosed ailment if individual is off-colour. Has no scientific meaning. See shiverer.

Chinese pony Similar to, and probably descended from, Mongolian. Up to 13 hands. Used for polo and Flat racing.

chiropractic therapy (chiro- + Gr. prattein, to do) Treatment by manipulation.

chloral hydrate Colourless crystals with pungent odour and bitter taste. Used as sedative or anaesthetic. Irritates locally so should not be injected sub. cut. Dose: sedative 3–6gms./50kg. body wt. with water by stomach tube; anaesthetic: 6–9gms./50kg. body wt. IV. Overdose can cause relaxation of voluntary muscles, staggering, dilation of pupils, subnormal temperature and death from respiratory failure.

chloramphenicol (trade names: Alficetyn, Chloromycetin) Fine white to greyish-white crystals with bitter taste. Obtained from Streptomyces venezuelae mould. Antibiotic effective against E.coli, Salmonella, Klebsiella. Used in gram-negative infections of alimentary tract and joints. Dose: 15–50mg./kg. body wt., twice daily, by mouth, IM or IV or used locally in ointment, paint or aerosol. **c. sodium succinate** Sodium salt of **c.** Antibiotic used on foals. Dose: 10mg./kg. body wt. IV.

chlorhexidine hydrochloride (trade name: Hibitane) White crystalline odourless powder with bitter taste. Potent antiseptic, effective against wide range of gram-positive and gram-negative organisms. Used for disinfecting wounds and burns (in 0.02–0.05% aqueous solution) and uterus in pessaries or solution.

chlorinated lime Chloride of lime. Dull white powder with characteristic odour resembling chlorine. Powerful bactericide and deodorant, acts by combining with organic material; used to disinfect and clean stables, drains etc at 6oz. per gallon of water.

chloroform Colourless heavy liquid with characteristic odour and sweet burning taste. Used as anaesthetic; may cause period of excitement. Can be given by mouth in tympanitic colic. Dose: 4–8ml. Overdose causes poisoning. See anaesthesia.

Chloromycetin Trade name. See chloramphenicol.

chlorpromazine/c. hydrochloride (trade names: Largactil, Thorazine) White or cream-coloured powder with slight odour and bitter taste. Used to tranquillise excitable or aggressive animals for handling, minor surgery, induction of general anaesthesia (or dishonestly as stopper dope). Dose: 1mg./kg. body wt. IM—never IV. Overdose causes paralysis of hindquarters, staggering, inco-ordination.

chlortetracycline hydrochloride (syn. aureomycin hydrochloride) Yellow odourless crystals with bitter taste; antibiotic produced from Streptomyces aureofaciens. Given by mouth, used in ointment or eye drops. Dose: by mouth, 60mg./kg. body wt. For action and uses see tetracycline.

choke Completely or partially obstructed gullet (oesophagus), caused by hay, straw, dry grain, partially chewed wood. Symptoms: distress with repeated arching of neck, anxious facial expression, saliva mixed with food drooling from mouth and nostrils. Recovery usually spontaneous if horse is transquillised by acetyl promazine or similar drug.

chol- Combining form meaning relationship to bile.

cholagogue (chol- + Gr. agogos, leading) Drug or substance which stimulates flow of bile from liver.

cholesterol (chole- + Gr. stereos, solid) Fat-like substance in animal fats and oils, bile, blood, brain and milk. Deposited in arterial walls as atheroma.

choline Vitamins in animal and vegetable tissues. See acetylcholine.

cholinergic Of choline (acetylcholine). Also applied to nerve fibres which liberate acetylcholine at junction where nerve impulse passes.

cholinesterase Substance (an esterase) in body tissues which splits acetylcholine into choline and acetic acid.

chondo-/chondro- (Gr. chondros, cartilage) Combining form meaning relationship to cartilage.

chondritis Inflamed cartilage.

chondroblast (chondro- + Gr. blastos, germ) Cell which produces cartilage, qv.

chondrocyte (chondo- + Gr. kytos, hollow vessel) Cartilage cell.

chorda (L., Gr. chorde, cord) Cord or sinew, eg **c. tendinese cordis** Tendinous cord connecting cusps of valves which guard entrance of ventricles of heart.

chorion Outermost membrane of embryo; nourishes and protects it and fuses with allantois to form placenta. See allantois, gonadotrophin, placenta.

chorionic Produced by placenta, eg **c.** hormone such as **c. gonadotrophin** (trade names: Antuitrin S, Chorulon, Lutormone, Physostab, Pregnyl, Prolan) Sterile white water-soluble powder obtained from urine of pregnant humans. Stimulates gonads. Given to mares IV to induce ovulation and to stallions to stimulate secretion of testosterone. Dose: 1,500–5,000 units. See oestrous cycle.

Chorulon Trade name. See chorionic gonadotrophin.

chromatin (Gr. chroma, colour) The portion of cell nucleus most easily stained. Carries genes in inheritance, **sex c.** Mass of **c.** at edge of nucleus. Present in normal females, but not normal males. See intersex.

chromatography (chromato- + Gr. graphein, to write) Chemical analysis in which different substances in solution produce bands of colour. Basis of method used for analysing saliva and urine samples in dope test, qv. See also electrophoresis.

chromic catgut See catgut.

chromosome (chromo- + Gr. soma, body) Structure, in nucleus of cell, which carries hereditary material, ie genes; constant number in each species—domestic horse (Equus caballus) 64. Evolutionary trend may be loss of **c.**'s (reference: Roger Short, Cambridge, 1965) as Przewalski (qv), probably most recent of domestic horse's antecedents, has 66 **c.**'s. Short found the following **c.** figures: donkey (Equus asinus) 62; Nubian wild ass (Equus asinus africanus) and Somali wild ass (Equus asinus somalicus) 62; Onager (Equus hemionus onager) 54; Grevy's zebra (Equus grevyi) 46. **C.**'s usually paired and animal with odd number likely to be infertile, eg mule has 63 (mean average of its parents' **c.** numbers—male donkey: 62, female horse: 64). Laboratory examination of tests of such hybrids shows odd **c.** unable to find a partner, plus paternal and maternal **c.**'s which differ in size and shape. Fertile crosses such as Przewalski/horse inherit from each parent **c.**'s so alike that they can fuse and overcome the odd **c. Sex c.** One concerned with determining sex and designated X (female) or Y (male). Normal male mammals have an XY pairing; normal females XX. Abnormal forms may have XXY, XYY (ie triploid numbers) or XX and XY cells, 2 sorts of cells in same individual (mosaicism). See gene.

chronic (L. chronicus from Gr. chronos, time) Continuing over long period, eg disease. Opp. acute.

chyle (L. chylus, juice) Lymph fluid which travels from intestine, in lymph ducts, to enter veins in chest.

CI See contra-indicated.

cicatrix New tissue formed in healing of wound.

cilia Pl. of cilium.

cilium Minute hair-like filament attached to free surface of a cell and which, with others, moves fluid and matter over area. See epithelium. Cf flagellum.

circulation (L. circulatio) Movement of fluid through vessels, eg blood and lymph **c.** **collateral c.** Fluid which is diverted; eg if blood vessel is obstructed, blood will find **c.c.** as other vessels open up. See heart; arteries, table of; lymphatic system.

cirrhosis (Gr. kirrhos, orange-yellow) Liver disease characterised by destruction of liver cells which are replaced by fibrous tissue. Liver becomes hard, enlarged and cuts like cardboard. See liver, ragwort poisoning.

cisterna (L., pl. cisternae) Space in which lymph or other body fluid accumulates, eg **c. magna** Space at base of skull. See occiput.

citrate Salt of citric acid. See sodium citrate.

Citrazine Trade name. See piperazine salts.

clamp Device for causing compression, eg preventing bleeding during operation, reducing hernia, qv.

claudication (L. claudicatio) Limping or lameness. **intermittent c.** Lameness of hindlimbs due to cramp-like pains after exercise, caused by thrombus in iliac arteries. See iliac thrombosis.

clay Hydrated aluminium silicate. Used in drugs, ointments, poultices. **China c.** See kaolin.

cleft palate Congenital lack of complete roof to mouth allowing abnormal opening between mouth and nasal passages. Roof of mouth fails to develop in embryo. Should be noticed in first 24 hours when milk runs out of nostrils and foal coughs after sucking. Cause: unknown, possibly inherited, but may be due to viral infection of mare or to drugs given in first 6 weeks of pregnancy. Treatment: plastic surgery (unlikely to succeed if defect extends to soft palate, qv). Not advisable to breed from affected horses.

Cleveland Bay Strong but light horse developed in Yorkshire. Only small white head-marking permissible on bay coat. Often crossed with Thoroughbred to produce hunter though pure-breds still popular; they provide some Royal carriage horses, probably because breed has Yorkshire Coach horse blood. Many exported, especially to USA. Assn: **C.B.** Horse Soc., c/o J. F. Stephenson, York Livestock Centre, Murton, York YO1 3UF (Dunnington 731).

clitoris Female counterpart of penis, in floor of vagina just inside vulva. Made up of corpus and glans clitoridis and prepuce. Has capacity to become erectile and extends to about 4cm. long and 2cm. wide. Exposed during eversion (winking) of vulva.

cloak fly See tabanid fly.

Clostridia Pl. of Clostridium.

Clostridium (Gr. kloster, spindle) Genus of bacteria which are gram-positive, spore-bearing, rod-shaped and live only without oxygen. See bacteria.

clot Coagulated mass, eg blood **c.** See thrombosis, blood.

clover Plant which can cause poisoning, eg mouldy hay of yellow sweet **c.** produces dicoumarol, which prolongs clotting time of blood and may cause internal bleeding. **C.** can aggravate photosensitisation, laminitis, bloat, liver disease and tympany. See food.

cloxacillin sodium (trade name: Orbenin) White odourless crystals with bitter taste. Antibiotic particularly useful against penicillin-resistant Staphylococci. Used to treat pneumonia, abscesses, skin infections. Dose: 2–4mg./kg. body wt. twice daily.

club foot Abnormal conformation of foot in which angle of wall of hoof with ground is greater than 60°; may affect one or both feet. May be inherited, due to incorrect use of foot, or nutritional deficiency. May cause lameness and eventual separation of pedal bone from horn of hoof.

Clydesdale Scottish draught breed founded in C. (now Lanarkshire);

112

possibly descended from Scottish mares and a Belgian stallion imported about 1700. **C.** has more white than other 3 main draught breeds of
Britain: Suffolk (which has none), Percheron and Shire. Assn: **C.**
Horse Soc., c/o R. Jarvis, 19 Hillington Gardens, Glasgow SW2
(041 882 4071).

coagulation (L. coagulatio) Forming of blood clot by process which
occurs only if blood is in contact with roughened surface or damaged
tissue. Blood contains about 12 factors which, under certain circumstances, react in 3 stages to produce clot (ie fibrin). (1) Damaged blood
platelets and tissues release thromboplastin. (2) If thromboplastin and
calcium are in contact with prothrombin (inactive thrombin) they form
thrombin. (3) If thrombin is in contact with blood protein (fibrinogen)
it forms fibrin.

coat (L. cotta, tunic) (1) Outer covering of organ. (2) Hair covering
horse's skin. **c. colouring** Colour of horse's hair; determined by inheritance and sometimes age (grey horse can be born black and coat
gradually turn grey, until in old age is it pure white). Some breed
societies recognise only those horses of a particular colour, eg Suffolk
Punch must be chestnut. Others, eg Albino, Appaloosa, Palomino, are
more a colour than a breed. Colours include: Albino (qv); Appaloosa
(usually white with black/brown spots and perhaps striped hooves), cf
Knabstrup; bay (any shade of brown from dark—mahogany—to pale
—sandy—but must have black mane and tail and often has black points
(hocks, knees downwards) with white on face and around feet. Pony
breeds sometimes have dark dorsal stripe. Can be picked to breed true,
as in Cleveland Bay, though some produce chestnut or another colour);
black (body no lighter than mane and tail but white markings allowed,
usually breeds true, though 2 blacks can produce bay foal); blue roan
(roaned black, ie black with sprinkling of white hairs); brown (almost
black but lighter areas around eyes, muzzle and legs); chestnut
(golden red or reddish/brown—liver chestnut—without black points of
bay, 2 chestnuts can produce only a chestnut foal. Cf Palomino);
dappled grey (barely perceptible spots in lighter grey coat, may be
equivalent of hammer spots in dark coat. Common in some breeds, eg
Percheron); dun (sandy cream, ie dark palomino, but with dark mane
and tail and often dorsal stripe. Dun reflects sunlight so horse able to
tolerate heat better than some colours. Common in native types, eg
Highland, Mustang); grey (seems particularly susceptible to melanotic
growths (see growth) around anus and is especially suspicious (see

113

behaviour). Those whose sire or dam were other than grey produce about 75% grey foals when crossed with another grey); grey roan (grey with sprinkling of white hairs in darker coat, colouring similar to dappled grey, but more evenly distributed); palomino (qv); piebald (black and white patches); pinto (qv); skewbald (patches of white and anything except black); sorrel (pale chestnut); spotted (see Appaloosa, Knabstrup); strawberry roan (roaned chestnut); striped (see zebra). See also marking.

cob Type of horse rather than breed, though may be similar to Welsh cob (q.v.) Up to 15.2 hands, usually used as heavyweight hack. Shown with hogged mane and docked tail in the past, but docking now illegal. Sometimes driven, when action is higher than in ridden horse. Assn: British Show Hack & C. Assn, National Equestrian Centre, Kenilworth, Warwickshire, CV8 2LR (Coventry 27192).

cobalamin Cobalt complex of vitamin B_{12}.

cobalt chloride Red slightly absorbant crystals contained in vitamin B_{12}. Minute quantities are essential. Deficiency not know in horses, though **c.c.** included in most supplements and tonics. Dose: 10–25mg. daily. Also available as oxide or sulphate.

cocaine Drug used as a local anaesthetic (or stimulant dope). Toxicity causes excitement, then depression, which ends in unconsciousness and death from respiratory paralysis. Treatment ineffectual, but oxygen and artificial respiration may help.

coccus (pl. cocci; L., Gr. kokkos, berry) Round bacterial cell. See bacteria, Streptococcus, Staphylococcus.

codeine phosphate Colourless crystals or white odourless powder derived from morphine. Actions similar to morphine. Used to treat cough. Dose: 0.2–2gms. daily.

codex Official formula of medicines. See British Veterinary C.

coffin Joint between second and third phalanges and navicular bone. See navicular disease.

Coggins test (after Dr Leroy C. of Cornell University, USA) Laboratory test to diagnose swamp fever (equine infectious anemia). Test takes 24–8 hours and is based on detecting antigen and antibody in infected horse's blood, by special technique (agar-gel-immunodiffusion).

coital exanthema (syns. spots, pox) Infectious disease of mares and stallions caused by equine herpesvirus. Transmitted by coitus, insects, personnel handling mares and stallions and without obvious contact. Not thought to affect fertility. Causes small blisters (vesicles) on mare's vulva and stallion's penis. Blisters rupture, leaving ulcerated, inflamed areas which may be round or joined to form irregular patches. Scabs form on ulcers, which may persist up to 3 weeks. Individual may refuse food, suffer malaise and rise in temperature. Condition may leave areas without pigment. Treatment not essential. Ulcers heal spontaneously, but may be helped by ointment or lotion containing antibiotics or corticosteroids. Horse should be sexually rested.

coitus (colloq. covering, mating, service) Sexual intercourse. See behaviour, fertility.

cold Low temperature. Also colloq. for catarrhal disorder of upper respiratory tract. See snotty nose.

cold-blooded Colloq. for horse tracing to prehistoric type of central Europe. Most heavy, slow horses are **c.b.** Cf hot-blooded.

colibacillosis Diseases caused by Escherichia coli. See septicemia of the newborn, diarrhoea.

colic Pain in tubes or ducts of abdomen. 3 main types: (1) **biliary c.** Disturbance in bile duct. Rare in horses; caused by growth or parasites blocking duct. (2) **renal c.** Disturbance in ureter (duct carrying urine from kidneys to bladder). Rare in horses, may be due to kidney stones (calculi). See stones. (3) **alimentary c.** Disturbance in alimentary tract; only type common in horses. **impacted c.** Simple stoppage due to dry food material, usually in colon at pelvic or diaphragmatic flexure (bend) in caecum, or at point where small intestine enters caecum. **sand c.** Form of impacted **c.** due to accumulation of sand in caecum; occurs in horses grazing on sandy soil: **spasmodic c.** Excess activity of gut, causing spasm. May include diarrhoea. **twist c.** (volvulus) Acutely obstructed small intestine due to its becoming twisted or due to larger organs, such as caecum, rotating on suspending membrane. **tympanitic c.** Fermentation of food so that gas accumulates, usually in stomach, caecum or colon. **verminous c.** That due to blood clots in arteries supplying small or large intestines so that blood supply to part of gut is cut off. The clot (thrombus) occurs because blood vessel is damaged by migrating redworm larvae (see aneurysm). Pain in **c.** caused by (1) gut wall distended by gas or food, causing stretched peritoneum (membrane) in which there are many pain receptor cells; (2) inflamed peritoneum; (3) spasm of muscle in gut wall. Symptoms: refusal to eat, sweating, looking round at flanks, pawing ground, getting up and down, rolling, lying on back, anxious expression (see plates 8–10). In tympanitic **c.** horse may straddle its limbs or crouch. In impacted **c.** it may show signs of full bladder and straddle in urinating position. Pulse rate may increase and temperature rise, according to severity of pain. Diagnosis: on symptoms plus absent or increased gut sounds (borborygmi). Rectal examination is useful to determine type of **c.** Prognosis: poor if pain fails to respond to treatment, if pulse is fast and weakens, hematocrit rises (above 50%) and mucous membranes of mouth and eye are red or purple. Treatment: (1) impacted **c.,** liquid paraffin and purgative drugs by stomach pump; (2) tympanitic **c.,** antispasmodic drugs by injection or by stomach tube; (3) twist, surgical operation essential. In all types, pain is relieved by injection of pethidine, Buscopan, antispasmodic and tranquillising drugs.

colitis Inflamed colon **c.X** Disease of unknown cause (possibly toxins from E. coli germ) characterised by acute pain, diarrhoea, shock and death in 1–2 days. At post-mortem: massive hemorrhage in wall of colon.

collagen (Gr. kolla, glue + gennan, to produce) Main protein of skin, tendon, bone, cartilage and connective tissue.

collapse (L. collapsus) Prostration and depression, usually applied to heart. **c. of lung** (atelectic lung) Airless state of lung. See emphysema.

collateral (L. con, together + latus, side) Secondary, not direct. See circulation.

Collovet Trade name. Iron tonic to treat anemia.

collyrium (L., Gr. kollyrion, eye salve; pl. collyria) Lotion or wash for eyes.

Colonial Quarter-Pather Old name for American Quarter horse, qv.

colony (L. colonia) Bacterial growth, as seen in laboratory study.

colorimeter (color + Gr. metron, measure) Laboratory instrument for measuring difference in colour.

colostrum (colloq. first milk) Thick milk secreted by mammary glands at birth, characterised by high protein content, especially globulin, which gives newborn foal its immunity. Close to birth drops of **c.** may exude from teats and form wax-like beads when mare said to be waxing-up. See tetanus toxoid, running of milk, hemolytic jaundice.

colour (L. color) See coat colouring.

colt Non-castrated male up to 4-5 years. Cf stallion.

column (L. columna) Grey matter of spinal cord. See cord.

coma (Gr. koma) Unconsciousness from which it is difficult or impossible to arouse sufferer. See neonatal maladjustment syndrome.

comatose Affected by coma.

commensal (L. com-, together + mensa, table) Organism living on or in another but not damaging host. Cf parasite.

commissure Site of meeting of parts, eg **c.** (angle) of lips.

compensation (L. compensatio from cum, together + pensare, to weigh) Counterbalancing of defect in structure or function, eg heart muscle can thicken to compensate for faulty valves so that heart's efficiency as pumping organ is not impaired. See heart valves.

complement Complex substance in blood serum, probably formed by white blood cells. Necessary for antigen/antibody reaction and used in laboratory in **c.** fixation test for diagnosis of some bacterial and other diseases, eg brucellosis and hemolytic jaundice in newborn foal.

compound (L. componere, to place together) Any substance composed of two or more materials.

compress (L. compressus) Pad of linen, cotton wool or other material applied with pressure; may be hot or cold. Used to treat inflammation, qv.

concave (L. concavus) Having rounded, depressed surface resembling hollow, eg profile of typical Arab.

concentrate (L. con, together + centrum, centre) Strength, as in medical preparations.

concentrated vitamin A solution Obtained from oils of fish liver and vegetable (arachis). Vitamin necessary for healthy epithelial tissue, bone growth and formation of pigment (visual purple) in retina. Minimum daily requirement: 20 IU per kg. body wt.

concentrated vitamin D solution Consists of suitable fish-liver oil or blend of oils and calciferol. Vitamin necessary for absorbing calcium and phosphorus from gut. Deficiency may cause rickets. Minimum daily requirement: 10 IU per kg. body wt.

concussion (L. concussio; syns. jar, shock, trauma) Stress caused by knock. Word used of head injury where consciousness is impaired or lost; or of damaged skeleton, especially legs. More likely to affect forelegs (which bear 65% of horse's weight) than hindlegs. See bucked shin, bowed tendon, foot.

condom (L. condus, a receptacle, or possibly after Condon, the inventor) Sheath or cover for penis applied to stallion before coitus to collect semen for laboratory examination. Cf artificial vagina, semen.

condyle (L. condylus, Gr. kondylos, knuckle) Rounded projection of bone, eg **c.** of humerus.

conformation Anatomical arrangement and proportion of parts of body. A major factor in soundness of legs. Poor **c.** may predispose to sprains of joints, ligaments, tendons, bone injuries and navicular disease. **C.** of limbs determines shape of feet and distribution of weight. **C.** of body varies between breeds, eg Arab has short back compared with Thoroughbred. American Quarter horse has heavy body. **functional c.** The way horse uses its legs (in contrast to static **c.**, seen in standing horse). They do not necessarily match each other. **faulty c.** Includes base-narrow, base-wide (legs set on to body too close together/too far apart), toe-narrow, toe-wide (feet too close/too far apart), long and upright pasterns refer to slope and affect angle of hoof. **c. of foot** Sole should be concave, bars well developed, frog large and in centre of sole. Front feet more rounded (less narrow) than hind. Angle formed by ground surface of hoof and front of wall should be 45–50° in front and 50–55° behind (see foot). **c. of vulva** Should be vertical line between anus and lower angle of vulva. Poor **c.** encourages infection. See Caslick.

congenital Present at birth, eg **c.** abnormality such as hare lip, cleft palate, contracted tendons, club foot.

congestion (L. from congerere, to heap together) Excessive accumulation of blood or other fluid in a part. **passive c.** That caused by obstructed blood flow. See inflammation, sprain.

conjunctiva Membrane lining eyelids and covering exposed surface of eyeball.

conjunctivitis Inflamed conjunctiva. May affect one or both eyes; characterised by red, perhaps swollen, eyelid, pus flecks and tears which run down face causing scalding and loss of hair. Spasm of eyelids and closure of eye is common. Cause: bacterial or viral infection, foreign body, injury, allergy, irritation from flies. Treatment: antibiotic and hydrocortisone eye drops. See also eye.

connective tissue One of 4 basic tissues in body (cf. epithelial, muscular and nervous). So called because it holds other tissues together and to the skeleton. Special property of **c.t.** cells is that they produce non-living substances to lie between cells. Some of these are hard, eg bone. C.t. is subdivided into (1) ordinary, including fat and soft tissue, binding skin to underlying muscles, bone etc; (2) special, including blood-forming cells and supporting structures composed of bone and cartilage.

Connemara pony Native breed of the C. and surrounding district in W Ireland. Hardy type, thrives on poor land. Now most often grey, must be 13–14 hands to be eligible for stud book, though taller examples exist after introduction of Thoroughbred blood. Breed's origin obscure, could be Celtic type (like Norwegian, Highland etc) tracing to Mongolian; could have developed from Oriental horses who swam ashore from wreck of Spanish Armada; or could trace to Irish

119

Hobby (qv). Some **C.** ponies tend to amble (see gait). Assns: English **C.** Pony Soc., c/o Mrs Barthrop, The Quinta, Bentley, Farnham, Surrey (Bentley 3159); **C.** Pony Breeders' Soc., c/o J. Killeen, 4 Nuns' Island, Galway, Eire (Irish Republic 091 32 77).

constipation (L. constipatio, a crowding together) Infrequent defecation due to dry or hardened dungs. See colic; meconium, retention of.

constitution (L. constitutio) Make-up or functional basis of body.

contagious (L. contagiosus) Able to spread from one animal to another as in disease, eg influenza. See veterinary rules (Ministry of Agriculture).

contra- Combining form meaning against.

contracted heels Heels that are too narrow. They should be wide, compared with the toe. May be partially corrected by increasing pressure on frog. Can be done by using T or bar shoes and by increasing flexibility of hoof wall by grooving at quarters. See shoeing. **c. tendons** (syn. hyperflexion of leg) Condition of newborn foals and yearlings. Flexor tendons and suspensory ligament are too short and cause permanent flexion of fetlock and sometimes knee, in one or both forelegs; may also affect hindlegs. Animal knuckles over at fetlock and, in severe cases, may walk on front of joint. Congenital cases may result in dystocia due to inability of forelegs to straighten normally to pass through birth canal. Some foals born normal, then develop condition at any age up to 2 years. Mild cases are described as being straight and upright. Cause unknown, probably inherited or result of abnormal inherited material, ie chromosomes. Other possible causes: infection, malnutrition and dietary deficiency. Treatment: fit splints and special boots to counteract abnormality. Severe cases might be helped by surgical cutting of flexor tendon and ligaments behind knee. Cf hypoflexion.

contraction (L. contractus, drawn together) A shortening as in muscles, ligaments, tendons of fore- or hindlegs of foal or yearling. Can often be surgically corrected. Also muscle in sustained **c.**, ie tetanic.

contra-indicated (CI) Not advisable, usually used about drugs, eg phenylbutazoine **c.i.** in heart, liver or kidney disease.

convalescence (L. convalescere, to become strong) State of recovering from illness.

convection (L. convectio from convehere, to convey) Route by which heat is lost through circulation of air or fluid. See temperature.

convex (L. convexus) Having rounded, elevated surface. Cf concave.

convolution (L. convolutus, rolled together) An elevation caused by structure folded on itself, eg intestine, brain surface.

convulsant Producing convulsions, eg drug. **anti-c.** Drug controlling convulsions, eg phenytoin, primidone.

convulsions (L. from convellere, to pull together) Violent involuntary muscle contractions. **clonic c.** Jerky movements due to alternate contracting and relaxing of muscles. **epileptic c.** Jerky movements accompanied by loss of consciousness, does not occur in horses. **general c.** Inco-ordinated movements, eg when foal lies on ground making galloping movements or throwing itself about. **tetanic c.** Spasms, as in lockjaw. See neonatal maladjustment syndrome.

convulsive Of convulsions.

cooling Reducing temperature; general, as in foals suffering illness immediately after birth, or local, as in treatment of injured tendons. See neonatal maladjustment syndrome, temperature, bowed tendon.

Coopane Trade name. See piperazine salts.

Cooper's liquid phenothiazine Trade name. See phenothiazine.

co-ordination Harmonious function of parts, especially movement of legs. Cf inco-ordination.

copper sulphate Blue odourless crystalline powder with astringent taste. Used in lotions to reduce proud flesh.

coprophagia Feeding on dung. See appetite, depraved; behaviour.

cor See heart.

121

coramine See nikethamide.

cord (L. chorda, Gr. chorde) Long, rounded body or structure. **genital c.** Formed in embryo by union of mesonephric and mullerian ducts. **c., rupture of** Usually refers to umbilical **c.** which breaks naturally as foal struggles or mare stands up. See birth. **spermatic c.** From abdomen, through inguinal ring to testis. Contains vas deferens, testicular artery, pampiniform plexus, nerves and muscle, enclosed by fine membrane. **spinal c.** Tissue made up of white matter (column) which extends from brain to level of third lumbar vertebra. Lodges in vertebral canal and gives off nerve branches to various part of body. See nerve. **umbilical c.** Connects umbilicus (navel) of foal to placenta and contains two arteries, one vein and urinary duct (urachus). See plates 13 and 14.

corium Modified vascular tissue inside horn of hoof. Divided into 5 parts all of which nourish horn: (1) **perioplic c.** Narrow band above coronary border and merging with skin. (2) **coronary c.** Together with (1) forms coronary band. Responsible for growth, bleeds easily when damaged. Can be likened to bed of human nail. (3) **laminar c.** Membrane attached to surface of pedal bone, bears sensitive laminae. (4) **sole c.** Membrane lining ground surface of pedal bone. (5) **frog c.** Membrane nourishing frog. See plate 18.

corn (L. cornu, horn) (1) Bruise of sensitive and insensitive laminae of sole of foot. Most common at seat of **c.** in angle formed by wall and bar. Causes: poor shoeing, stones, improper trimming when heels are too low. Symptoms: lameness, evidence of pain on pressure, especially when turning. **dry c.** Due to hemorrhage on inner surface of horn, ie between the sensitive and insensitive laminae. **moist c.** Dark brown, moist area seen at seat of **c.** **suppurating c.** Due to infection of corn. Treatment: cut area of **c.** and dress with astringents, antibiotics and, if severe, bandage. Special shoes can be used. See shoeing. (2) Type of food, qv.

cornea (L. corneus, horny) Transparent structure forming part of eye, qv.

corneal Of cornea.

cornu (L., horn; pl. cornua) Anatomical term meaning horn-shaped. **uterine c.** One of horns of uterus.

corona (L., Gr. korone; pl. coronae, coronas) Anatomical term meaning crown-like or encircling. **dental c.** Part of tooth crowned with enamel.

coronary (L. corona, Gr. korone) Of the heart, especially its vessels. See heart; arteries, table of. **c. band** Band at top of hoof and lower part of pastern, seat of horn growth. See corium, quittor.

corpus (L., body; pl. corpora) Main part of a structure, organ or part. **c. cavonosum penis** Vascular structure forming greater part of penis. **c. luteum** See yellow body.

corpuscle Small mass or body, eg red or white blood **c.**

Corsican Pony of Italian island of Corsica, similar to Sardinian, qv.

Cortelan Trade name. See cortisone acetate.

cortex (L., bark, rind, shell) External layer. **adrenal c.** Outer layer of adrenal gland which secretes the hormones corticosteroids. **renal c.** Consists of filtering units (glomeruli) and secretary ducts of kidney. See adrenal gland, corticosteroids, kidney, urine.

cortical (L. corticalis) Of cortex.

corticosteroids Hormones produced by adrenal cortex. (See adrenal gland.) Three classes: glucocorticoids (affect carbohydrate metabolism and have anti-inflammatory action), mineralocorticoids (affect mineral/salt balance), sexcorticoids (affect male and female characteristics).

corticotrophic Having specific effect on cortex of adrenal gland, eg hormone produced by pituitary gland. See adreno-cortico-trophic hormone.

corticotrophin (trade names: Acthar, Actos, Adrenocorticotrophin) Hormone (obtained from anterior lobe of pituitary gland) which stimulates adrenal cortex to secrete cortisol. Used as adjunct to cortisone therapy. Dose: 200–600 units IM. See adreno-cortico-trophic hormone.

Cortisol Trade name. See dexamethasone.

cortisol Hormone produced by adrenal cortex. See hydrocortisone.

cortisone/c. acetate (trade names: Cortelan, Cortistab, Cortone acetate) Small white odourless crystals with bitter taste. Hormone affecting carbohydrate metabolism and with anti-inflammatory action, converted by body into hydrocortisone. Causes rise in glycogen in liver and sugar in blood. May affect water and mineral metabolism and modify growth of fibrous tissue; reduces resistance to infection and suppresses inflammation. Used with an antibiotic, to treat arthritis, allergies and other inflammatory processes, such as in sprained tendons. Dose: 2–10mg./kg. body wt. IM. See adrenal gland, corticosteroids, betamethasone, dexamethasone.

Cortistab Trade name. See cortisone acetate.

Cortone acetate Trade name. See cortisone acetate.

Cortril Trade name. See hydrocortisone.

Corynebacterium (Gr. koryne, club + bakterion, little rod) Genus of gram-positive bacterium of family Corynebacteriacae; straight or slightly curved rod and generally aerobic. **C. equi** Causal organism of pneumonia in foals. Infection tends to stay in lungs and antibiotics have little effect. At post-mortem **C. equi** typified by abscesses (filled with cheese-like pus) in lymph nodes and body of lungs. See pneumonia; newborn foals, diseases of.

coryza (Gr. koryza) Acute catarrhal condition of mucous membranes. See strangles, snotty nose.

costal (L. costalis) Of a rib.

Costeno (syn. Criollo of Peru) See Criollo.

cotyledon (Gr. kotyledon) Subdivision of surface of placenta in which union between that organ and uterus is particularly close; microscopic in horses.

cough Reflex movement controlled by nervous pathways to and from brain. Analysed as: (1) closing of glottis (larynx entrance) by epiglottis; (2) deep inhalation when abdominal muscles push against diaphragm until air pressure in lungs is enough to expel mucus, dust, etc; (3) opening of larynx to allow sudden gush of air. **C.** caused by inhaling dust, pollen or other irritant, structural change in lung (eg emphysema) or viral infection especially with A/equi or herpesvirus. May be accompanied by rise in temperature except if caused by lungworm. Should never be treated lightly, especially in Thoroughbred. **Hoppengarten c.** Originally disease in Germany of which **c.** was main symptom, now syn. for influenza. **Newmarket c.** Syn. for influenza, qv.

count (L. computare, to reckon) Numerical index of composition. **blood c.** Number of cells in measured volume of blood (red or white cells per cu.mm., see blood tests). **egg/dung/fecal/parasite c.** Numbers of strongyle (red) and ascaris (white) worm eggs per gm. of feces.

counter-irritant Drug or chemical causing increase in blood flow to a part. See blister.

cover Colloq. to serve; have coitus/sexual intercourse. See plates 4 and 5.

covering disease See dourine.

cowbain (Cicuta virosa) Plant which, if eaten, causes nausea, dilated pupils, colic, convulsions and death from asphyxia. No obvious changes at post-mortem.

cow hocks Poor conformation, best seen from behind horse, in which hocks are too close together and feet splayed wide. Tends to produce bog spavin, qv.

coxa Hip or hip joint.

Coxiella Genus of micro-organisms of Rickettsieae.

coxitis Inflamed hip joint.

cranium (L., Gr. kranion, upper part of head) Bones of head except lower jaw; those surrounding brain. See skull.

creatinine phosphokinase (syn. CPK) Enzyme responsible for releasing energy in muscle during contraction. Serum (SCPK) level normally fewer than 40 IU/100ml.; may be raised to 60–4,000/100ml. in setfast or other muscle damage, including heart disease.

creosote Strong-smelling liquid, colourless or pale yellow when neat. Distilled from wood tar. Acts as bactericide, parasiticide and deodorant Should not be applied to skin as may be absorbed causing toxic symptoms. Active principle: phenol, qv.

crepitus/crepitation (L. crepitare, to crackle) Grating noise made by ends of fractured bone rubbing together. Likely to be serious if **c.** can be heard with naked ear.

crest (L. crista) Anatomical term meaning ridge.

cribbing/crib-biting Vice in which animal grasps manger or other object with front teeth, arches neck and usually swallows air. Regarded as vice, qv. Diagnosed on sight and by noting worn front edge of teeth and marks on manger, box door. Cf wind-sucking.

cricoid (Gr. krikos, ring + eidos, form) Resembling a ring, eg **c.** cartilage.

Criollo Argentinian pony noted for endurance. Usually dun or skewbald, about 14 hands. Developed from Andalusian horses imported into S America in 1530s, which escaped captivity and bred freely. Now under auspices of Argentine government which keeps stud book. Virtually same as Peruvian **C.** or Costeno.

Crioulo Hardy, Brazilian breed similar to Criollo and with many local names, eg Mangalarga, Campolino, Nordestino, Courraleiro.

crofton weed (Eupatorium species). If eaten causes Numimbay horse sickness of New South Wales. Symptoms: acute oedema of lungs, followed by hemorrhage.

cross-firing Condition in which inside of toe or wall of a hindfoot strikes inner quarter or undersurface of opposite forefoot. Cf forging.

crossing over (1) Used in embryology to describe exchange of genes between chromosomes, qv. See embryology. (2) Used to describe action of hindlegs, eg in brain disorders such as encephalomyelitis and spinal cord disorders, eg wobber syndrome, segmental myelitis.

cross-matching Process of testing blood from one individual against that of another; laboratory test: mix red blood cells from recipient with plasma from donor. Any incompatability is demonstrated by clumping together (agglutination) of red cells. Test used before blood transfusion. See blood tests, hemolytic jaundice.

crotalaria plants Various species in USA, Australia and S Africa are poisonous if eaten, including **C.** globifera (wild lucern). Symptoms: difficult breathing, rapid and weak pulse, collapse and death. **C.** retusa causes dullness, wasting, irritability, yawning, muscular spasms and aimless galloping (Kimberley horse disease). No known cure.

croup (1) Part of hindquarters from highest point to top of tail; varies from virtually flat to generous slope. See Dutch Draught. (2) Acute obstruction of voice box.

crown (L. corona) Upper part of organ or structure, eg surface of tooth; colloq. temporary premolars shed between $2\frac{1}{2}$ and $3\frac{1}{2}$ years (also known as caps). See teeth. **c. to rump** Measurement of fetus, qv.

cruciate Shaped like a cross, eg **c. ligament** Two strong, round bands in stifle attached between femur and tibia in form of X.

crypt (L. crypta from Gr. kryptos, hidden) Minute opening on surface, eg **c.**'s of Lieberkuhn glands in inner lining of small intestine.

Cryptococcus Old name for Histoplasma fungus which causes epizootic lymphangitis, qv.

cryptorchid (crypto- + Gr. orchis, testis) Male suffering from cryptorchidism. Cf anorchid. See rig.

cryptorchidism Defect in development when testes fail to descend into scrotum. See rig.

Crystapen Trade name. See benzylpenicillin.

cuboidal epithelium See epithelium.

cull To remove defective members of herd; term usually applied to mare with poor breeding record.

culture (L. cultura) Process of growing micro-organisms in laboratory, on media or in tissue cells. **c. medium** Substance or preparation used to cultivate bacteria, virus or fungus. Virus is cultivated in tissue culture as it will not grow without living cells (**c.** media include egg embryo and kidney cells). Bacteria and fungus are cultivated on blood agar and other substances.

cuneiform (L. cuneus, wedge + forma, form) Shaped like a wedge, eg **c.** cartilage, foot of voice box (larynx).

curare Dried extract of various species of Strychnos. Highly toxic, used in general anaesthesia and to reduce spasm in lockjaw (tetanus.) Overdose causes complete paralysis and death. Treatment: artificial respiration.

curarization Producing paralysis with curare.

curb Enlargement at seat of **c.**, ie at back of upper end of cannon, about 6 inches below point of hock. Causes include conformation (sickle hocks, curby hocks), putting strain on ligaments. May be result of trauma or sprain. Symptoms: soft, sometimes painful, swelling on upper end of cannon. Best seen standing at right angles to hock. Horse may be lame. Treatment: reduce acute inflammation, eg with cold water application, corticosteroids, irradiation.

curettage (Fr.) Removal of growth or other tissue from wall of cavity or skin surface using instrument known as curette. Used to treat barren mares (by scraping surface of uterus) so that new lining forms.

cusp (L. cuspis, point) Triangular segment of cardiac valve. See heart valves.

cut Colloq. to castrate, qv.

cutis Outer covering of body. See skin.

cyacetazide White tasteless odourless powder. Used against lungworm, rendering parasites inert so they can be coughed up. Dose: 17.5mg./kg. body wt., 3 consecutive days.

cyanide poisoning (including hydrocyanic acid, prussic acid) Occurs in contact with fertilisers or plants including family Sorghum, certain clovers and linseed meals. Acid is liberated when plant tissue is damaged or decayed. Symptoms: convulsions, paralysis, stupor and respiratory failure, followed by quick death. Diagnosis: on chemical analysis of stomach contents. Treatment: (where possible) solution of 3gms. sodium nitrate, 15gms. sodium theosulphate in 20ml. water, sub. cut.

cyanosis (Gr. kyanos, blue) Bluish colour of mucous membranes due to blood's abnormally low oxygen content. Causes: heart failure, severe pneumonia. Sign of impending death, best seen in gums.

cycle (Gr. kyklos, circle) Events recurring regularly and in same sequence, eg oestrous **c.**, qv.

cyclitis (Gr. kyklos, ciliary body + -itis) Inflamed ciliary body of eye. See eye, diseases of: moon blindness.

cyst Abnormal sac lined with epithelial cells and coated with fibrous cells. Contains fluid or other matter; several varieties, eg dermoid **c.**, qv. **distention c.** Normal spaces are distended by excessive fluid, eg tendon sheath, bursa. **ovarian c.** One in ovary. **retention c.** Blockage in normal escape route of fluid.

cystitis Inflamed urinary bladder. Symptoms: repeated urination, possibly red-coloured urine. May accompany stones, qv.

cytology Study of structure and function of cells.

cytopenia (cyto- + Gr. penia, poverty) Deficiency of cells in blood. **erythro-c.** Deficiency of erythrocytes in blood, as in anemia. **leuco-c.** Fewer than normal white cells, as in viral infections. See anemia, virus.

cytoplasm (cyto- + Gr. plasma) Protoplasm of cell outside nucleus. See cell.

D

Dales Pony of N England, similar to Fell pony (qv) but with some cob and Clydesdale blood. Originally used to ferry weight in mines, now popular for pony trekking. Up to 14.2 hands with fine mane, tail and feathers (long hairs around pastern). Often black, also bay or grey, but not chestnut or mixed colours. Assns: **D.** Pony Soc., c/o G. H. Hodgson, Ivy House Farm, Yarm-on-Leer, Yorkshire. See veterinary rules (Ministry of Agriculture): pit ponies.

Danish horse Originally thick-set pony type, later crossed with horses from Spain, Turkey and England. These, bred with Neapolitan and Andalusian horses, were forerunners of Frederiksborg and Knabstrup breeds.

danthron (trade names: Altan, Istin) Orange odourless tasteless powder. Purgative acting on involuntary muscle of large intestine, given in food or by stomach tube. Acts in about 12–24 hours; more effective if mixed with water. May produce red-coloured urine. Dose: 10–30gms. depending on age and size.

dapple grey See coat colouring.

Dartmoor Hardy pony, up to 12.2 hands, of **D.** district of SW England. Long-lived type, usually handled only at round-up and breeding times. All colours except piebald and skewbald. Domesticated **D.** is popular child's pony. Assn: **D.** Pony Soc., c/o D. W. J. O'Brien, Chelwood Farm, Nutley, Uckfield, Sussex (Chelwood Gate 251).

data (L.; pl. of datum) Collection of facts or information.

davitamon-E See tocopheryl acetate.

dawn horse (syn. Eohippus) See evolution.

DDT/DDT poisoning See dicophane.

deadly nightshade. See nightshade poisoning

deaf Impaired or lost sense of hearing.

death End of life shown by lack of heart beat and respiration. **fetal d.** Abortion. **early fetal d. D.** of fetus in early pregnancy, ie before 100 days. See post-mortem, rigor mortis.

decalcification Loss of calcium salts from bone.

decay (de-+L. cadere, to fall) Decomposition of organic matter.

decidua (L. from deciduus, falling off) Loss of tissue; usually applied to that from uterus, thrown off with placenta after birth in most mammals, but not in mares.

decongestant Drug or substance that reduces congestion or swelling.

decubitus (L., a lying down) Ulcers or sores formed by prolonged lying down. Common sites: point of hip, stifle region, elbow, prominences of head.

deep heat Colloq. for treating injury with heat. See physiotherapy.

defecation (L. defaecare, to deprive of dregs) Act of voiding rectum. See behaviour, colic, diarrhoea.

defect Imperfection. **acquired d.** Result of accident or disease after birth, eg loss of eye. **congenital d.** Present at birth, may be inherited or due to faulty environment in uterus, eg parrot jaw, contracted tendons. **septal d.** Hole in heart wall between opposite chambers. See bladder, rupture of; contracted tendons; parrot jaw; unsoundness.

deficiency Lack of nutrient, eg vitamin **d.**

deformity Abnormal development. See defect.

degeneration (L. degeneratio) Pathological term meaning death or deterioration of cells. **hyaline d.** Tissue tranformed into translucent material.

deglutition (L. deglutitio) Act of swallowing; may be strained in, eg, grass sickness, some colics.

degree (1) Unit to measure arc, angle or temperature. (2) Grade of learning. See temperature, veterinary surgon, weights and measures.

131

dehydration Condition in which more water is lost from body than is absorbed; causes reduced circulating blood and relatively dry tissues. Caused by decreased water intake and/or excess fluid loss through sweating, diarrhoea or urination. As water content of body decreases, fluid is drained from tissue spaces, cells and blood; hemoconcentration is recognised by increase in packed cell volume (hematocrit). Dry skin loses its pliability, so if pinched it stays raised instead of sliding back normally. Eyeball recedes into socket (especially noticeable in dehydrated foal); there is weight-loss, small dry feces, decrease in urine; blood may become increasingly acid (acidosis); pulse becomes small, there is depression and, in extreme cases, coma. Treatment: give fluids IV, sub. cut. or by mouth. See blood, diarrhoea, fluid balance. Cf drycoat.

Deli See Batak.

delivery Expulsion of foal through birth canal. **premature d.** Premature birth. See birth, immaturity, plate 12.

Deltacortril Trade name. See prednisolone.

Deltastab Trade name. See prednisolone.

Demavet Trade name. See dimethyl sulphoxide.

demodectic Of Demodex.

Demodex (Gr. demos, fat+dex, worm) Genus of mite. See mange, demodectic.

demulcent Soothing, bland drug or substance.

dendrite (Gr. dendron, tree) Part of nerve cell, qv.

denervate To remove nerves to a part, eg horse's foot can be denerved by cutting volar nerves at level of fetlock. See neurectomy. Cf nerve block.

dental (L. dentalis) Of dentistry, tooth or teeth. See teeth, gag.

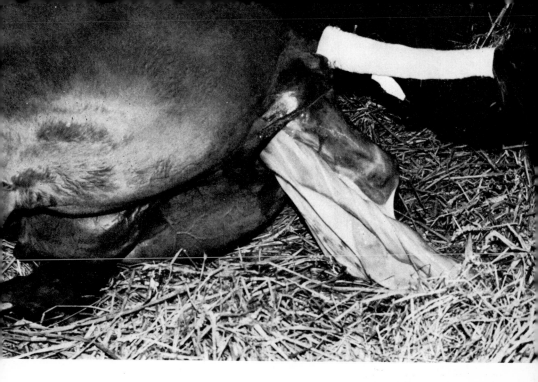

11 The foal's muzzle and forelegs emerge; the amnion is still intact

12 Final delivery: the foal's muzzle and forelegs have broken the amnion

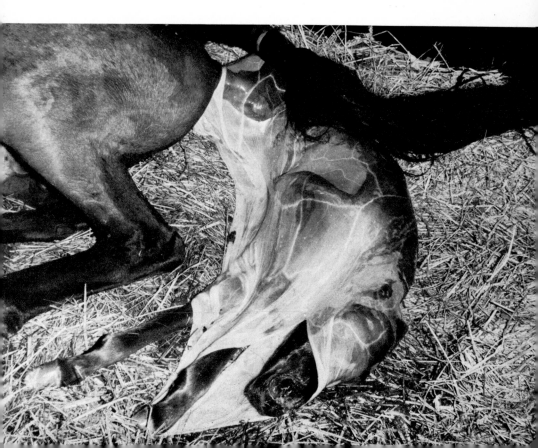

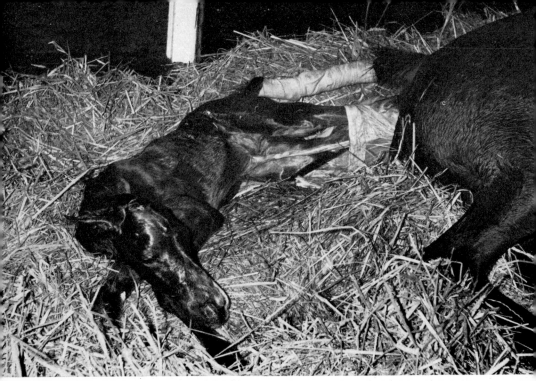

13 Umbilical cord is fully stretched during last stages of delivery

14 A few minutes later, it has ruptured leaving a wet stump

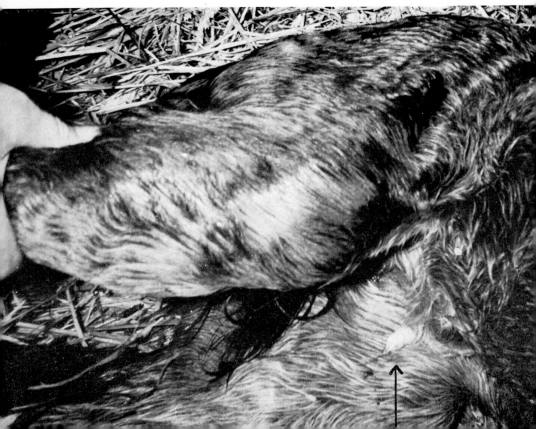

dentigerous (denti-+L. gerere, to carry) Bearing teeth. **d. cyst** See dermoid cyst.

dentin/dentine (L. dens, tooth) Chief substance surrounding tooth pulp and covered by enamel and cement. See teeth.

dentition (L. dentitio) See teeth.

deodorant (L. de, from+odorare, to perfume) Substance that destroys strong or offensive odours, eg chlorinated lime, creosote, hydrogen peroxide solution. See also foster.

Depo-Medrone Trade name. See methylprednisolone acetate, cortisone.

deposit (L. de, down+ponere, to place) Sediment, qv.

depraved appetite See appetite.

depression (1) Concave area in organ or body, eg prophet's thumb mark (**d. in muscle of neck**). (2) Dull state of health, often present with fever conditions of central nervous system, infections, liver disease.

Dermacentor Genus of tick, qv.

dermatitis (Gr. derma, skin + -itis, pl. dermatitides) Inflamed skin caused by bacteria, fungus, virus, allergy or chemicals. Types include acne, nettle rash, eczema, Queensland itch, photosensitisation, ringworm, mud fever, dermoid cyst. See separate headings.

dermatophilosis See mud fever.

Dermatophilus Genus of micro-organism with bacterial and fungal characteristics. **D. congolensis** Causal organism of mud fever, qv.

dermatosis (pl. dermatoses) Any skin disease.

dermis See skin.

dermoid cyst Egg-shaped growth with thick walls and cavity containing yellowish, greasy matter and, sometimes, a tooth (dentigerous cyst). Can occur anywhere on body, but usually on head, eg in nostril, eye, below ear. Often opens on to skin surface. Treat surgically.

derris Dried resin and roots of **D.** elliptica and other plant species of Burma, Thailand and Malaysia. Active principle: rotenone. Widely used as dusting powder or wash to control parasites, especially warble fly, qv.

descent of testes (testicles) In fetal life testes develop in upper part of abdomen, close to kidneys. Towards full term, each testis migrates down inguinal canal into scrotum. Testes have usually descended by birth but one or both may be retained in inguinal canal or abdomen. Migration is not clearly understood, the ligament known as gubernaculum testis, from tail of epididymis to inguinal ring, may exert traction. Retention of testis is cryptorchidism; absence of both testes: anorchidism or bilateral cryptorchidism. See rig.

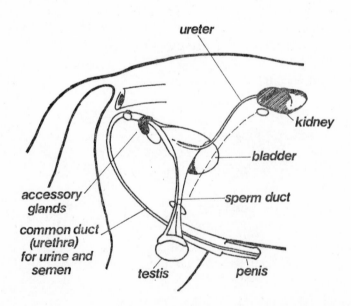

8 Male horse seen from off-side, showing route of descending testes

desmitis Inflamed ligament. See sprain.

desoxycorticosterone acetate (DOCA) Crystalline steroid, same as corticosteroid except hydroxyl group is replaced by hydrogen atom. Has marked effect on metabolism of water and electrolytes. See cortisone.

deterioration (L. deterior, worse, poorer) Becoming worse. See degeneration.

dexamethasone (trade names: Cortisol, Opticorten) White crystalline odourless powder with slightly bitter taste. Dose: 10–50mg. Actions and uses similar to cortisone, qv.

Dextran Trade name. Synthetic plasma expander; used in blood transfusions.

dextro- (L. dexter, right) Combining form meaning relationship to right-hand side.

dextrose (1) White odourless crystals or grains with sweet taste. Given in solution by mouth or IV to treat shock, blood-loss, severe dehydation. (2) Product of digested carbohydrate in alimentary tract.

diabetes (Gr.) Faulty metabolism. **d. insipidus** Increased production of urine (polyuria). It is of low specific gravity and free from protein and sugar. Associated with growths of pituitary gland in man, but in horses occurs after eating mouldy hay or oats, in glanders or tuberculosis. **d. mellitus** Condition in which sugar cannot be stored in body. Causes increase in blood sugar (hyperglycemia) and excessive discharge of sugar in urine (glycosuria). Rare in horses. Symptoms: thirst, abnormally high blood sugar concentration, weight-loss and coma.

diagnose To identify disease or condition.

diagnosis (dia- + Gr. gnosis, knowledge) Nature of disease deduced by observing, examining, special tests and laboratory measures. May or may not be specific, eg colic or certain type of colic, such as twist. **clinical d.** One based on signs. **differential d.** Distinction between diseases with similar symptoms, eg cough caused by influenza or broken wind. **laboratory d.** Based on lab. tests, eg hemolytic jaundice of newborn foal. **D.** can be based on departure from normal, eg lameness, eating, movement, stance, defecation, urination. **D.** by physical examination includes palpation (feeling part) and percussion, qv.

diagnostic Of diagnosis.

diaphragm Broad, domed, muscular partition between chest and abdomen. Chest side is covered by pleura, abdominal side by peritoneum. **D.** is attached to ribs, cartilage of sternum and lumbar vertebrae. It can change volume of chest to help breathing and can exert pressure on abdomen, eg during foaling (see birth). **D.** forms complete membrane except for 3 openings through which pass an artery (aorta), gullet and a vein (posterior vena cava).

diarrhoea (syns. scour, purge and, in foal, wet tail) Loose, runny feces. Symptom of increased water in feces due to disturbed fluid exchange between body tissues and gut contents. Often associated with increased gut movement (peristalsis) and inflamed intestinal mucous membrane (enteritis). Caused by (1) dietary factors such as composition and quantity of milk (foal **d.** more likely when dam is in oestrus) or, in adult, excessive protein in fast-growing grass; poor quality food; imbalanced diet; (2) bacteria (certain strains of E. coli, Salmonella), fungus or virus; (3) antibiotics—they may disturb natural flora of bacteria in gut; (4) purgative drugs and poisons taken by mouth. Symptoms: dung of cow-like consistency, sometimes bloodstained; relaxed anus, allowing air into rectum; dehydration, qv. Treatment: correct the diet, give antibiotics if cause is bacterial, or antifungal drugs if fungal, plus soothing drugs such as kaolin, chalk, sodium bicarbonate.

diathermy Treatment using frequent electric discharge to heat body tissues, eg sprained tendons. See physiotherapy.

Dibencil Trade name. See benzamine penicillin.

dichlorvos (trade name: Equiguard) Drug used to treat most worms and botfly larvae. Should not be used in horse with broken wind, diarrhoea or constipation; chickens etc should not be allowed to forage in dung of treated horse, as drug can kill birds. Dose: 0.036mg./kg. body wt. Antidote: atropine.

dicophane (syn. DDT) First synthetic insecticide, once widely used against external parasites but now replaced by more effective preparations. Kills stable flies and mosquitoes but not necessarily ticks. Non-toxic at recommended concentrations; poisoning produces nervous symptoms, inco-ordination, convulsions and death.

dicoumarol Substance produced in fermentation of sweet clover. Interferes with prothrombin formation and prevents blood clotting. Antidote: vitamin K. See coagulation.

Dictyocaulus Genus of lungworm, qv.

diethylcarbamazine citrate (trade names: Caritrol, Dicarocide, Franocide) White crystalline odourless powder with acid taste. Used to control lungworm, qv.

diethylstilboestrol See stilboestrol.

digestion (L. from dis, apart + genere, to carry) Process of converting food into materials fit to be absorbed through lining of alimentary tract so that they enter blood stream. From here they are transported to organs and tissues of body (eg hay is converted into the simpler carbohydrate, fat and protein). D. starts in mouth as food is mixed with saliva (which contains digestive enzyme), continues in stomach (which contains enzyme pepsin). But main organs of d. in horse are caecum and large colon. See alimentary canal, food.

digit Finger or toe. See evolution.

digital cushion Fibro-elastic fatty pad at back of foot, above frog and below second phalanx. Forms bulbs of heel and reduces concussion. See foot.

digitalis Green powder with slight odour and bitter taste, from dried leaf of D. purpurea (foxglove). Used in heart conditions. Prolongs time taken by nervous impulse to travel through heart muscle. This enables force of heart contraction to be increased while rate of beat is decreased. Dose: 1–4gms. Effects are cumulative and may cause toxicity. See heart impulse, neonatal maladjustment syndrome.

digitigrade (L. digitus, finger or toe + gradi, to walk) Walking on toes, when only digits touch ground. Horses are permanently on their toes. Cf plantigrade. See evolution.

digitoxin White crystalline odourless powder with bitter taste; prepared from digitalis and given by mouth or injection. See digitalis, alkaloid.

digoxin (trade name: Lanoxin) Colourless odourless crystals with bitter taste, obtained from leaves of Digitalis lanata. See digitalis.

dilatation/dilation Being dilated or stretched beyond normal. **d. of cervix** Before birth or at mating. **d. of pupils** See eye. **d. of heart** Enlargement of chambers with thinning of walls and therefore weakened beat. **d. of stomach** See colic.

dimethyl sulphoxide (abbr. DMSO; trade name: Demavet) Drug used to treat muscular pain. Unusual in that it can penetrate skin and carry other drugs into underlying tissue. Used alone, it has anti-inflammatory and some antifungal and antibacterial action. Dose: 10–15cc rubbed in 2/3 times a day. Used to treat bucked shins, qv.

diminazene aceturate Yellow odourless powder effective against parasites Trypanosoma and Babesia, also bacteria Brucella species and Streptococci. Dose: 3.5mg./kg. body wt. IM or sub. cut.

dimorphism (di- + Gr. morphe, form) Having two forms. **sexual d.** With characteristics of both sexes (hermaphrodite). See intersex.

diphenhydramine hydrochloride White odourless bitter-tasting powder. Used as antihistamine. Dose: 0.5–1mg./kg. body wt. Also applied externally in cream or lotion. See antihistamine.

diplococcus Spherical bacterium occurring in pairs; does not generally cause disease. See bacteria, streptococcus.

diploid (Gr. diplous, twofold) Having full set of paired chromosomes, ie 32 pairs for a horse. Opp. haploid. See chromosome.

Diptera (Gr. dipteros, two-winged) Order of insects including flies, gnats and mosquitoes. All can trouble horses and carry disease. See tabanid fly.

Direma Trade name. See hydrochlorothiazide.

dirty Colloq. for mare discharging catarrhal fluid from vulva. See endometritis. **d. nose** See snotty nose.

disc (L. discus, Gr. diskos) Flat, circular plate, eg **optic d.** See eye.

discharge Exudate or outpouring of matter. **catarrhal d.** From nose in horses suffering from strangles or herpesvirus infection. See catarrh, snotty nose, virus.

disease (Fr. des, from + **aise**, ease) Any abnormal process associated with characteristic signs; may affect whole body or any part. Its cause, consequences, outlook may be known or unknown. See various organs, also bacteria; fungi; virus; newborn foal, diseases of. **D.'s of Animals Act** See veterinary rules (Ministry of Agriculture).

dish (1) Shallow vessel as in culture **d.** or Petri **d.** used in laboratory. (2) Faulty action when foreleg below carpus (knee) is thrown outwards (syn. paddle). **d.-faced** Face with concave profile, as in typical Arab.

disinfectant Substance that reduces or destroys infective micro-organisms, eg cetrimide, chlorinated lime, potassium permanganate, phenol, sodium hydroxide.

disk See disc.

dislocation (dis- + L. locare, to place) Displacement of part, especially a joint.

dispensary (L. dispensarium from dispensare, to dispense) Place where medicines and remedies are dispensed. See also veterinary hospital.

distress (L. distringere, to draw apart) Difficulty or suffering, as in distressed breathing.

distressed breathing (syn. dyspnoea) May be due to obstructed air passages, including nasal cavities, voice box, windpipe; diseased lung using extra effort to compensate; biochemical disturbance in blood, affecting breathing centres of brain. Occurs in growths in nostrils, paralysed vocal cords, pneumonia, hemorrhage of brain, acute infection causing high fever, broken wind. Symptoms: anxious facial expression, dilated nostrils, laboured movements of chest and abdomen, stentorious or wheezing sound.

diuresis (Gr. diourein, to urinate) Process of passing urine. See behaviour.

diuretic (Gr. diouretikos, promoting urine) Substance which promotes excretion of body fluids by increasing urine flow. May help treat Monday morning leg, fever. Natural **d.**'s include potassium salts, alcohol, hay-tea, small amounts of caffeine, turpentine oil, oil of juniper. Digitalis and strychnine, which increase blood pressure, have **d.** side-effect. See hydrochlorothiazide.

diurnal (L. dies, day) During day. Opp. nocturnal.

diverticulum (L. divertere, to turn aside) Anatomical term meaning pouch or sac.

DMSO Abbr. dimethyl sulphoxide, qv.

DOCA Abbr. desoxycorticosterone acetate, qv.

dog-sitting posture Squatting on hindquarters with forelegs erect. Rare; symptom of bloat (see colic) or of nervous disease, eg encephalomyelitis.

dog's mercury (Mercurialis perennis) Plant, common in woods, which can poison. It contains mercurialin which causes acute irritation of stomach, diarrhoea, bloodstained urine. Chronic cases develop anemia, subcutaneous oedema and nettle rash.

dolor Pain; one of main signs of inflammation, qv.

domed forehead Forehead with convex profile; often occurs with roman nose.

dominance See gene, Mendel's law.

donkey (Equus asinus/domesticated ass) Member of horse family which varies in different parts of the world; 4 heights often used to classify: minature (under 9 hands), small standard (9–10.1h.), large standard (10.2–12h.), Spanish (above 12h.). Colours from black through all shades of brown, grey and dun to white (**D.** Breed Soc. recognises 20 colours). Probably introduced to Britain by Celtic traders in Roman times; differs from most Equidae as it has large head, ears and eyes; short neck; small, boxy hooves; especially thick coat, often with dorsal stripe and stripe across shoulders. (Stripes rare in white **d.**'s and will not be visible in black ones, but these animals may have bands of particularly coarse hair.) Tail is usually short-haired with tufted end; ergots and chestnuts are absent (site of chestnut is a hairless patch); male has vestigal teats on sheath. **D.** has 62 chromosomes (qv) and is aged from 1 Jan. of year born. It may be willing pack animal or live up to reputation for stubbornness; seems particularly susceptible to glanders, strangles, influenza and lungworm, so should not graze with horses unless checked. Only minimum dose of tranquillisers should be given, as **d.** likely to suffer inco-ordination. (See plate 24.) Assns: **D.** Breed Soc., c/o Mrs Walter Greenway, Prouts Farm, Hawkley, near Liss, Hampshire (Hawkley 289); **D.** Sanctuary, c/o V. Philpin, Springfield, Fosters Lane, Woodley, Berkshire (Sonning 3015).

dope test Colloq. for laboratory analysis of fluid collected from horse to discover presence of drug (dope). Official Jockey Club **d.t.** performed on saliva and/or urine (see urine sample, veterinary rules). Blood or, less commonly, feces can be used. Methods include electrophoresis and chromatography, in which substances in fluid are split by special process which causes each to travel at differing speeds on paper. Presence and quantity of non-normal nutrient can be determined because separation of particular substance is specific and typical of that substance. Difficulties are: (1) body metabolises drugs, so they may be excreted in another form, eg phenylbutazone (bute) as oxyphenbutazone; (2) individual may excrete drug faster or slower than average; (3) large numbers of drugs available and **d.t.** can be used only for known drugs (search is limited to those likely to have been used).

dorsal (L. dorsalis from dorsum, back) Of the back, eg **d. position** Normal position during birth, ie foal's back uppermost. **d. stripe** Band of colour, darker than majority of body, along line of backbone from poll to tail. Often seen in donkeys, mountain and moorland breeds.

dose (Gr. dosis, a giving) Quantity of medicine given at one time. **lethal d.** Sufficient to kill. **toxic d.** Amount causing toxic signs. **sensitising d.** First d. of protein or antigen, second of which will cause allergic reaction. **skin d.** Amount of radiation at surface of skin, eg where radiation therapy is applied to deeper structures as in treating carpitis. See allergy, anaphylaxis, poisoning, radiation, toxicity.

dourine (syns. equine syphilis, covering disease, genital glanders, mal de coit) Contagious disease caused by Trypanosoma equiperdum parasite; transmitted by coitus and characterised by inflamed genital organs, skin lesions and paralysis. Occurs in Africa, Asia, SE Europe, S America; kills 50–70% of infected animals. Treatment: see quinapyramine salts, homidium bromide.

dram (also drachm) Unit of weight equal to 60 grains or $\frac{1}{8}$oz. **fluid d.** Unit of capacity: 60 minims or 3.697ml. See weights and measures.

Drapolene Trade name. See benzalkonium chloride solution.

draught Dose of liquid medicine. **d. horse** Originally one used to pull vehicle (colloq. cart horse), now also any heavy, shire type, usually cold-blooded. Does not thrive in hot climates; is particularly susceptible to flies, ticks, etc.

draw Colloq. to unsheath penis. See behaviour, masterbation.

dressing (1) Applying materials, eg gauze, bandage, to a wound. (2) The material used. **antiseptic d.** One impregnated with antiseptic. See wounds.

drill Rotating instrument for boring holes in hard substances, eg bone. Used in surgery, qv.

Dr Med Vet Abbr. Doctor of Veterinary Medicine; followed by (Bern) or (Zurich) depending on which university awarded degree. See veterinary surgeon.

dropped elbow (syn. radial paralysis) Condition when horse cannot take weight on affected foreleg due to paralysed triceps muscle supporting elbow joint. Causes: injured radial nerve, fracture of humerus or olecranon (point of elbow) or possibly of 1st rib due to lying down too long. Elbow drops, fetlock joint is flexed and horse cannot advance leg. Partial recovery possible, but chronic cases are incurable. **d. sole** Occurs in laminitis and, to lesser extent, seedy toe. See plate 16.

dropsy (L. hydrops from Gr. hydor, water) Abnormal accumulation of fluid tissues or body cavity. See oedema.

drug Chemical compound given to help treat, diagnose or prevent disease or abnormal condition.

dry-coat (syns. anhidrosis, non-sweating syndrome, puff disease) Failure to sweat. Occurs in hot, humid climates such as India, Ceylon, Malaysia, Trinidad, Australia. May be due to repeated sweating, causing insensitivity of sweat glands. Results in reduced heat loss and rise in temperature, especially on exercise; difficult breathing and death from heart failure if exercise is not restricted. Horses usually recover capacity to sweat when returned to cool climate. Cf ichthyosis, sweat.

ductus arteriosus Blood vessel connecting pulmonary artery to aorta; open in fetus, closes during first 4 days of life when murmur can be heard on left side of chest, over position of line from shoulder joint to intersection with edge of triceps muscle. See muscles. **d. deferens** See vas deferens. **d. venosus** Fetal vein in liver; connects umbilical vein direct to posterior vena cava, allowing by-pass of liver. Closes in equine fetus at about 4th month so that all blood returning from placenta has to find its way through liver.

dull (1) not resonant on percussion, qv. (2) Lacking brightness, spirit. Dullness is symptom of most diseases, especially those connected with fever.

dummy/d. syndrome See neonatal maladjustment syndrome.

dung Colloq. feces, qv.

dupp Syllable representing second heart sound, which is short and high-pitched. Caused by closure of pulmonary and aortic valves. Complete beat termed lubb-dupp. See heart.

Durabolin Trade name. See nandrolone phenylpropionate.

Duracillin Trade name. See procaine penicillin.

dura mater (L., hard mother) Outermost and toughest of 3 membranes covering brain and spinal cord. Cf pia mater. See brain.

Dutch Draught Possibly heaviest breed in Europe. Carefully controlled by Royal Netherlands Draught Horse Soc. Distinguished from other breeds by particularly sloping croup and low-set tail. Colours: bay, grey, chestnut, occasionally black.

Duvaxyn 1 E Trade name; influenza vaccine (prepared in Holland) without an adjuvant.

D Vet. Med. Abbr. Doctor Veterinary Medicine (London).

DVH Abbr. Doctor of/Diploma in Veterinary Hygiene.

DVM Abbr. Doctor, Veterinary Medicine.

DVMS/DVM&S Abbrs. Doctor of Veterinary Medicine and Surgery.

DVS Abbr. Doctor of/Diploma in Veterinary Science/Surgery.

DVSM Abbr. Diploma in Veterinary State Medicine (RCVS). Same initials followed by (Edin) or (Vict) indicate diplomas from Edinburgh or Victoria University, Manchester. See also veterinary surgeon.

dysentery (L. dysenteria from Gr. dys- + enteron, intestine) Acute diarrhoea, qv.

dysphagia (dys- + **Gr.** phagein, to eat) Inability to swallow caused by pain, presence of foreign body in throat, or nervous inco-ordination. Occurs in shock, fracture of skull, grass sickness.

dysplasia (dys- + Gr. plassein, to form) Abnormal development, eg **epiphyseal d.** Faulty growth of epiphysis (growth plate, qv).

dyspnoea Distressed breathing, qv. Cf apnoea.

dystocia/dystokia (Gr. tokos, birth) Impeded birth. **fetal d.** That caused by abnormal size, position, presentation or posture of fetus so that it lodges against mare's pelvis at entrance to birth canal. Common **d.** includes flexed legs, head turned backward, foal presented backward or in upside-down position. May be result of deformity, eg contracted tendons (preventing forelegs extending in normal manner) or fetal illness, so that muscular tone is lost. **maternal d.** Caused by subnormal strength of uterine contractions (uterine inertia) or lack of voluntary straining. Treatment: realign fetus by manipulation (usually with mare standing, with help of muscle relaxants injected intravenously or intramuscularly or with spinal anaesthesia to abolish straining). If possible, fetus is aligned to lie in normal manner for delivery (see birth); if not, caesarean section (or possibly embryotomy) is performed. **D.** occurs in about 2% of severe abnormalities and 3% of minor ones.

dystrophy (L. dystophia from dys- + Gr. trephein, to nourish) Wasting of organs or tissues. **muscular d.** Wasting of muscles; can be caused by lack of vitamin E or lack of selenium.

dysuria Difficulty in passing urine. Usually associated with bladder stones and inflamed bladder (cystitis). Symptoms: repeated attempts to stale, with grunting, swishing of tail, kicking at belly. See stone.

Dyvon Trade name. See metriphonate.

E

ear Organ of hearing; consists of external, middle and internal e. **external e.** Funnel-like movable organ which collects sound waves and conveys them to e. drum. Formed of skin and cartilage, controlled by muscles. **middle e.** Comprised of e. drum, an air cavity containing 3 small bones (auditory ossicles), the malleus, incus and stapes, plus eustachian tube including the gutteral pouch. Bones form a chain by which sound vibrates from e. drum to internal e. **internal e.** Membraneous sac containing fluid and supporting sensitive cells which convey nervous messages to brain in auditory nerve; and series of cavities in skull containing semicircular canals and other structures concerned with balance.

earth Any easily pulverised mineral. See fuller's e.

earwax (syn. cerumen) Waxy secretion in ear canal.

ecchymosis (Gr. ekchymosis; pl. ecchymoses) Abnormal splash of blood under mucous membrane or skin, eg inside nostrils in allergy or infection. Cf petechia.

ECG Abbr. electrocardiogram, qv.

E. coli Abbr. Escherichia coli, qv.

ecraseur (Fr., crusher) Surgical instrument used instead of knife (causes less bleeding), eg in removing ovary.

ectoderm (ecto- + Gr. derma, skin) Outermost of 3 main layers (germinal layers) of embryo; it develops horn (of hooves), hair, skin, nervous system, external sensory organs (ear, eye) and mucous membranes of mouth and anus. Cf endoderm, mesoderm.

ectodermal Of ectoderm.

ectoparasite Parasite which lives on outside of body, eg tick, mite, louse.

ectopia (Gr. ektopos, displaced) Displacement, especially of part when congenital.

ectopic Of ectopia; not in usual position. **e. beat** See heart impulse.

eczema (Gr. ekzein, to boil out) Any non-specific inflammatory skin disease. See dermatitis, Queensland itch.

edathamil calcium disodium See sodium calcium edetate.

edema See oedema.

Ef-cortelan Trade name. See hydrocortisone.

efferent Conveying away from a centre, eg e. nerves pass messages from central nervous system. Cf afferent.

effusion (L. effusio, a pouring out) Escape of fluid into cavity, part or tissue, eg blood blister. **pleural e.** Presence of fluid around lungs. Likely in septicemia, pneumonia, abortion caused by equine herpesvirus 1.

egg (L. ovum) (1) Female sex cell containing hereditary material in haploid (qv) form. See ovum, embryology. (2) **E.** of parasite. See redworm, stomach worm, whiteworm.

EHV See equine herpesvirus.

Einthoven, William. Dutch physiologist 1860–1927. Developed string galvanometer with basis for such instruments as ECG (electrocardiogram, qv).

ejaculate (L. ejaculatio) To expel semen. See behaviour, male sexual; semen.

ejaculatum (Colloq. ejaculate) The fluid (semen) expelled at ejaculation.

elastic (L. elasticus) Having elasticity; capable of stretching then assuming original shape. Certain body tissues contain elastin, eg **e.** cartilage (see cartilage).

elbow (L. cubitus) Hinge joint between humerus and radius. See capped **e.**, dropped **e.**

electricity (Gr. elektron, amber) Fundamental form of energy. **faradic e.** See physiotherapy.

electrocardiogram (ECG, electro- + Gr. kardia, heart + gramma, mark) Graphic tracing of electric impulse passing through heart during each beat. Wave form of **e.** represents change of electric potential in heart muscle as it contracts and relaxes. The waves are designated P, Q, R, S and T. Record is formed by attaching electrodes of apparatus (electrocardiograph) to skin, usually on legs and chest. **E.** leads labelled I, II, III, aVl, aVf. (Chest leads usually designated VI-4, CR.LA, CL.LA, CF.LA.) Deviations from normal pattern indicate damaged heart muscle. **E.** particularly helpful in diagnosing general irregular heart beat (arrythmia), fast, irregular movements of first chambers (atrial fibrillation) and beat originating outside usual starting point (ectopic beat). See heart impulse, telemetry.

electrocardiograph Instrument for recording electrocardiogram.

electrocardiophonogram Tape recording of heart sounds (so they can be studied later or translated into visual record, ie graph).

electrocardiophonograph Instrument for recording electrocardiophonogram.

electrocautery Apparatus for cauterising tissue, usually platinum wire or iron which can be heated directly or by electricity. Used for firing, qv.

electrode (Gr. elektron, amber + hodos, way) Medium between electric conductor and object to which current is applied, eg electrical impulse passing through heart when it beats. Can be picked up by placing **e.** on body surface and connecting it to instrument known as electrocardiograph. Special conducting jelly is placed between **e.** and skin. See electrocardiogram, physiotherapy.

electroencephalogram Graphic record of electrical impulse passing through brain.

electroencephalograph Instrument for making electroencephalogram.

electrolyte (from Gr. lytos, soluble) Any solution which conducts electricity by its ions. In horses, usually a salt of body, eg sodium.

electron Unit or atom of negative electricity. Constitutes an electric current when flowing in a conductor.

electuary (L. electurium from e, out + legere, to select) Medicine in semi-fluid form with basis such as honey or butter and given by placing dose on tongue, gums and teeth. Used especially as cough **e.**

element (L. elementum) Main part or constituent. In chemistry, simple substance made up of similar atoms, which cannot be changed by a chemical.

emasculate (L. emasculare, to castrate) See castrate.

embolism (L. embolismus from Gr. en, in + ballein, to throw) Sudden blocking of artery or vein by clot carried in blood stream. Common site of **e.** is branch of anterior mesenteric artery, ie that supplying small intestines; often result of redworm damage to blood vessel at junction with aorta. See aneurysm, redworm, thrombus, colic.

embolus (Gr. embolos, plug; pl. emboli) Blood clot carried in blood stream from large vessel to smaller one, which it obstructs.

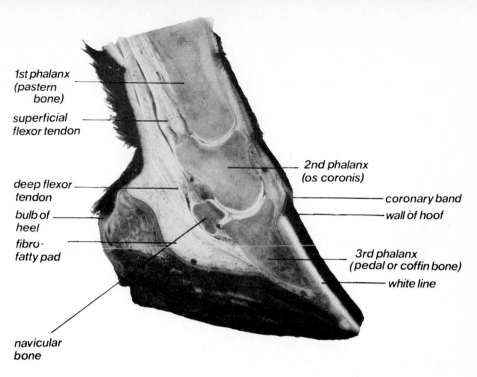

1st phalanx (pastern bone)

superficial flexor tendon

2nd phalanx (os coronis)

deep flexor tendon

coronary band

bulb of heel

wall of hoof

fibro-fatty pad

3rd phalanx (pedal or coffin bone)

white line

navicular bone

15 Section through normal foot. Cf laminitis pictures

16 Section through foot, showing abnormal position of the pedal bone. See *laminitis, dropped sole* and normal foot (above)

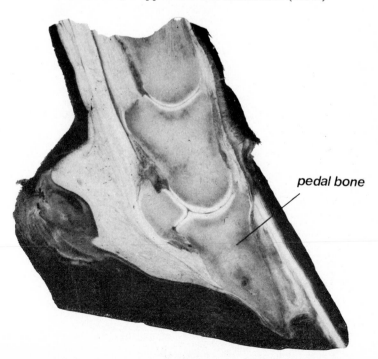

pedal bone

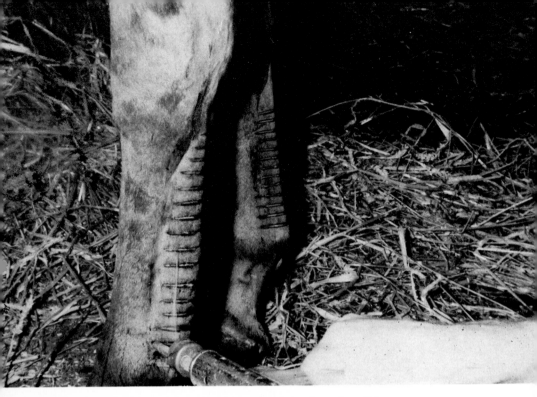

17 Line firing. See *bowed tendon, firing*

18 Hoof seen from above, after separation from foot. Insensitive laminae is immediately inside wall. See *foot, corium*

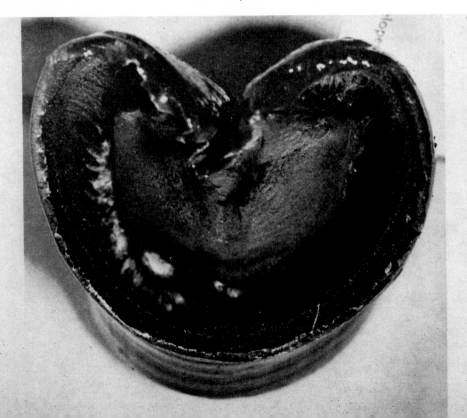

embryo (Gr. embryon) Fetus up to approx. 40 days. After this, it is called fetus.

embryology Science of development of fertilised egg to fully-formed fetus (developing foal). Individual begins as a single cell (zygote or fertilised egg) formed by fusion of spermatozoon and egg (2 gametes, one from each parent). This cell contains all inherited material (chromosomes and genes) which give foal its individuality. Zygote divides repeatedly until it is a ball of cells (blastula). A cavity (blastocoele) develops inside. A process (gastrulation) follows, in which primitive gut cavity and 3 germ layers are formed, ie ectoderm, mesoderm and endoderm from which skin, organs and linings of internal passages (nose, alimentary tract) develop. Then, brain, body cavity, organs of sense, alimentary canal, kidneys, gonads, arteries and veins and soft (cartilaginous) skeleton are formed. Amnion and placenta grow from embryo to surround it and placenta becomes attached to wall of uterus, so it can exchange nourishment for waste material. E. is not limited to precise period (see embryo). Most organs are formed by about 30th day of pregnancy, although development of bone from cartilage occurs much later and hair forms only in last 8 weeks. Congenital abnormalities, eg cleft palate, probably occur in first 30 days. See plate 6.

embryotomy (embryo- + Gr. tome, a cutting) Dismemberment of fetus. Generally replaced by caesarian section, qv. See dystocia.

emetic (Gr. emetikos, L. emeticus) Drug that causes vomiting—not normally given to horses as they are unlikely to vomit, qv.

emollient Drug which softens and allays irritation.

emphysema (Gr., an inflation) Swelling due to air; applied to abnormal distension of air sacs (alveoli) of lung, also to skin lifted by air entering through wound. See broken wind, percussion, wind.

empyema (Gr.) Accumulation of pus in body cavity, especially chest; may occur in foals due to bacteria. See newborn foal, diseases of; guttural pouch.

emulsion (L. emulsio, emulsum) One liquid distributed in small globules throughout a second liquid, eg paraffin emulsified in water, used as laxative in foals. See meconium retention.

enamel White, compact, very hard substance that covers and protects crown of tooth. See teeth.

encephalitis Inflamed brain.

encephalo- (Gr. enkephalos, brain) Combining form meaning relationship to brain.

encephalomyelitis (syn. equine e.) Inflamed brain and spinal cord, caused by virus; 3 strains important because they can affect man, viz., Western (WEE), Eastern (EEE) and Venezuelan (VEE). Disease is spread by blood-sucking insects, contaminated instruments, direct contact and infected bedding. Occurs June–November and usually dies out when frost kills mosquitoes. Horses of all ages susceptible, though older ones may develop resistance. Symptoms: fever, depression, restlessness, excitement, walking in circles, wandering into obstacles, refusing food and water, sleepiness, adopting strang postures, eg sitting on quarters (dog-sitting posture), possibly with forelegs crossed, pressing head against wall. Paralysis, collapse and death occurs in 2–4 days. Diagnosis: on symptoms and lab. innoculation of guinea pigs with blood from suspected case. Treatment: hyper-immune serum may help, also supportive measures, eg feeding by stomach tube. Control: vaccines are available and TC 83 (containing live virus grown in fetal guinea pig cells) was used for first time in 1971 outbreak in N America. Insects should be kept down if possible and horses stabled at night. Pathology: damaged nerve cells of brain, but there are no inclusion bodies, which helps distinguish e. from borna disease and rabies.

endarteritis (from Gr. arteria, artery + -itis) Inflamed inner lining of an artery. Caused by migrating redworm larvae. See redworm, thrombus.

endemic (Gr. endemos, dwelling in a place) Disease or condition present in area but affecting only a small number of animals at one time.

endocarditis Inflamed lining (endocarduim) of heart chambers and/or valves (valvular e.). Caused by bacteria, usually Streptococci, or migrating larvae of Strongylus vulgaris (redworm). Nodules and cauliflower-like growths cause leaking valves, heart murmurs.

Associated with intermittent fever, loss of body condition and lack of stamina.

endocardium (endo- + Gr. kardio, heart) Membrane lining heart chambers and their valves. Formed of endothelium, qv.

endocrine (from Gr. krinein, to separate) Any gland which secretes hormones into blood or lymph stream, eg pituitary. (Hormone then carried to organ or part to exert influence.) Cf exocrine. See gland.

endocrinology Study of endocrine glands and their hormones.

endoderm (endo- + Gr. derma, skin) Epithelium (qv) of throat, respiratory and digestive tracts, bladder and urethra. Cf ectoderm, mesoderm. See embryology

endogenous (endo- + Gr. gennan, to produce) Developing or originating inside organism. Cf exogenous.

endometritis Inflamed lining of uterus. Caused by infection with bacteria, fungus and possibly virus. Predisposing causes: hormonal influences, poor conformation of vulva, pregnancy, birth, coitus. Phagocytic and other inflammatory cells collect close to surface and mix with secretions of glands to produce catarrhal fluid that drains to outside through cervix and vagina (colloq. dirty mare). Treatment: antibiotics injected and infused into uterus.

endometrium (endo- + Gr. metra, uterus) Mucous lining of uterus.

endothelium (endo- + Gr. thele, nipple; pl. endothelia) Layer of epithelial cells lining cavities of heart, blood and lymph vessels.

endotracheal tube See tube.

enema Liquid put into rectum with syringe or gravitated from container; rarely used on adult horses but frequently on newborn foals to help passage of meconium, qv. May be paraffin and water or soap and water at blood temperature; quantity about 600ml. (1 pint). Blunt, soft rubber tube should be used to avoid damaging anus and rectum.

energy (Gr. energeia) Source of power. **nutritional e.** That from food, qv.

Entacyl Trade name. See piparazine salts.

Entavet Trade name. See streptomycin.

enter-/entero- (Gr. enteron, intestine) Combining form meaning relationship to intestines.

enteric Of intestines.

enteritis Inflamed intestines (strictly small intestines). Used non-specifically in cases of diarrhoea or inflamed alimentary tract. Caused by agent which disturbs natural flora in intestine, eg fungus, excess protein, antibiotics, bacteria. Can be fatal, especially in foals. See newborn foals, disease of; dehydration. Cf ulcerative **e.**

Enterobacteriaceae (enteric bacteria) Rod-shaped, gram-negative organisms. **E.** family contains Escherichia, Aerobacter, Klebsiella, Proteus, Shigella.

entero-toxemia Infection of alimentary tract by organisms of toxin-producing Clostridia, which poison blood. Causes severe enteritis and diarrhoea. Not common in horses but well recognised in lambs, calves; may account for sudden death in horses and foals.

enterovirus Group of viruses infecting alimentary tract and discharged in dung. Includes Poliovirus, Coxsackie. Horses not known to be affected by **e.** but infection probably occurs.

entropion (Gr. en, in + tropein, to turn) Inversion of an edge, eg eyelid. Result of dehydration (qv) when eyeballs sink into sockets, or of rubbing head on straw. Common in foals. Treatment (essential to prevent serious damage to eye): stitch lid parallel to its edge.

enuresis (Gr. enourein, to void urine) Urinary incontinence; more common in old mares (with weak sphincter muscle at bladder exit) than in geldings. Hindquarters may be lightly scalded by continual dribble of urine.

enzootic (Gr. en, in + zoon, animal) Old English for endemic, qv.

enzyme Organic compound, frequently a protein, acting as catalyst and producing a specific change. Cf hormone, pheromone.

Eohippus (syns. dawn horse, hyracotherium) Fox-sized animal of Eocene period about 55 million years ago. Ancestor of today's horse. See evolution.

eosin (Gr. eos, dawn) Rose-coloured stain or dye used in laboratory for histological sections.

eosinophil (eosin + Gr. philain, to love) Special blood cell belonging to white cell type but containing granules which stain red with eosin in lab. work. See white blood cell.

eosinophilia Abnormally large number of eosinophils in blood or accumulating in tissues.

Epanutin Trade name. See phenytoin.

ephedrine Colourless odourless crystals with bitter taste and action similar to adrenaline, qv.

Ephynal Trade name. See tocopheryl acetate.

epicardium (epi- + Gr. kardia, heart) Layer of the pericardium (qv) on outer surface of heart.

epicondyle Rounded projection of bone, above condyle, which does not articulate with another bone, eg medial e. of femur (thigh bone).

epidemic (Gr. epidemios, prevalent) Any disease affecting many animals in a region at same time. **e. cerebrospinal nematodiasis** See filaria.

epidemiologist Person concerned with epidemiology. Horserace Betting Levy Board appointed its first **e.** (Dr David Powell) in 1971 to study equine virus disease in UK.

epidemiology The study of epidemics.

epidermal Of epidermis.

epidermis (epi- + Gr. derma, skin) Outermost, non-vascular part of skin, qv.

epididymis (from Gr. didymos, testis; pl. epididymides) Tubes attached to testis. Has head (consists of 12 or more small coiled tubes), body (single tube) and tail (where tube joins vas deferens, qv). **E.** stores spermatozoa prior to ejaculation.

epidural anaesthesia See anaesthesia.

epiglottis Small flap of cartilage which covers entrance to voice box. See wind.

epilepsy (Gr. epilepsia, seizure) Type of convulsion, qv. Does not occur in horses.

epinephrine (adrenaline) Hormone secreted by middle (medulla) of adrenal gland. Synthetic **e.** given to increase blood pressure and heart rate.

epiphysis (Gr., an ongrowth; pl. epiphyses) End of long bone. See growth plate.

epiphysitis Inflamed epiphysis (growth plate) caused by infection, trauma or imbalanced diet (excess protein, incorrect calcium/phosphorus ratio). Most common during rapid growth, in lower end of radius (bone immediately above knee) at 12–24 months and in lower end of cannon at 6–8 months. May also occur at lower end of second thigh bone (tibia) at 12–24 months. Symptoms: swelling, usually above and inside fetlock, knee and/or hock, pain, lameness. Treatment: reduce protein in diet, correct calcium/phosphorus ratio (qv), give vitamin D and confine to large loose box, preferably on soft bedding.

epistaxis (Gr.) Nosebleed. See bleeder.

epithelium (epi- + Gr. thele, nipple) Cells which form covering of internal and external surfaces of body, including lining of vessels and small cavities. Classified by shape and structure. **ciliated e.** Bearing cilia on free surface; lines air passages. **columnar e.** Tall, narrow cells; lines digestive tract. **cuboidal e.** Square cells; covers ovaries. **germinal e.** Lines ducts of gonads and produces germ cells, ie ovum and spermatozoon. **glandular e.** Cells of glands or secreting cells. **scaly e.** Forms horn of hoof. **squamous e.** That of skin. **transitional e.** That of bladder.

epizootic lymphangitis (syns. pseudo-glanders, mycotic lymphangitis, equine blastomycosis) Chronic contagious disease causing inflamed lymphatic vessels and glands, skin ulcers and pneumonia. Occurs in Asia, Africa and Mediterranean countries as epidemics with death rate of about 15%. Important because it is similar to glanders and because it incapacitates victim for up to a year. Cause: fungus Histoplasma farciminosum (*ex* Cryptococcus or Blastomyces). Horses under 6 are most susceptible and fungal spores enter through small wounds and are carried by bedding, grooming utensils, blankets, harness etc. Symptoms, after 2/3 months' incubation: ulcer at site of entry, lymph vessels nearby thicken and develop nodules. These rupture, discharging thick, creamy pus; abscesses form in lymph nodes (especially around hocks, back, sides, neck, vulva/scrotum). Horse may also suffer inflamed eyes and nostrils and pneumonia. Recovery may be spontaneous after 3–12 months. Diagnosis: on laboratory examination of pus containing fungus cells. Must be distinguished from glanders, strangles, and Corynebacterium infection. Control: observe strict quarantine, destroy or disinfect bedding, saddlery, etc.

epsom salts See magnesium sulphate.

Equidae (L. equus, horse) Family of mammals containing single genus Equus (qv) which includes horse, ass, zebra.

Equiguard Trade name. See dichlorvos.

equilenin An oestrogen hormone. See sex.

equilin Oestrogen hormone produced by fetus and passed in mare's urine from about 120 days' pregnancy to full term. Used in human medicine as hormone treatment and additive for cosmetics.

equine (L. equinus, relating to horses) Of horse family Equidae. **e. behaviour** See behaviour. **e. blastomycosis** See epizootic lymphangitis. **e. cutaneous papillomatosis** See milk warts. **e. encephalomyelitis** See encephalomyelitis. **e. flu** See influenza. **e. herpesvirus** (EHV, syn. rhinopneumonitis) Virus which causes abortion, coital exanthema, snotty nose. (See separate headings and virus.) **e. infectious anemia** See swamp fever. **E. Influenza Vaccine** Trade name. See Grippequin. **e. sounds** Divided into vocal and internal. George Waring (S Illinois University, 1971) named categories: squeal, nicker, whinny, groan (all

159

vocal) and blow, snort and snore (non-vocal). Squeal: high-pitched, typically used as threat, noted during aggression; sexual rejection; when mare running milk is touched near flank or mammary gland. Nicker: low-pitched and pulsating, used before being fed; by stallion investigating mare; by mare concerned for foal. Whinny: one of the loudest sounds, begins as squeal and ends as nicker; used for calling, especially between mare and foal at weaning. (Some members of Equidae, eg donkey, bray instead of whinny. Bray is harsh, rasping sound, almost a bark.) Groan: used during pain, especially when horse is lying on side. Blow: expulsion of air through nostrils (horse cannot breath through mouth), used before being fed; when suspicious. Snort: strong, pulsating blow, used to clear nasal irritation; after cough (in which case cough thought less serious) during colic; occasionally if in conflict situation. (Some consider snort sign of contentment.) Snore: rasping sound when inhaling, sometimes used before blow sound of alarm; during colic. Other sounds include cough, chew, flatus, hoof beats and movements in male sheath. Internal sounds, sometimes audible with naked ear, include borborygmi, heart and lung noises. See separate headings. Other references: Von Maday (1912), Frank Odberg (Ghent University, 1969). **e. syphilis** See dourine. **E. Veterinary Journal** Published quarterly by British Equine Veterinary Association, qv. **e viral arteritis** (EVA) Acute virus disease of respiratory tract. Symptoms: fever, thick, nasal discharge, inflamed mucous membranes of eyes, respiratory and alimentary tracts, oedema of eyelids and legs, reduced circulating white cells (leucopenia), abortion. Was once confused with influenza, qv. Virus causes degeneration of middle layer (media) of small arteries (arterioles) and is present in nasal secretions, saliva, blood, feces, urine and occasionally semen. Diagnosis: not always possible due to number of forms, but signs described appear in an outbreak. Incubation: 2–10 days; virus can be recovered from nasal swabs during fever, blood serum can be tested in acute and convalescent phases. Abortion occurs simultaneously with symptoms, which distinguishes it from abortion due to herpesvirus. Treatment: no vaccine available, but antibiotics can suppress secondary infection. Horse should be rested and isolated 4–6 weeks.

Equi-Palazone Trade name. See phenylbutazone.

equisetum See horsetails.

Equizole Trade name. See thiabendazole.

equorum medicus Ancient Roman for veterinary surgeon. Succeeded mulomedicus and preceded veterinarius.

Equus (L., horse) Genus of horse family (Equidae) which includes all living members of family and their immediate ancestors and close relatives during Ice Age. Genus is followed by species name, eg **E.** asinus (donkey). **E. caballus** Species which includes all breeds of domesticated horse and those feral or wild relatives so closely related that they can, or could, inter-breed and produce fertile offspring. See chromosome, wild.

ergometrine maleate (trade name: Ergotrate) White crystalline odourless powder. Alkaloid drug which promotes contraction of uterus. Given, by mouth or injection, after birth to help restore uterus to non-pregnant size. Dose: 10–20mg.

ergot (Fr., L. ergota) Small, horny area in tuft of hair behind fetlock joint. May be vestige of another hoof (see evolution). Cf chestnut.

Ergotrate Trade name. See ergometrine maleate.

Erythrocin Trade name. See erythromycin.

erythrocyte (erythro- + Gr. kytos, hollow vessel) Red blood cell, qv. **e. sedimentation rate** (ESR) See blood tests, hematology (7).

erythrocytosis Increase in number of red blood cells, qv.

erythromycin (trade names: Erythrocin, Ilotycin) White crystalline odourless powder with bitter taste. Produced from Streptomyces erythreus. Antibiotic with bacteriostatic and bactericidal activity against gram-positive and some gram-negative bacteria. Given to foals with conditions caused by bacteria, eg joint-ill, pneumonia. Dose: 2–6mg./kg. body wt. twice daily by mouth.

Escherichia Genus of gram-negative micro-organisms of tribe Escherichieae, family Enterobacteriaceae, order Eubacteriales. Have motile or non-motile short rods. **E. coli** Intestinal flora (mainly in caecum, large and small colon, rectum) connected with digestion. Strains can cause diarrhoea, septicemia. See newborn foal, diseases of.

Escherichieae Tribe of family Enterobacteriaceae, order Eubacteriales; non-motile or motile rods that ferment glucose and lactose, producing acid. Comprises coliform bacteria including 5 genera: Aerobacter, Alginobacter, Escherichia, Klebsiella and Paracolobactrum.

eserine Syn. physostigmine, qv.

Esmarch bandage (after German surgeon Johann von E.) Rubber bandage used to reduce blood flow to an area before surgery.

esophagus See oesophagus.

ESR Abbr. erythrocyte (red cell) sedimentation rate. See blood tests, hematology (7).

esterase Body substance which breaks link between biological compounds such as esters and fatty acids, eg choline e. of blood, which destroys acetyl-choline.

Estonian Klepper See Klepper.

estr- See words beginning oestr-.

ether Clear colourless volatile liquid with characteristic odour and sweet, burning taste. Used as anaesthetic; less effective than chloroform.

ethics (Gr. ethos, manner and habits of man or animal) Rules or principles laid down by professional body to guide conduct of members. See Royal College of Veterinary Surgeons, veterinary rules.

ethmoid (Gr. ethmos, sieve) Sieve-like, eg e. turbinate bones of nasal passages.

ethological Of ethology. **E. Society** c/o R. Ewbank, Liverpool University Veterinary Field Station, Leahurst, Neston, Wirral, Cheshire.

ethology Study of animal behaviour. **equine e.** Study of horses' behaviour. See behaviour, equine sounds.

ethyl chloride Volatile liquid with pleasant odour and burning taste. Occasionally used as fine spray to freeze skin, producing short-term anaesthesia.

etorphine hydrochloride (trade name: Immobilon/Revivon) Fast-acting immobiliser/pain killer used in surgery, eg castration. Action rapidly reversed by diprenorphine hydrochloride.

eugenics (eu- + Gr. gennan, to produce) Study of ways of improving hereditary characters in a breed.

euthanasia Mercy killing or humane destruction. May be necessary in cases of fractured leg, pelvis, vertebrae or painful conditions with no apparent chance of recovery. Carried out by IV injection of drug or humane killer (eg Greener) consisting of bolt placed against forehead (at intersection of lines drawn from base of ear to opposite eye), then hammered home. Gun and bullet require great care because of danger of accident/ricochet.

EVA See equine viral arteritis.

evisceration (L. evisceratio from e, out + viscus, inside of body) Disembowelment; rare congenital fault in which floor of abdomen is not formed.

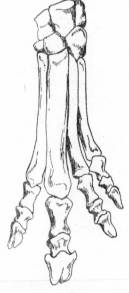

9 Eohippus (the dawn horse): skeleton of lower part of foreleg shows the first horse-like animal had 4 toes on each forefoot

evolution (L. evolutio from volvere, to roll) A rolling out, continual change and development; generally of a species over a long period. That of horse family (Equidae) can be traced from Eocene (Gr. dawn, new) period, which began approx. 55 million years ago. Animal living then, Eohippus (scientific name Hyracotherium), considered forerunner of today's horse. It was fox-like with arched back; 4 horn-covered toes (padded underneath) on each forefoot and 3 on each hindfoot. It had small, primitive brain, 44 teeth and browsed on shrubs. (Usual number of teeth now: 40 in male, 36 in female. See teeth.) Eohippus (syn. dawn horse) developed (via Orohippus and Epihippus) into Mesohippus, pad-footed animal with 3 toes on each foot. It lived in Oligocene period (which began 35 million years ago) and its brain was much larger than Eohippus's. Mesohippus gradually evolved (via Miohippus and Parahippus) from pad-footed animal into spring-footed one (Merychippus) better adapted for running fast to escape enemies. It had 3 toes but outer 2 (dew hooves) had shortened leaving middle one to take most weight. Ulna and radius bones of leg had fused and lengthened and Merychippus looked much like today's pony— perhaps striped or patchy for camouflage.

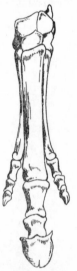

10 Merychippus

Merychippus was a grazer, so its teeth were longer (hypsodonty, cf brachydonty); it had grown (probably to 10 hands) and its eyes were farther back in skull (so that it could see horizon when grazing). After Merychippus came Pliohippus (of Pliocene period which began 10 million years ago). This had lost dew hooves (see chestnut, splint, ergot) and it evolved into today's Equus by continual streamlining.

Today's domestic horse belongs to kingdom Animalia, phylum Chordata, class Mammalia, order Perissodactyla, family Equidae, genus Equus (cf ass, donkey, zebra), species Equus caballus, qv. See also chromosome, hippus, Przewalski.

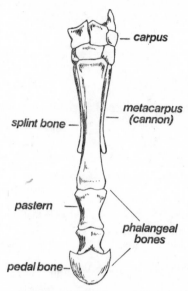

11 Equus, the present-day horse

ewe-neck Neck in which line along mane is concave. (Bones of neck—cervical vertebrae—are concave, but flesh usually hides this.) See neck.

examination (L. examinare) Investigation. **clinical e.** Looking for abnormality; listening to chest and abdomen; recording of heart, pulse and breathing rates and rectal temperature; watching behaviour; palpation (feeling) of legs, poll, back, withers; inspecting mouth. **cardiac e.** Listening to heart and making electrocardiographic (ECG) recordings of heart beat before (possibly during) and after exercise. **genital e.** (mare) Rectal palpation of ovaries and uterus; visual inspection of cervix, vagina, by speculum inserted through vulva. **insurance e.** One on behalf of underwriters to ascertain health and fitness for insurance of a horse's life or, in certain cases, its fitness to work. **laboratory e.** Tests on blood, feces, urine, abdomnial fluid; and material collected from cavities, discharges and tissues, for bacteriological, histological, biochemical and hematological analysis. **laryngo-scopic e.** Passing of a special instrument (laryngoscope). This is tube containing mirrors and lights which is inserted into nostril so that throat and voice box can be seen. **ophthalmological e.** Inspecting internal structures of eye using opthalmoscope, inspecting eyeball surface and feeling to ascertain pressure in eyeball. **post-mortem e.** (PME) See post-mortem. **radiographic e.** X-ray photography of bones, joints and other tissues with evidence of abnormality. See radiation. **rectal e.** Feeling of abdominal contents by inserting arm into rectum. **soundness e.** See soundness.

exanthema (Gr.) Eruption under skin or mucous membrane. See coital e.

excipient (L. excipiens, from ex, out + capere, to take) Inert substance acting as vehicle for drug, eg in pessary or pill.

excitation (L. from ex, out + citare, to call) Stimulation, eg of a muscle, as in faradism. See physiotherapy.

excretion (L. excretio) Act of voiding waste material, especially feces, urine. See behaviour.

Exmoor Possibly oldest-established of England's mountain and moor-land types; roams **E.** district in Devon and Somerset, SW England. Extremely hardy and strong. Will carry full-grown man hunting or make good child's pony. Has prominent 'toad' eyes and mealy (ie light-coloured) muzzle, eyelids, insides of ears and belly. Colours: bay, brown or dun, without markings except those mentioned. Mares up to 12.2 hands, stallions up to 12.3. Cf Dartmoor. Assn: E. Pony Soc., c/o Mrs J. Watts, Quarry Cottage, Sampford Brett, Williton, Somerset (Williton 539).

exocrine (exo- + Gr. krinein, to separate) Any gland which secretes outwardly or externally, ie its products act locally, eg salivary gland. Cf endocrine. See gland.

exogenous (from Gr. gennan, to produce) Developing outside organism.

ex-ophthalmic goitre See hyperthyroidism.

exostosis (ex- + Gr. oesteon, bone) Bony growth on surface of bone; usually follows inflammation. See osselet, ringbone, splint.

exotoxin Toxin formed by bacteria and having its effect at a distance.

expectorant (ex- + L. pectus, breast) Drug or substance which promotes coughing up of mucus from lungs and air passages, eg ammonium chloride.

experiment (L. experimentum, proof from experience) Procedure which might discover or confirm fact. See examination, gnotobiota, temperature.

expiration (ex + L. spinare, to breathe) Act of breathing out. See breathing, wind.

expression (L. expressio) Facial appearance. **anxious e.** Seen in painful conditions, eg colic. **mask e.** Seen in lockjaw.

extension (L. extensio) Movement which straightens body part, eg. leg, head.

extensor Any muscle or tendon which extends joint. Opp. flexor. See contracted tendons.

extirpation (L. extirpare, to root out) Removal of a part.

extrasystole/extra-systolic beat See heart impulse.

extravasation (extra- +L. vas, vessel) Escape of blood or fluid, from vessel into tissues. Types include hemorrhage, oedema, petechia, ecchymosis.

extremity Any part far from body centre, eg ear, hoof.

exudate (L. exsudare, to sweat out) Mixture of fluid, cells and cellular debris which has escaped from blood vessel into tissues or on to surface of mucous membrane; result of inflamation.

eye (L. oculus, Gr. ophthalmos) Organ of sight, one either side of face in e. socket (orbit) in skull. Provides mainly monocular vision (not binocular vision as in human eye) except when looking at close objects. Consists of ball, flattened on front surface with tough, fibrous coat (sclera) modified in front to form cornea. Bordered by angle (canthus) at either side of e. lid. Inside, lens divides ball into front and back chambers. Pupil is formed by iris, which dilates to admit more light and constricts

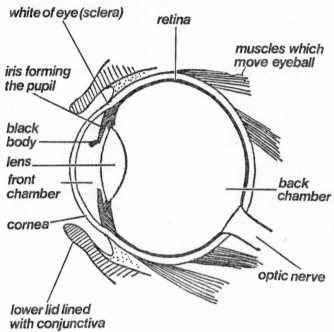

white of eye (sclera) *retina*

muscles which move eyeball

iris forming the pupil

black body

lens

front chamber

back chamber

cornea

optic nerve

lower lid lined with conjunctiva

12 Section through eye

to cut out light. Light falls on retina, a sensitive nervous membrane lining inside of e. and conveying messages to brain. Optic disc is pale area in retina where optic nerve and blood vessels leave and enter e. **e., diseases of: amaurosis** Blindness resulting from fault in nervous mechanism of brain; unrelated to abnormality in e. Occurs suddenly, usually after shock. Signs include rapid ear movement, reluctance to move from dark into light, or to pass through gate or doorway. **cataract** Opacity (scarring) of lens or its capsule, caused by trauma or occasionally inherited or congenital; varies in size from pinpoint to complete coverage of lens, so interference with sight varies. Types include those in centre of lens and those in capsule. **conjunctivitis** See under heading. **corneal perforation** Penetration of cornea by foreign body (eg straw), trauma (eg kick) or ulcer, allowing escape of aqueous humor (fluid in front chamber) and collapse of eyeball due to lowering of internal pressure. **dermoid cyst** (qv) Wart-like growth on cornea, contains hairs up to 1in. long. Surgical removal necessary. **glaucoma** Abnormally increased pressure in eyeball causing changes in retina and blindness. Common only in injury. **hypopyon** Pus in front chamber of e. Result of inflamed cornea (keratitis), ulcer on cornea or complication after infectious disease, eg strangles. **keratitis** Inflamed cornea; result of trauma, foreign body, turning in of lids (entropion), viral or bacterial infection. Symptoms: white spot on surface of cornea, blood vessels growing towards area. Ulcer may develop and, in severe cases, penetrate front chamber, resulting in prolapse of fine membrane lining inside of **e.** As healing takes place, blood vessels disappear, white scar (opacity) remains and eventually disappears. Treatment: antibiotic drops of ointment, weak astringent, eg silver argentum, corticosteroid (use sparingly because it may cause ulcer to penetrate deeper). **luxation of lens** Displacement of lens, usually as result of blow. **moon blindness** (syn. periodic ophthalmia) Inflamed ciliary body and iris (iridocyclitis). Affected horses suffer recurring attacks, each of which is increasingly severe until eventually internal structures of **e.** are irreversibly damaged. **E.** loses tension and collapses. Signs: spasm of lids when exposed to light (photophobia), inflamed surface of **e.** (scleritis) and membranes. Lids may swell, tears run down face and pupils constrict. Cause unknown, but infections with leptospira bacteria, virus and parasites have been blamed. Treatment: keep horse stabled in dark during attack, drop corticosteroids and atropine into **e.** to dilate pupil. Condition unlikely to improve. **retinitis** Inflamed retina; often occurs after moon blindness or infections such as arteritis and purpura.

eyelid (syn. palpebra) One of 3 membranes: 2 main (upper and lower) and third lid (syn. nictitating membrane) which sweeps across **e.** from inner to outer angle. See plate 30.

F

F. (1) Abbr. fahrenheit, qv. See also temperature, weights and measures. (2) Abbr. Fellow (of Royal College of Veterinary Surgeons, qv). More often written FRCVS.

face (L. facies) That part of head comprising forehead and bridge of nose. Conformation differs with breed (see Arab).

facelessness (aprosopia) Rare congenital fault in which eyes, nostrils and mouth have not formed. Foal usually dies immediately after birth.

facial (L. facialis) Of the face. **f. expression** Can show pain/distress (eg in colic, grass sickness), anxiety, fear, anger, etc. See flehmen posture. **f. paralysis** See paralysis.

facultative Ability to adjust, as in **f. anaerobe** an organism which can live without air. See anaerobe.

fahrenheit (abbr. F., after German physicist Gabriel Daniel F.) Scale of temperature in which freezing point of water is 32° and boiling point 212°. To convert f. to centigrade subtract 32° and multiply by $\frac{5}{9}$. See temperature, weights and measures.

Falabella Miniature breed, about 7 hands, developed in South America by down-breeding from Thoroughbred.

Falapen Trade name. See benzylpenicillin.

fallopian tube (after Italian anatomist Gabriele Falloppio; syn. oviduct) One of two ducts joining the two ovaries to uterus. Conveys eggs to uterus (spermatozoa swim up tube to meet and fertilise egg). 20–30 cm. (8–12in.) long and about 3mm. wide.

faeces See feces.

family Group of related living things (ie animals, plants, micro-organisms). Horse **f.**: Equidae, qv.

Famous and Celebrated Colonial Quarter-Pather Old name American Quarter horse, qv.

faradic Of faradism.

faradism (after English physicist Michael Faraday) Treatment using electricity to produce a rhythm of contractions in muscle. See physiotherapy.

farcy See glanders.

Faroe Isles pony Similar to Iceland pony, except usually chestnut, brown or sometimes black.

fascia (L., band) White fibrous sheets beneath skin or between muscles.

fat/f. tissue (syn. adipose tissue) White or yellowish material laid down around, or in, various organs and muscles of body.

Fe ++   See ferrous.

Fe +++   See ferric.

feathers Colloq. for long hairs around pasterns of most heavy breeds and some ponies.

febrile (L. febrilis) Characterised by fever.

feces (L., pl. of faex, refuse; syns. dung/s, droppings) Excreta passed from intestines through anus; may be formed or soft, depending on feed. Adult horse of 500kg. passes 10–25kg. of **f.** in 24 hours. Hard, mucus-covered **f.** indicate stoppage in gut; diarrhoea suggests bacterial infection. See behaviour; colic; appetite, depraved.

fecundate (L. fecundere, to make fruitful) To fertilise.

fecundity (L. fecunditas) Ability to produce offspring. See fertility.

feed/ing To eat or give food. Colloq. ration provided, typically grass, hay, oats. See also behaviour, eating; food. **artificial f.** See food by stomach tube.

Fell Native pony of Pennine hills in N England. Made to carry great weights in past, now popular for pony trekking. Originally similar to Dales pony, but few inches smaller and unchanged by influence of other breeds. Most commonly black without any markings, also bay, and less commonly grey or dun. Assn: F. Pony Soc., c/o Miss P. Crossland, Packway, Windermere, Westmorland (Windermere 3152).

female genital organs Consist of 2 ovaries which produce eggs (ova) and secrete hormones, oestrogen and progesterone; 2 fallopian tubes (oviducts) in which egg is fertilised; uterus in which foal develops; cervix (neck of uterus) which guards contents of uterus and separates it from vagina; vulva, which acts as a valve preventing air entering genital tract; mammary glands (udder). See under separate headings. Diseases and conditions: see birth, hazards of; virus; bacteria; Caslick operation; cervicitis; endometritis; hemorrhage; mastitis; metritis.

femoral (L. femoralis) Of the femur.

femur (syn. thigh bone) Large bone between hip joint above and stifle joint below.

fenestra (L., window; pl. fenestrae) Anatomical term meaning window-like opening, eg **f.** cochleae, round opening in middle ear.

feral Free-roaming; animal whose ancestors have escaped from captivity. **F.** breeds include Camargue. Cf wild.

fermentation (L. fermentatio) Decomposition of carbohydrate by enzyme action. See colic.

ferric (L. ferrum) Iron in trivalent form, Fe $^{+++}$

ferrin Iron-containing substance found in bile pigment.

ferritin Form in which iron is stored in body.

ferrous Iron in divalent form, Fe $^{++}$

fertile (L. fertilis) Capable of causing pregnancy or becoming pregnant. Male usually **f.** at $2\frac{1}{2}$ years, female at 2 years, although colts and fillies under $1\frac{1}{2}$ years have been known to be **f.**

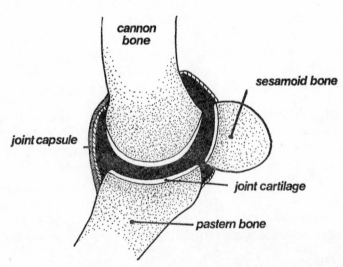

13 Fetlock joint, from left—normal

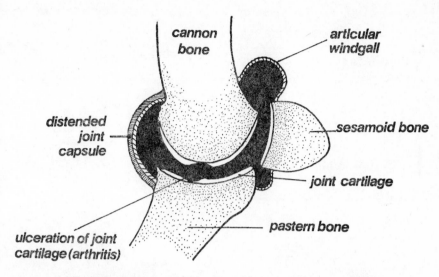

14 Fetlock showing arthritis and articular windgall; cf plate 22

fertilisation Process when spermatozoon fuses with ovum (egg); results in restoration of diploid number of chromosomes and establishes inherited characters of new individual. Occurs in upper part of fallopian tube. See embryology.

fertility Ability to conceive or fertilise. **f. rate** (1) Percentage of mares particular stallion gets in foal. In captivity usually 60–80%; claimed (but unsubstantiated) to be higher in the wild. (2) Percentage of mares producing foals in any given season. (Thoroughbred Breeders' Association figure, using all known results, in UK in 1972—75.3%, compared with Weatherbys' figure, including mares for which no return was made—63.6%.) Cf infertility.

fetal Of fetus. **f. membrane** See after-birth.

fetlock Foreleg or hindleg joint formed by cannon (metacarpal or metatarsal), pastern (first phalanx) and sesamoid bone. Joint capsule surrounds bones and bursa is between capsule and extensor tendons on front of joint. Behind, a thin-walled pouch extends between cannon bone and suspensory ligament (see windgall). Joint often develops arthritis, with distension of joint capsule due to excess joint oil (synovia), pain on flexion and lameness. May become dislocated or affected by fracture of pastern bone if break extends to joint surface. See osselet, joint mice.

fetus (L.) Unborn foal. Measured by weight and length (crown to rump—just in front of poll to top of tail).

Age in days	Weight	Length
60	10 – 20gms.	4 – 7.5cm.
120	700 –1,000gms.	15 – 20cm.
180	3 – 5kg.	35 – 60cm.
240	12 – 18kg.	60 – 80cm.
300	25 – 40kg.	70 –130cm.
340 (full term)	30 – 50kg.	100 –150cm.

See embryology, gestation, plates 6 and 7.

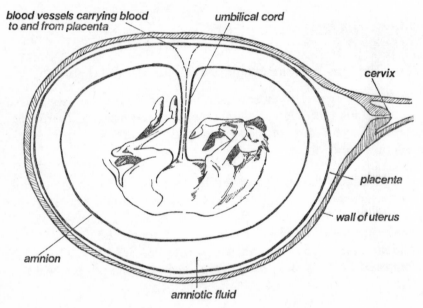

15 Position of fetus before it revolves ready for birth

fever (L. febris) Abnormally high temperature, ie above 39°C. (102.2°F.). Accompanied by fast pulse and breathing, rise in skin temperature and, possibly, patchy sweating. Symptom of infection by bacteria or virus, eg strangles, influenza, septicemia. See temperature.

fibre Elongated structure, usuallly refers to nerve cells. See nerve.

fibrillation Rapid contraction as in atrial **f.**, qv.

fibrin Whitish protein formed from thrombin. See coagulation.

fibrinogen (fibrin + Gr. gennan, to produce) Plasma protein converted to fibrin by action of thrombin; also called coagulation factor 1. See coagulation.

fibrocartilage Type of cartilage, qv.

fibroma Benign tumour of fibrous tissue. See growth.

fibrosis Laying down of fibrous tissue in organs where not normally present, eg cardiac **f.** follows inflamed heart muscle infected with virus or affected by bacterial or other toxins.

fibrous tissue (syn. gristle) Densely or loosely arranged elongated cells (fibroblasts). They produce inert substance collagen, which forms basis of tendons, joint capsules, ligaments and scars.

fibula Small slender bone attached at upper and lower ends to tibia.

filament (L. filamentum) Delicate fibre or thread, applied to nerve fibres and cells such as spermatozoa, bacteria, fungi.

filaria (pl. filariae) Nematode (roundworm parasite) of order Filarioidea. It is long and thin, resembling thread. Genus Onchocerca cervicalis lives in a ligament of the neck (ligamentum nuchae) of horse and mule and may cause poll evil and fistulous withers. Parasites live in blood from which they are sucked up by midges. Genus Onchocerca reticulata similar—and some experts believe identical—to cervicalis. Genus Setaria equina lives in abdomen, scrotum or lungs and is not known to cause disease. Setaria digitata is natural parasite of cattle but can infect horses and, in Japan, the migrating larvae have been found to cause disease of central nervous system known as epidemic cerebrospinal nematodiasis. Can also affect eye.

filariasis Infection by filariae. See filaria.

filling (1) Blood's entry into heart chambers during relaxation (diastole). (2) Colloq. oedema of limbs or soft swellings on body. See oedema; joints, filled.

film Thin layer, as in blood smeared on to glass slide for examination under microscope. **X-ray f.** See radiation.

filter (L. filtrum) (1) Device for straining liquid. (2) In radiation, f. permits passage of some wavelengths but absorbs others. (3) Used to separate virus from bacteria (which are larger). **Wood's f.** Glass containing nickel oxide which allows only ultraviolet waves to pass and which causes hairs infected with some types of ringworm to fluoresce.

firing Traditional treatment, usually for leg injuries, now dying out in face of claims that it is cruel. Skin over flexor tendon, splints, fetlock and knee joints, ringbone or curbs is burned with red-hot iron. Penetration varies from superficial to underlying tissues and causes scar tissue to form, hardening the area; carried out under general or local anaesthesia. **line f.** Lines or bars burned into skin surrounding flexor tendons and continuing at intervals for length of cannon bone. **pin/ point f.** Individual puncture marks made around joints or over tendons. (Most common f. now in use.) All cases need rest after treatment—up to a year or more depending on severity of injury and whether horse is required to do fast work.

first aid The help any attendant should be able to give to injured horse. **f.a. kit** Should include: bandages (cotton and elastic), cotton wool, gauze, poultices, oiled silk, disinfectant, detergent, petroleum jelly, liquid paraffin, gentian violet, fly repellent, wound powder, wound ointment. **f. breath** See breath. **f. dung** See meconium. **f. milk** See colostrum, running of milk.

fistula (L., pipe) Abnormal passage connecting internal structures or between these and body surface. See recto-vaginal f., pervious urachus.

fistulous withers Abscess in region of w., bursts to discharge pus. Caused by wound at top of spine, infected with Brucella or other bacteria. See filaria.

fixation (L. fixatio) Act of holding or fastening, eg internal f. of fractured ends of bone. **complement f. test** See complement.

fixative Substance used to preserve sample, eg skin or organ, to study later in laboratory; eg 10% formalin in saline solution.

Fjord/ing (syns. Westland, Vestland) Stocky, good-tempered Norwegian pony of Celtic or Baltic type. Often dun with black dorsal stripe; widely used for farm work.

flagellum (L., whip) Whip-like thread on some rod-shaped bacteria which moves the bacterium. Cf cilium.

flap Detached or partially detached piece of skin, as in injury or surgery.

flat-foot walk See gait.

flatulence (L. flatulentia) Distension of alimentary tract with gas.

flatus (L., a blowing) Gas in alimentary tract. See colic.

flatworm Internal parasite belonging to phylum Platyhelminthes including the classes Trematoda (fluke, qv) and Cestoda (tapeworm, qv).

flea Parasite insect belonging to order Siphonaptera. Does not normally live on horses although two genera may attack those in tropical regions, viz., stick-tight f. of poultry and chigger (or jigger) of S America, Africa and West Indies.

flehmen posture (after German, Flehmen) Extended neck and curled upper lip. Seen in sexually aroused male, during colic and in mare in 1st stage labour. See behaviour, male sexual; birth.

flexor Muscle or tendon that flexes joint. Opp. extensor.

floating (syns. filing, rasping) Removing sharp edges on molar teeth with a rasp. See teeth.

flu See influenza.

fluid (L. fluidus) Liquid or gas; elements or particles which change position without separating, eg allantoic f. (see allantois). **f. balance** Proportion of water in the 2 major compartments of body, ie in blood stream (intravascular) and in tissues (extravascular); extravascular fluid is further divided into that inside, and that outside, cells (interstitial and intracellular). The water in compartments relates to salts of the body and is therefore a measure of salt concentration, eg shortage of water (dehydration) may reduce cellular, intercellular or intravascular water (see hemoconcentration). Body weight is normally 70% water (intracellular 50% body wt., intercellular 15% body wt. and blood 5% body wt.).

fluke (Fasciola hepatica) Parasite of liver belonging to class Trematoda. (The **f.** of sheep and cattle can live in other animals, including horses.)

It is leaf-shaped with conical projection at front, measures up to 26mm. (about 1in.) by 13mm. ($\frac{1}{2}$in.), is hermaphrodite (having male and female tissue) and is without alimentary canal—its simple excretory system consists of small canals. Life cycle: adult lives in bile ducts of liver where it lays eggs that pass, with the bile, into the small intestine. Eggs are then passed out in the feces. The larva (miracidium) develops in warm, moist conditions then hatches and swims in water until it penetrates an intermediate host. In Britain this is mud snail (Limnaea A. Truncatula). A second larva (sporocyst) then develops. Each sporocyst produces 5 to 8 radiae and finally a cercaria, a young fluke that can infect main host. The cercariae take about 6 weeks to develop in snail, then make their way to the outside, where they form a cyst and are swallowed by the main host. They penetrate intestinal wall and make their way to the liver, causing chronic disease with anemia, unthriftiness and diarrhoea. F.'s of family Schistosomatidae live in tropical areas. They are elongated, worm-like and live in blood vessels. S. japonicum lives in veins of liver and abdomen causing schistosomiasis. Worms can penetrate skin, causing dermatitis, and will inflame intestines or other organs. S. indicum affects horses and camels in India. S. nasalis affects horses in India and America (especially Louisiana) causing inflamed nostrils (snoring disease). Control: remove intermediate host, the snail. Treat with carbon tetrachloride, qv, hexachlorophane, qv and hexachlorethane.

fluorescein Orange-red odourless tasteless powder. **f. sodium** Used as solution for detecting ulcers on cornea. If drops, of 10% solution, are put into eye, ulcer will look green if studied in sunlight 5–10 minutes later. See eye.

fluorine poisoning May follow misuse of sodium fluoride as anthelmintic against roundworms. Symptoms: gastroenteritis, abdominal pain, diarrhoea, muscular weakness and, in severe cases, collapse and death. Horses are relatively resistant. Can also occur near industries, eg aluminium, glass, enamel, stone, steel and metal works and potteries. Plants collect f. dust on leaves which horses then eat. F. is deposited in bones and teeth and, in high concentration, causes bony outgrowths in skeleton. Symptom: lameness, which may shift from one leg to another and there may be spontaneous fractures which take 2 or 3 months to heal. Diagnosis: best on bones from dead animals. Over 5,000 p.p.m. (parts per million) of f. confirms poisoning. In life, urine values of 15 p.p.m. and above indicate poisoning.

Fluothane Trade name. See halothane.

Fluvac-Equine Trade name; influenza vaccine with oil-water adjuvant. Prepared in USA.

Fluvet DMSO Trade name. See flumethasone.

fly Two-winged insect belonging to order Diptera. See bot, tabanid f., warble f.

foal Young horse from birth (newborn f.) to weaning time (weanling) or 1 year old (yearling). **f., diseases of** See newborn foal.

focus (L., fireplace) Chief centre of disease, eg foci of infection in strangles are the lymph nodes. See strangles.

foetus See fetus.

follicile Small fluid-filled sac or gland. **hair f.** Sac at root of hair. **graafian f. of ovary** F. developing round egg during oestrus. Eventually ruptures when 2½–6cm. (ovulation) to allow escape of egg; lined by cells which secrete fluid and help to form yellow body, qv. **f. stimulating hormone** (FSH) Hormone produced by part (anterior lobe) of pituitary gland of both sexes. In mare it acts on ovaries, causing increase in size of f. and production of hormone oestrogen. As level of oestrogen in blood rises, pituitary stops producing FSH and liberates luteinising hormone (LH) which causes ovulation. FSH in male stimulates production and growth of spermatozoa in testes.

follicular (L. follicularis) Of a follicile.

Folligon Trade name. See serum gonadotrophin.

food Amount and type varies with age and status, ie barren or pregnant mare, horse in training or resting, stallion, horse during long sea voyage, illness or convalescence. General considerations: (1) Digestion. Poor-quality f. less digestible than good quality. (2) Fibre. Plant material of carbohydrate nature gives necessary bulk; heavy work demands some concentrates but horse's digestive system cannot deal with these alone and requires some coarse fodder such as hay. Daily minimum: about 0.7lb. per 100lb. body wt., though double this is usually fed. (3) Protein. Essential for building muscle. Mature horse needs about 250gms. of digestible protein per day; about 8% of diet. Pregnant mare needs 14% during the last third of pregnancy and in the first three months of lactation. Weaned foal or yearling needs 15–20% protein; 2-year-olds, 12–15%. (4) Energy. Supplied by cereal grains such as oats; usually fed rolled, flaked or cracked. (5) Minerals. Typical ration of grass, hay and grain is usually deficient in calcium, adequate in phosphorus and deficient in salt and iodine. On average, horse eats about 3oz. of salt daily, according to work and temperature. Calcium/phosphorus should be given in a ratio of 1.5:1.0–1.2:1.0 (see calcium and phosphorus). (6) Vitamins. Necessary for growth, health and reproduction. Rarely deficient in grazing horses but stabled ones may suffer vitamin A, D and E deficiency. Lack of vitamin E (alpha tocopherol succinate) may contribute to infertility. Recommended amount: 600–1,000 IU daily. (7) Water. Essential; average adult horse consumes 5–10 gallons daily depending on amount of work and weather conditions. Horses should always have free access to water. (8) Specific requirements: brood mare—when barren should not be allowed to get fat, when pregnant, must have adequate protein, minerals, vitamins, in last third of pregnancy and during lactation. Stallion—balanced ration that discourages obesity. Foal and yearling—adequate protein. Foal with access to spring grass may get too much protein. Avoid overweight. If possible use scientifically formulated ration to ensure proper balance. Adult's f. should include carrots and bran mashes. Adult in light work: $\frac{1}{2}$lb. grain, $1\frac{1}{2}$lb. hay per 100lb. body wt.; in medium work: $\frac{3}{4}$lb. grain, $1\frac{1}{4}$lb. hay per 100lb. body wt.; in hard work: 2lb. grain, $\frac{1}{2}$lb. hay per 100lb. body wt. F. should be given in 3 or 4 equal feeds. (Horses are continuous feeders, unlike, say, dogs, whose digestion is tuned to occasional large meals.) The dungs are a guide to feeding; small hard feces indicate too little water. Can be counteracted by mashes and more salt, causing horse to drink more. Pellet (cube) f. is cleaner, needs less storage space and labour and is a balanced diet. (Feces of pellet-fed horses are softer than those on traditional feeds.) Horses at pasture show preference for the following grasses and herbs: crested dogstail, perennial ryegrasses, sceempter, melle, petra, midas S.23 and S.321, Timothy S.48 and S.50, dandelion, chicory, yarrow, ribgrass, burnet, sainfoin and, particularly, wild white clover (but not red clover). Grasses which should not be sown for horses: perennial ryegrass S.24, creeping red fescue, brown top, meadow foxtail, red clover. **f. by stomach tube** (qv) Should be given if foal has lost suck reflex. Pass tube, lubricated with water or liquid paraffin, when foal is standing or lying. Push end gently into one nostril, but not past entrance to throat. After feeding, flush tube with saline so that milk is not left in nostrils. (Foal can be fed by bottle if suck reflex present but ability to suck from mare is absent.) F. can be colostrum, mare's milk, skimmed cow's milk or dried milk. Feed mare's or skimmed cow's milk at 80–100ml./kg. body wt. per day, divided into a minimum of 10 equal feeds. Foal of 50kg. would then be fed 4–5 litres per day. Ensure cleanliness and give milk at 38°C. (100°F.) or below—never above.

foot (L. pes; syn. hoof) Horny box surrounding third phalanx (pedal bone), navicular bone, ligaments, tendon (insertion of the deep flexor), digital cushion, sensitive laminae, corono pedal joint, blood vessels and nerves. Hoof consists of wall divided into toe and quarters, with sole, bars and frog underneath.

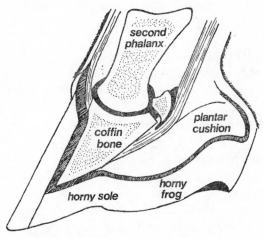

16 Section through foot

Hoof wall is about 25% water and is modified skin or nail. Outer layer (periople) helps protect wall from evaporation; middle layer forms dense portion of wall and contains pigment; inner layer or laminar layer forms insensitive membranes (laminae) which bind hoof to pedal bone. (Hundreds of thin primary laminae, each of which bears a hundred or so secondary laminae, intermesh with sensitive laminae lining pedal bone.) Hoof wall grows approx. ¼in. per month, taking 9 months to grow from coronary band to toe. See also bars, frog, white line, corium, contracted heels, evolution. **f., abscess of** May be caused by imbedded stone, etc. See abscess. **f. anti-concussion mechanism** Frog represents most elastic structure of **f.** When this strikes ground,

181

heel expands and forces of concussion are distributed. Digital cushion expands outward putting pressure on cartilages of pedal bone. The blood in veins and vascular bed of **f.** adds to the efficient cushioning. **f. blood supply** Comes from the medial and lateral digital arteries, which arise from common digital artery at lower end of cannon bone. See arteries, table of; corium. **f., diseases of** See dropped sole (plate 16), contracted heels, club foot, laminitis, pedal osteitis, abscess, corn, bruised sole, sand crack, navicular disease, quittor, side bones and seedy toe. **f., nerve supply** Comes from medial and lateral volar nerves (see nerve block, neurectomy). **f., weight-bearing structures** Wall, bars and frog contact the ground. The sole does not bear weight, except for a strip about ¼in. wide inside the white line. Bottom of wall should be level with frog to distribute weight evenly. See plates 15 and 18.

foramen (L., pl. foramina) Anatomical term for natural opening, especially into or through bone.

forceps Instrument with two blades and handles used in surgery for grasping or compressing tissue. **artery f.** Used to clamp artery to reduce bleeding during surgery. **dental f.** Used to extract teeth.

Forgastrin Trade name. See bismuth.

forging Action when toe of a hind foot strikes bottom of front foot of the same side as it leaves ground. Cf brushing, cross-firing, over-reaching, interfering.

formaldehyde solution Colourless liquid with characteristic, pungent, irritating odour and burning taste. Powerful antiseptic, reacts with proteins. Used to treat proud flesh, to fumigate after infectious disease and in laboratory to preserve specimens.

foster To raise young other than natural offspring. Foals can be reared on a f.-mother if their dam has died, has insufficient milk or attacks foal. Foal can be transferred to the f.-mother at any age but it is increasingly difficult after one month. Some mares accept orphan foal better than others. Methods include (1) confusing f. mare by rubbing strong-smelling ointment on to nostrils before introducing orphan foal; (2) clothing orphan in amnion or skin of f.-mother's foal. Restraint of mare, injection of tranquillisers, and careful, patient handling of foal to avoid injury can usually make fostering successful.

182

foxglove See digitalis.

fox trot See gait.

fracture (L. from frangere, to break) Break in bone; may be hairline (minute), greenstick (bending of young bone), spiral (corkscrew-like), comminuted (many pieces), impacted (one end driven into other), compound (bone exposed by skin wound). See lameness, sclerosing agent.

Franocide Trade name. See diethylcarbamazine citrate.

FRCVS Abbr. Fellow of the Royal College of Veterinary Surgeons, qv.

Fredericksborg Denmark's best-known breed developed by King Frederick II, in 1560s from Andalusian and Neapolitan horses. Breed related to Lipizzaner, now usually chestnut and about 15.3 hands.

fremitus Thrill or vibration which can be felt, eg in extremely loud heart murmur, by placing fingers on chest. See heart murmur.

frenulum (L. dim of fraenum; pl. frenula) Small fold of mucous membrane that curbs movement of an organ or part. **f. linguae** Fold of membrane beneath tongue attaching it to floor of mouth.

Friesian (syn. Harddraver) One of Europe's oldest breeds, descended from horses which survived Ice Age. Reared in F. district of Holland and breed society given Royal title by Queen Juliana. F. popular for willingness, especially in harness. Usually about 15 hands, often with jet-black coat and exceptionally long mane.

frog Wedge-shaped mass in central back part of undersurface of hoof, ie bounded by bars and sole. Contains about 50% water; shaped as narrow triangle with point (apex) and base; and part of weight-bearing structure of foot, particularly suited to absorb concussion. See foot.

frontal sinus Cavity in skull from line in front of eye sockets (orbits) to back of skull, in front of cranium. See sinus.

fructose (L. fructus, fruit) Carbohydrate or sugar in fetus and newborn foal, which disappears from blood stream after two days.

frusemide (trade name: Lasix) White odourless tasteless powder; increases flow of urine (diuretic drug) and excretion of sodium potassium and chloride from kidney; used to treat filled joints and other types of oedema. Dose: 2mg./kg. body wt. IM or slow IV.

FSH See follicle stimulating hormone.

Fulcin Trade name. See griseofulvin.

fuller's earth An impure aluminium silicate used in dressings.

fundus Bottom or base of organ, eg **f.** of bladder, **f.** of eye. See bladder, eye.

fungal abortion See abortion.

fungi (L., singular fungus) Organisms belonging to vegetable kingdom but different from plants in that they do not contain chlorophyll. Composed of mycelium and a reproductive portion of spores. 4 main classes: (1) phycomycetes, (2) ascomycetes (containing the yeasts), (3) basidiomycetes (including mushrooms, toadstools), (4) hyphomycetes (containing pathogenic fungi). The following are caused by yeast and fungi:

Condition	Causal organism
epizootic lymphangitis	Histoplasma farciminosum formerly Cryptococcus farciminosus) yeast family
ringworm	Microsporum and trichophyton
fungal abortion (see abortion)	Aspergillus species
broken wind	Aspergillus species Alternaria species Hormodendrum species
mud fever	Dermatophilus species
guttural pouch mycosis	Aspergillus species
See separate headings.	

fungicide Drug or substance that destroys fungi. Can cause poisoning if treated food is given to horses. Symptoms: skin irritation, inflamed windpipe and urinary tract. May also affect central nervous system, causing inco-ordination.

Furacin Trade name. See nitrofurazone.

furazolidone (trade name: Neftin) Yellow odourless powder. Antibiotic effective against many types of bacteria, especially Salmonella; poorly absorbed from gut and sometimes used to treat diarrhoea in foals.

G

G. Abbr. of gram, also written gm.

gag Device for holding mouth open. Useful in dentistry, anaesthesia etc. Popular type: Haussman (colloq. American). Half-moon pieces fit on to front teeth of upper and lower jaws and join crossbars on either side. Crossbars, held in place by strap over horse's poll, have ratchet (with quick release) to hold mouth open.

gait Sequence of leg movements, usually forward. First effectively recorded in 1880s by British photographer E. J. Muybridge. (Before this horses were thought to gallop as depicted in old paintings, ie with forelegs outstretched together and hindlegs back together, which does not occur.) Horses move similarly to other 4-legged animals (quadrupeds) and are 3-gaited (walk, trot, canter) or 5-gaited (walk, trot, canter, plus rack and a slow **g.**). However, there are many variations (Dr Milton Hildebrand of California University recognises 104 support sequences theoretically possible for most quadrupeds, 55 of which might be used by horses). Of these about 7 are identifiable as **g.**'s viz., walk, trot, canter, gallop, (natural **g.**'s); amble, similar to rack and running walk, and pace (either natural or false **g.**'s). **amble:** 4-beat, walking speed **g.** Legs move in lateral pairs, ie near-fore and near-hind virtually together. No period of suspension (when all 4 feet off ground); classed as slow **g.** See Connemara, Spanish Jennet. **asymmetrical g.** One in which either pair of feet, fore or hind, move in uneven time, eg gallop. **backing** Usually at diagonal 2-beat **g.** of trot. **canter** 3-beat **g.** (may be 4-beat in some horses); puts greatest wear on leading foreleg and opposite hindleg. Horse usually leads with same foreleg but may change legs negotiating a bend (if left-hand bend it should lead with near-fore; if right hand, with off-fore). **flat-foot walk** Similar to walk, but looser. Natural to Tennessee Walking horse, qv. **fox-trot** Classed a slow **g.** A slow, broken trot, usually with nodding of head. **gallop** Fastest **g.** virtually an uncollected canter—so may be 3 or 4-beat. Fastest breed (Thoroughbred) can gallop at more than 40 miles per hour over short distances. **pace** Fast, 2-beat lateral **g.** seen mainly in Standardbreds that race in harness (as it is unnatural to most horses, pacers usually race in hobbles). Pace slightly faster than trot (trotters also race in harness). Devotees of Peruvian Paso (qv) name one of that breed's **g.** a pace. Considered unnatural in most horses (a natural pacer is the camel). **paso** (normal and marching) **G.**'s of laterally-gaited Peruvian Paso. Similar to pace. **rack** (syns. singlefoot, broken amble) Exaggerated, regular 4-beat walk. Comfortable for rider but tiring on horse. See American Saddle horse. **running walk** 4-beat **g.** between walk and rack. Hindfoot oversteps print left by forefoot in smooth, gliding motion. Accompanied by bobbing of head; easy on horse and rider. A **g.** of Standardbred (as well as pace). See also American Saddle horse. **symmetrical g.** One in which fore or hindfeet are evenly timed, eg walk, trot. Other names for **s.g.**'s include jog, parade **g.**, stepping pace, pacing walk, but meanings vary enormously. **trot** 2-beat **g.** in which opposite fore- and hindfeet meet ground virtually together. Can be slow or extended (when forging is common in some horses). Cf pace. Hackney (qv) renowned for particularly high-stepping trot. **walk** 4-beat **g.** slower than flat-foot walk and running walk. See lameness. Cf cross-firing, brushing, forging, over-reaching, interfering.

galactagogue (galact- + Gr. agogos, leading) Drug or substance that promotes flow of milk.

Galiceno Mexican pony with characteristic running walk. Probably descended from Minho ponies imported from Portugal.

gall-bladder Reservoir, in species other than horse, for storing bile, qv. See liver.

gallon Measure of volume. See weights and measures.

gallop See gait.

Galloway Extinct strain of Highland pony which influenced Lundy pony.

galvanism (after Luigi Galvani) Uninterrupted current of electricity. Cf faradism.

galvanometer (galvanism + **Gr.** metron, measure) Instrument for measuring current by electromagnetic action. See Einthoven, electrocardiogram.

gamete (Gr. gamete, wife; gametes, husband) Male (spermatozoon) and female (ovum) sex cells which unite to form new individual (zygote). See embryology.

gamma Third letter of Greek alphabet. See globulin, radiation. **g. benzene hexachloride** (trade names: Gammexane, Lorexane) White crystalline powder with slight odour. Effective against fleas (rare in horses), ticks, mites, lice.

Gammexane Trade name. See gamma benzene hexachloride.

ganglia Pl. of ganglion.

ganglion (Gr., knot) Any group of nerve cells found outside spinal cord (central nervous system). See nerve cell.

gangrene (L. gangraena, Gr. gangraina) Death of tissue because it is separated from blood supply. Rare in horses, but may occur in severely damaged foot, artery blocked by clot, strangulated blood supply (possibly if wound is bandaged too tightly). Part becomes cold, decayed and foul-smelling. Treatment: cut away dead tissue. Amputation or destruction may be necessary in severe cases.

Garrano See Minho.

Garron See Highland pony.

gas Colloq. for flatus. See flatus, colic.

gaskin (syns. second thigh, calf) That part of hindleg between stifle and hock.

gastric (L. gastricus, Gr. gaster, stomach) Of the stomach. **g. dilatation** Flatulence associated with colic or grass sickness, qv. Symptoms:

depression, excessive sweating, tendency to crouch in dog-sitting position, or extend fore- and hindlegs, vomiting (rare in horse and usually sign of impending death or rupture of stomach). Condition often eased **by** passing stomach tube. See colic.

gastritis Inflamed stomach.

gastrocnemius (gastro- + Gr. kneme, leg) Muscle acting on hock. See muscles, table of.

gastroenteritis Inflamed stomach and intestines. See colic, diarrhoea.

gastrula Early stage of embryo after blastula. See embryology.

gastrulation Process by which blastula acquires three tissue types (germ layers). See embryology.

gauze Open-mesh muslin or similar material. Can be impregnated with antiseptic and used for dressing, qv.

Gayoe Pony bred in hills in N of Sumatra and similar to Batak.

gelatin (L. gelatina from gelare, to congeal) Product of bones and other animal tissues, used as food and to make capsules in which drugs can be given by mouth.

Gelderland Developed in **G.** province of Holland last century by crossing native mares with many types of imported stallion. Equally good for riding, driving, or light agricultural work. Often bright chestnut marked with white and usually about 15 hands.

gelding Gelded (castrated) male. See castration. Cf stallion.

gene (Gr. gennan, to produce) Hereditary unit in definite position on chromosome. **allelic g.'s** At corresponding places on pair of chromosomes. **dominant g.** One which produces effect regardless of state of corresponding allele, ie if one parent possesses **d.g.** that characteristic will appear in progeny (cf. recessive **g.**). **lethal g.** One that kills individual. **recessive g.** One effective only when transmitted by both parents. **sex-linked g.** One carried on X or Y chromosome. See chromosome, embryology.

genetic Of inheritance.

genital (L. genitalis, belonging to birth) Of reproduction or reproductive organs.

genitalia Reproductive organs. Mare: two ovaries, fallopian tubes, mammary glands; one uterus, cervix, vagina. Stallion: two testes, epididymi, vas deferentia, seminal vesicles and bulbo-urethral glands, one penis, scrotum, prostate gland. **external g.** Organs outside body, eg testes. See descent of testes.

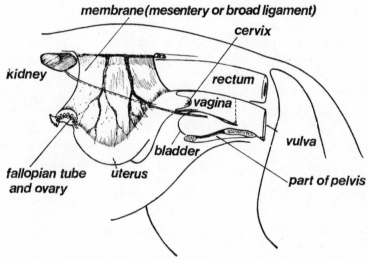

17 Mare's reproductive organs (genitalia)

genotype (geno- + Gr. typos, type) Hereditary material; genes passed on through gametes (spermatozoon and ovum) at mating. See embryology, gene. Cf phenotype.

gentian Light or yellowish-brown powder with characteristic odour and taste, from root of Gentiana litea. Used to improve appetite. Dose: 8–30gms. **g. violet** Antiseptic dye used alone or with antibiotic on wounds and proud flesh.

genu (syn. stifle) Joint between femur (thigh) and tarsus (gaskin). See stifle.

germ (L. germen) Micro-organism capable of causing disease. See bacteria, fungi, virus. **wheat** g. Embryo of wheat containing tocopherol, thiamine, riboflavin and other vitamins. Cf bran. **g. layers** 3 types of body cells, originating in embryo. See embryology.

germicidal (L. germen, germ + caedere, to kill) Destructive to germs.

Germinol Trade name. See tocopherol acetate.

gestagen Any hormone with progesterone-like activity. See progesterone.

gestation (L. from gestare, to bear) Pregnancy; period of development of young inside uterus from fertilisation of ovum to birth.

gestational age Length of pregnancy at time fetus is expelled by abortion or birth. Usually measured from last date of service but should be from ovulation following last mating. Can also be measured by weight and crown to rump length (see fetus). **g. length** Average in Thoroughbred: 340 days, range 320–60. Foals have lived after only 287 days' gestation and after as long as 419 days. Pony breeds have shorter **g.l.** (315–35 days) and colts longer **g.l.** than fillies. See abortion, birth, dystocia, position, posture, presentation, prematurity.

gestyl See serum gonadotrophin.

ghost Laboratory term for red blood cell which has lost its hemaglobin. See hemolytic jaundice.

Gidran Large saddle horse of Hungary developed by covering local mares with English half-bred or Thoroughbred stallions; usually bay or chestnut. **G. Arabian** Hungarian breed developed from the Arab Siglavy-Gidran, imported in 1816. S and E European types have Arabian looks but mid-European is heavier. All types most often chestnut.

gingiva (L., gum of mouth) See gum.

gingivitis Inflamed gums.

ginglymus (L., Gr. ginglymos, hinge) Type of joint allowing movement in one plane, ie forwards and backwards. Also called hinge joint, eg elbow. See joint.

girdle (L. cingulum, Gr. zoster) A surrounding structure, eg pelvic **g.** See pelvis.

glacial acetic acid Clear colourless liquid with pungent odour. Applied to warts after protecting surrounding area with petroleum jelly. See milk warts.

gland (L. glans, acorn) Small organ or structure which produces fluids, eg homones, enzymes, mucus, milk, saliva. **endocrine g.** One which secretes directly into blood or lymph (rather than through duct) and is effective at a distance, eg pituitary. **exocrine g.** One which secretes through duct towards outside of body, eg salivary **g.**

Main **g.'s**

Endocrine	Exocrine
adrenal	gastric
liver	Lieberkühn (intestinal)
ovary	mammary
pancreas (islets of Langerhans)	pancreas
	prostate
parathyroid	salivary
pituitary	sebaceous
thyroid	sweat
testes	liver (bile)

Lymph **g.** (syn. node) not a true **g.**; see lymphatic system. Endocrine and exocrine **g.'s** further classified by their type of fluid, viz., apocrine, holocrine and merocrine. **apocrine g.** One that throws off part of cells with secretion, eg mammary **g. holocrine g.** One in which cells forming secretion come away with the fluid, eg sebaceous **g. merocrine g.** One in which cellls forming secretion remain intact, eg salivary **g.**

glanders (syn. farcy) Contagious, notifiable disease of horse and man. (See veterinary rules, Ministry of Agriculture.) First described by Aristotle 300 years BC. Causal organism: Loefflerella mallei (syns. Malleomyces or Pfeifferella) discovered by Loeffler and Schutz in 1882. Disease restricted to Eastern Europe, Asia and North Africa (eradicated in North America and not present in Britain since 1925). Infection is spread by contaminated fodder or utensils. Organism enters blood through gut wall and is localised in skin and mucosal surfaces, especially in nostrils. Symptoms, in acute form: high fever, cough, nasal discharge, ulcers and nodules which spread rapidly on nasal mucosa, legs and abdomen. Death occurs in a few days. In chronic form signs depend on where lesions occur, eg if in lungs there is chronic cough, nosebleeds and difficult breathing. Nodules in nostrils ulcerate producing bloodstained nasal discharge. Lymph nodes between angles of the jaw swell. Affected horse may be ill for several months then appear to recover, but remain a carrier. Eventually it relapses and dies. Diagnosis: on mallein test or complement fixation test on blood and isolation of germ from ulcers. There is no specific treatment. **genital g.** See dourine. **pseudo-g.** See epizootic lymphangitis.

glandular Of a gland.

glans (L., acorn) Small, gland-like body. **g. clitoridis/clitoris** Tissue at end of clitoris. **g. penis** (syn. rose) Cap-shaped tip of penis.

glauber's salt See sodium sulphate.

glaucoma (Gr. glaukoma, opaque lens) Condition of eye characterised by increased pressure inside eyeball. See eye, diseases of.

gleet Pus-like discharge, sometimes bluish colour. **nasal g.** Chronic catarrhal discharge. See snotty nose, sinusitis.

globin Protein constituent of hemoglobin, qv.

globulin (L. globulus, globule) Class of protein insoluble in water but soluble in saline. Several types: alpha 1 and 2, beta, gamma. The latter contains antibodies which form basis of immunity, qv.

globulinuria (globulin + Gr. ouron, urine) Abnormal presence of globulin in urine.

glomeruli Pl. of glomerulus.

glomerulonephritis Inflamed kidney (nephritis) in which capillary loops in glomeruli are affected. See kidney, diseases of.

glomerulus (L. from glomus, ball; pl. glomeruli) Cluster, eg of blood vessels, nerve fibres or kidney (renal) g.

gloss-/glosso- (Gr. glossa, tongue) Combining form meaning relationship to tongue.

glossitis Inflamed tongue.

glossopharyngeal Of tongue and pharynx.

gluck Abnormal clucking noise made by soft palate, qv.

gluco- (Gr. gleukos, sweetness) Combining form meaning relationship to sweetness.

glucocorticoid One of several hormones secreted by adrenal cortex, affects body's metabolism, such as build-up of glycogen and blood sugar (process known as glyconeogenesis/gluconeogenesis). See cortisone, mineralocorticoid.

glucose Carbohydrate which body can convert to dextrose (for absorption from gut) faster and more easily than sugar. Colourless crystals or white powder, up to 2kg. sometimes given to Thoroughbreds night before race or up to 0.2kg. to foals suffering from maladjustment. Can cause diarrhoea in adult horse.

glycemia (Gr. glyks, sweet + haima, blood) Presence of sugar in blood. See hypoglycemia, hyperglycemia.

glycerin (L. glycerinum) Syrupy liquid used as softener or solvent for drugs. Given through stomach tube or as enema to foals. See meconium retention.

glycogen (glyco- + Gr. gennen, to produce; syn. animal starch) Body's main carbohydrate-storing substance. Formed by (and stored mostly in) liver, which releases it as glucose when necessary. Small amounts stored in tissues, especially muscles.

glycogenesis Formation of glycogen, qv.

glyconeogenesis/gluconeogenesis Accumulation of glycogen and blood sugar.

glycoprotein Chemical compound; a protein with a carbohydrate. Found in mucus, cartilage, synovia.

glycosuria (glyco- + Gr. ouron, urine) **Abnormally large amount of** glucose in urine; symptom of kidney disease, diabetes (rare in horses).

gm. Abbr. for gram (gramme). Also written G.

gnat Flying insect. In England colloq. for mosquito, in America insect smaller than mosquito. Can spread diseases, eg swamp fever, encephalomyelitis, by sucking blood of affected horse and feeding on another.

gnotobiota Sterile life free from germs, as in gnotobiotic foal, one taken by caesarian section and reared in environment free from microbes, for experimental study.

goitre Enlarged thyroid gland, qv.

gonad (L. gonas from Gr. gone, seen) **Sex gland of male (testes) or** female (ovaries). Grow large in fetus between 100 and 280 days' gestation, then reduced by full term.

gonadotrophin Substance stimulating gonads. 3 varieties: (1) those of anterior pituitary, (2) of fetus (chorionic), (3) of pregnant mare's serum. See follicle stimulating hormone, luteinising hormone, **pregnant mare's serum g.**

gone in the wind Colloq. for any respiratory unsoundness. See wind.

goneitis/gonitis Inflamed stifle joint.

GOT Abbr. for glutamic-oxalacetic transaminase. See serum g.o.t.

Gotland (syns. Russ, Skogsbagge) Swedish moorland breed in demand as child's pony, though some still feral. Appear to suffer rare brain condition similar to cerebellar degeneration, qv.

GPT Abbr. for glutamic-pyruvic transaminase. See serum g.p.t.

gr. Abbr. of grain. See weights and measures.

graafian follicle (after Dutch anatomist Reijnier de Graaf, 1641–73) Follicle in ovary, qv. See follicle.

graft (1) To implant skin or other tissue. (2) The skin etc so used. See skin graft.

grain (L. granum) (1) Central part of cereal plant. See food. (2) 20th part of scruple. See weights and measures.

gram (Fr. gramme) Basic unit of mass of metric system, equivalent to 15.432 grains. See weights and measures. **g.-negative bacteria** Those **b.** which, stained with dye, are decolorised by alcohol, eg Escherichia coli, Klebsiella pneumoniae, Proteus vulgaris, Salmonella. **g.-positive bacteria** Those that resist decolorisation by alcohol, eg Clostridium tetani, Corynebacterium equi, Staphylococcus. **G.'s stain** (after Hans Christian Joachim Gram, 1852–1938) Method used in laboratory to identify bacteria. Bacteria on slide are (1) stained with gentian violet or methyl violet dye, (2) immersed in iodine, (3) decolorised with alcohol, (4) re-stained with carbol-fuchsin dye.

granulation (L. granulatio) Forming of soft, fleshy mass (proud flesh) in base of wound; contains numerous blood vessels. See wound.

granule (L. granulum) Particle. See white blood cell, inclusion body, virus.

granulocyte (granular + Gr. kytos, hollow vessel) Cell containing granules, such as certain white blood cells, eg eosinophil. See blood.

granulosa cell Epithelial cells lining ovarian follicle and growing into blood clot after ovulation to form yellow body, qv (see ovary, follicle). **g.c. tumour** Abnormal growth of **g.c.**'s in ovary and formation of cysts containing bloodstained fluid. Affected ovary may be large, or small and inactive. Causes infertility. Treatment: surgical removal. See plate 37.

195

graph (Gr. graphein, to write or record) Diagram or curve representing clinical or experimental data.

grasses See food.

grass sickness Fatal condition of major disturbance of alimentary canal (not confined to horses at grass). First reported in Scotland in 1911 and most common there and in N England but occasionally occurs in S England, N France, Ireland and possibly USA. 4 types: (1) Para-acute—horse may die within 24 hours without previous attack. Symptoms: depression, fast pulse, absence of gut movement, regurgitation (vomiting) of green, evil-smelling fluid down nostrils, profuse sweating and sometimes pain. (2) Acute—death in 24-48 hours. Symptoms: similar to those in (1) plus jaundice, muscle tremor. On rectal examination hard feces can be felt in colon. (3) Sub-acute—death in 10-21 days. Symptoms: as (1) and (2) plus increased jaundice, muscle tremors near elbow and between hip and stifle (possibly staggering), variable appetite, rising hematocrit. (4) Chronic—death from exhaustion after 21 days. Symptoms: firm feces often turning to diarrhoea. Diagnosis: on symptoms, impacted masses in colon and hematocrit rising from 45% to 60 or 70%. On post-mortem: stomach and intestines distended with green fluid (amount varies with severity), abnormal change in nerve cells (possibly responsible for paralysed gut). Cause: unknown, possibly infection with virus. Treatment: unlikely to be effective, but saline IV and injections of neostigmine or physostigmine may help. Siphoning off fluid from stomach eases pain temporarily. Purgatives have little or no effect on impacted feces. Chronic cases occasionally live if given enough nourishment by stomach tube, but they are seldom capable of hard work again. Control: horse should be isolated to reduce risk of spread, but as cause is unconfirmed control is difficult. Infection might be carried by migrating birds.

gravel Black track in sole of foot, leading upwards into wall of heel. May be due to stone penetrating sole, more probably result of abscess or degenerating horn. See foot, abscess of.

gravid (L. gravida, heavy, loaded) Pregnant. See gestation.

gravida Pregnant individual. **g. I/II/III** etc. Describes first, second, third pregnancy etc. **primigravida** First pregnancy. **multigravida** Mare pregnant for second (or successive) time.

Greener Humane killer. See euthanasia.

grey/dapple g. See coat colouring. **g. matter** See brain. **g. roan** See coat colouring.

Griffin Colloq. Chinese pony.

Grippequin (syns. Equine Influenza Vaccine, TVL) Trade name: influenza vaccine with aluminium hydroxide-sodium alginate adjuvant. Prepared in France.

griseofulvin (trade names: Fulcin, Grisovin) White odourless bitter-tasting powder; antibiotic capable of destroying fungus in skin and effective against ringworm in cure and prevention. Dose 15–20mg./kg. body wt. daily for at least 14 days.

Grisovin Trade name. See griseofulvin.

Groningen Dutch farm, saddle or carriage horse now dying out. Similar to, but heavier than, Gelderland.

groove Shallow depression. Made in hoof to treat sandcrack, qv. See also bishop.

growth (1) Normal process of increase in size (height measured in hands, 1 hand = 4in. (approx. 10cm.) Most rapid in first 3 months of life, when gain is only slightly less than during whole of next 9 months. See also fetus and various breeds. (2) Abnormal formation of bone or tissue (syns. tumour, neoplasm). Arises from normal cells but different in behaviour and structure (leads useless existence, does not arise in response to normal body reaction). It may grow without regard for surrounding structures and can destroy them by infiltration or pressure. Known causes include virus, irritation and hormones. Classification based on clinical behaviour of g. (1) Benign or simple (those which grow slowly and rarely recur after removal, do not form seedlings (metastases) and are serious only if they press on surrounding tissues or ulcerate and bleed). (2) Malignant (grow rapidly, infiltrate locally and produce seedlings (metastases) in other parts of body, recur after removal and cause serious consequences by destroying normal tissue and organs). g. also described by its cells, eg epithelial or connective tissue. Epithelial g.'s include papilloma, (benign) and carcinoma (malignant). Connective tissue g.'s include fibroma (benign) and fibrosarcoma (malignant). Bone tissue g.'s include osteoma (benign) and osteosarcoma (malignant).

TABLE OF GROWTHS

Growth	Arises from	Character
adenocarcinoma	glands	malignant
adenoma	glands	benign
* carcinoma	an epithelial surface	malignant
fibroma	beneath skin	benign
fibroma	fibrous tissue	benign
fibrosarcoma	fibrous tissue	malignant
* granulosa cell tumour	ovary	benign
hemangioma	blood vessels	benign
hepatoma	liver	benign
interstitial cell tumour	testicle	benign
lymphoma	blood-forming tissues (lymph nodes)	malignant
(1) leukemic	raised white blood cell count	
(2) aleukemic	normal blood cell count	
lipoma	fat in abdomen	benign
melanoma	skin (especially around tail in grey horses)	benign
* melanosarcoma	skin	malignant
osteoma	bone	benign
osteosarcoma	bone	malignant
* papilloma (wart)	skin	benign
polyp (papilloma)	nasal passage or alimentary canal	benign
* sarcoid (Angleberry)	skin	**semi-malignant
* squamous cell carcinoma	skin, sinus	malignant
* teratoma	ovary, testicle, see cyst, dermoid, dentigerous cyst	benign

* relatively common

**grows rapidly, recurs after removal but does not form seedlings

gubernaculum (L., helm) Structure which guides, eg g. **testis** See descent of testes, rig, testis.

Gudbrandsdal Medium size Norwegian horse named after **G.** valley. Has influenced many Scandinavian breeds but now almost entirely merged with Døle.

gum (L. gummi; syn. gingiva) (1) Membrane of upper and lower jaw which covers lower part of teeth. Regarded as part of buccal membranes (those of cheek) and their colour helps diagnose anemia, internal hemorrhage (when they turn pale), disturbed blood system (purple) or shock (remain blanched after pressure of thumb removed). (2) Excretion of plants, some types used in drugs, eg tragacanth.

gurgling See wind.

gut Colloq. for intestine, bowel, alimentary canal. See alimentary canal, catgut.

guttural Of throat. **g. pouch** 2 large sacs (only in horses) connected to tube (eustachian) between ear and throat. Sacs (lined by mucous membrane) form triangle (Viborg's triangle) with apex at ear and sides bounded by lower jaw in front, upper part of neck behind, and beginning of windpipe below. Opens into throat and has capacity of about 300ml. May fill with pus (empyema) or bleed from ulcers in roof of pouch (often caused by fungus—g. pouch mycosis). See bleeder, fungus.

gyn-/gynaeco-/gyne-/gyno- (Gr. gyne, gynaikos, woman) Combining form meaning relationship to female sex.

gynaecology Branch of medicine dealing with diseases and conditions of female genital tract.

gyrus (L., Gr. gyros, ring) Tortuous convolution of surface of brain. See brain cortex.

H

Habronema (Gr. habros, graceful + nema, thread) Genus of nematode (roundworm) parasites, of order Spiruroidea; parasites of stomach and skin (**H.** microstoma and **H.** megastoma). See stomach worm.

habronemiasis (syn. summer sores) See stomach worm.

hack (1) To ride casually rather than in particular fashion. (2) Any horse used for riding, not a specific breed. Most popularly mixture of breeds such as cob, Thoroughbred, Anglo-Arab. Assns: Show **H.** & Cob Assn, National Equestrian Centre, Kenilworth, Warwickshire (Coventry 27192); British Driving Soc., c/o L. H. Chandler, 10 Marley Avenue, New Milton, Hampshire (New Milton 612901).

Hackney (Fr. haquenee) Harness horse: 14.3–15.2 hands, or pony: 12–14.2 hands. Descended from English trotting horses which had some Thoroughbred blood. Now characterised by particularly high-stepping trot. Assn: **H.** Horse Soc., c/o Maj. G. Worboys, 35 Belgrave Square, London SW1 (01 235 6431).

haem- Combining form meaning blood (English spelling). Frequently replaced by American hem-, qv.

Haflinger/Hafflinger Austrian mountain pony named after **H.** district. Origin obscure, now popular for pulling sleighs. Most often bay, chestnut or palomino-like with flaxen mane and tail. Assn: **H.** Soc. of Gt Britain, c/o Jane Evers-Swindell, Bron-y-Craig, Pwillglas, Nr Ruthin, Denbighshire.

half-bred Usually horse with Arab or Thoroughbred on one side of pedigree, but can mean any cross-bred horse. In British racing it is horse entered in Weatherbys' Register of Non-Thoroughbred Horses (which superseded **H.-B.** Stud Book, by Miss Florence Prior).

halothane (trade name: Fluothane) Colourless liquid with characteristic odour resembling chloroform. Has sweet burning taste. Used as volatile (gaseous) anaesthetic. About twice as potent as chloroform, four times as potent as ether. See anaesthesia.

haloxon White powder with slight odour. Drug given by stomach tube or in feed to kill whiteworms and seatworms. It may also kill redworms and botfly larvae. Dose: 75mg./kg. body wt.

hand 4ins. (10cm.) of horse's height. So called because width of human hand (about 4ins.) can be used to gauge distance between ground and highest point of withers (qv). Smallest Equidae is probably Falabella,

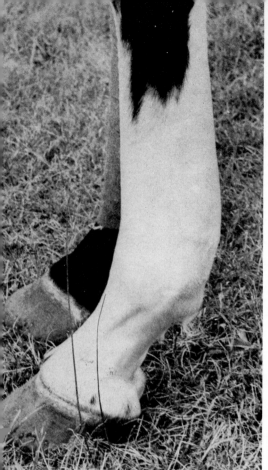

19 Bowed flexor tendon (the off-fore is bandaged). See *bowed tendon*

20 Bucked shin, qv

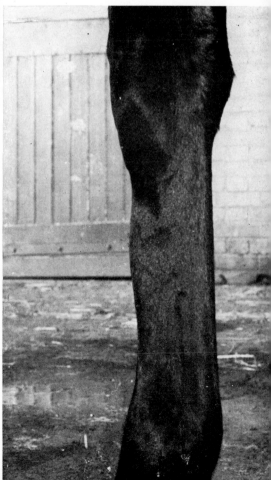

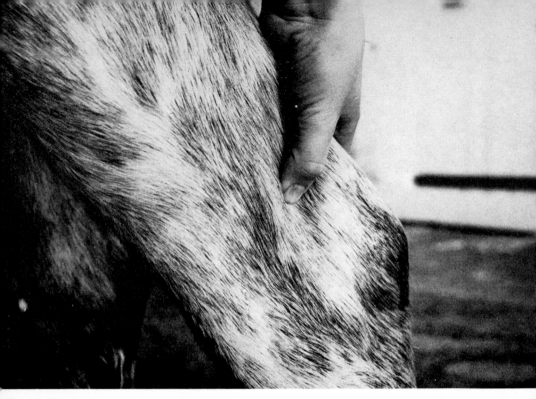

21 Feeling for thoroughpin, qv

22 Feeling for articular windgall. See *windgall*

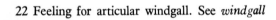

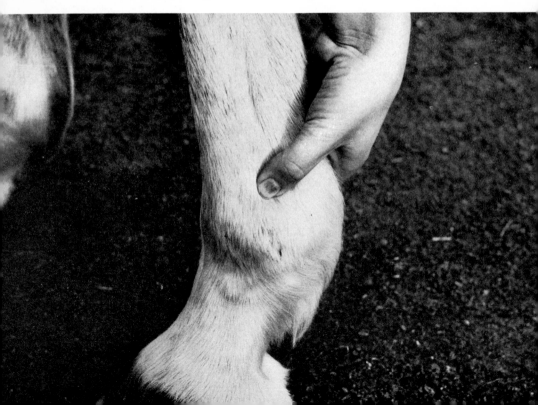

about 7 hands (28ins. or 70cms.) and tallest, eg Shire, may reach 18 hands. Forerunner of horse, Eohippus, which lived about 55 million years ago, varied from 2.2–5 hands. See evolution.

Hanoverian One of best-known German breeds. Traces to middle ages when English Thoroughbreds were crossed with heavy types such as German Great horse. In 17th and 18th centuries breed modified to lighter cavalry type, which fell into 3 main groups: **H.**, Danish and Mecklenburg. Now popular for riding, especially eventing, though some claim **H.** is deteriorating due to apparent inability to breed true.

haploid Cell containing single chromosomes (qv) as opposed to pairs. Cf diploid. Sex cells, eg spermatozoa and ova, are **h.**, containing 32 single chromosomes.

Harddraver See Friesian.

harelip Congenital defect in upper lip due to two sides of lip failing to unite during development. Uncommon in horses. Requires plastic surgery—seldom attempted and usually uneconomic.

harvest mite (Trombicula autumnalis; colloq. harvester, berry bug, orange tawney, red bug, chigger) Arthropod parasite belonging to family Trombiculidae. Has scarlet, red-orange or yellow velvety body. Adults and nymphs are free-living; parasitic larvae hatch from eggs laid on ground. They cling to host and use saliva to digest outer layer of skin, to suck fluid. They attack head and legs of horse, causing itchy dermatitis, loss of hair and scabbing. Most common in autumn when larvae, whose natural hosts are rodents such as mice, crawl on to horses grazing in low-lying fields. Diagnosis: on recovering larval mites in skin scrapings. Treatment: apply gamma benzene hexachloride (qv) to kill mites, then antiseptic lotion on sores. See also mange.

Haussman See gag.

headlessness (acephalia) Rare congenital condition in which skull has not formed. Fetus usually aborted or born dead.

healing Process of making good an injury, particularly skin wound. **h. by 1st intention** Skin which unites without granulation (proud flesh). **h. by 2nd intention** Filling of wound with granulation tissue before skin cells (epithelium) grow over. See wound.

heart (L. cor, Gr. kardia) Muscular organ with 4 chambers which pumps blood through system of vessels—arteries, veins, capillaries, etc. Weighs 8–15lb. and has walls of muscle (myocardium), lined on inside with membrane of epithelium (endocardium) and on outside (epicardium). **H.** is contained in tough sac (pericardium) and is divided into 2 sides, left and right. Each side has 2 chambers; the first (auricle or

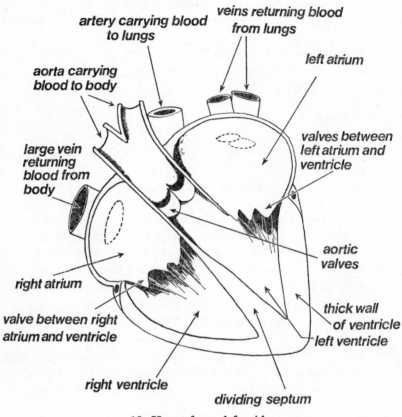

18 Heart from left side

atrium) has relatively thin walls, the second (ventricle), below, has thicker walls. The left ventricle pumps blood to all parts of body so has thicker walls than the right, which pumps blood through only the lungs. Between first and second chambers of both sides, there are valves (mitral on the left, tricuspid on right). These prevent blood returning to first chamber when the ventricles contract and force blood into aorta and pulmonary artery. These arteries have valves at their entrances; three cusps known as semilunar valves. They stop blood returning from arteries to the second chambers when heart relaxes and fills with blood from veins. See myocarditis, endocardium, pericardium, aorta, aortic semilunar valves, plate 36. **h., diseases of** Primary heart disease as in humans, uncommon in horses; they rarely suffer coronary thrombosis or heart attacks, nor is there evidence of angina. Secondary infection, from bacteria, virus or toxemia are frequent. Conditions fall into following categories:

1. Damaged heart muscle (myocardium) = myocarditis.
2. Damage to any one of 4 sets of valves = valvular endocarditis.
3. Hemorrhage from, or clot in, coronary arteries = coronary thrombosis.
4. Inflamed inner lining (endocardium) = endocarditis, outer lining (pericardium) = pericarditis.
5. Dilated chamber walls.
6. Rupture of wall of 1st chambers.
7. Abnormal increase in thickness of chamber wall = hypertrophy.

See myocarditis, pericarditis, thrombus, hemorrhage, endocarditis, heart failure.

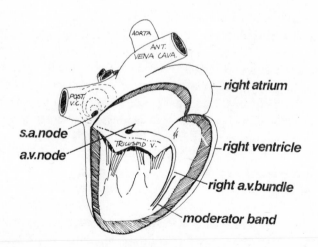

19 Right side of heart with walls of first and second chambers removed to show tricuspid valve

h. failure Stopping or reducing of **h.** action. Caused by defect in organ, eg damaged valve, or by excessive strain, eg raised blood pressure in lungs due to broken wind condition. **h. impulse** Electrical activity which spreads through **h.** muscle during each beat. Impulse starts at SA (sino-atrial) node and spreads into walls of first chamber, then to AV (atrio-ventricular) node. From there it travels in special bands of cells (bundle branches) to muscles of left and right second chambers (ventricles). Passage of impulse coincides with contraction of muscle and can be recorded in an electrocardiogram, qv. Abnormalities include ectopic beat (syns. extrasystole, extra-systolic beat, premature beat), one originating outside SA node. **h. murmur** Sound made by blood as it passes through **h.** May be set up by counter current (whirlpool effect). Classified according to pitch (low, high), quality (blowing, musical), area where most clearly heard (mitral, aortic, tricuspid) and place in relation to heart sounds (eg systolic or diastolic). May be benign result of condition which does not reduce **h.**'s efficiency, or pathological, when it indicates damage to heart valve. **ejection h.m.** One caused by forward-flowing blood being forced through relatively small opening. Intensity (volume) is graded from 1 (almost inaudible) to 6 (heard at a distance from chest). Most **h.m.**'s of grade 4 or over are pathological. **h. muscle** (syn. cardiac m.) One of 3 types of muscle. That which forms wall of **h.** chambers is not arranged in individual fibres, but composed of sheet of muscle which has rhythmic properties. Cf striped muscle, smooth muscle. **h. rate** Normal adult: 35–40 beats per minute. May be slower at rest; increases in excitement, fever, anemia. Foals at birth: 80–120 per minute, older foals: 60–80, yearlings: 40–60. **h. sounds** Movement of blood heard on auscultation, ie listening with ear against chest or with stethoscope. Sounds divide into 2 phases, when muscle is contracting (systole) and relaxing (diastole). First sound (termed lubb) is low-pitched and corresponds to heart muscle contracting and mitral and tricuspid valves closing. Second sound (termed dupp) has a higher pitch and occurs when semilunar valves close. Instruments such as the phonocardiogram can record parts of these sounds which are inaudible to naked ear. Sounds are described according to where they are most clearly heard when stethoscope is used, eg mitral region, aortic area, tricuspid area. An abnormal sound is usually termed a **h.** murmur, qv.

heat (L. calor, Gr. therme) (1) Colloq. for oestrus (see oestrous cycle). (2) Form of energy transferred by conduction, convection through air, or in electro-magnetic waves by radiation. See dry-coat, physiotherapy, radiation, temperature.

heaves Type of abnormal breathing. See broken wind.

heckbury Colloq. dark brown. See coat colouring.

heel (L. calx) One of 2 bulb-like areas either side of mid-line at back of foot. See foot, contracted heels, mud fever.

height Vertical measurement from ground to top of withers. Usually gauged with stick or rule. See hand.

helcoma Ulcer on cornea. See eye.

Helmezine Trade name. See piperazine salts.

helminth (Gr. helmins, worm) See tapeworm.

hemagglutination Agglutination (clumping) of red blood cells by serum, as a result of an antibody/antigen reaction. **h. inhibition test** Basis of blood pregnancy test (see pregnancy test).

hemagglutinin Antibody that causes clumping of red blood cells. See antibody.

hemarthrosis (hem- + Gr. arthron, joint) Bleeding into joint or synovial cavity; follows injury. Joint fills, causing pain.

hematocrit (hemato- + Gr. krinein, to separate; syns. packed cell volume, PCV) Percentage volume of red blood cells to blood plasma measured by centrifuging (spinning) column of blood containing anti-coagulant for 30 minutes, so that cells separate from plasma. Normal values 35–50% according to age, state of fitness, etc. Level rises with fitness, on excitement and in pathological conditions such as acute colic, grass sickness and dehydration. It falls in anemia, hemolytic jaundice, infections, especially those associated with fever, and severe hemorrhage. **micro-h.** That measured in very small (capillary) tube and spun for 5 minutes. See blood tests.

hematocyturia (hematocyte + Gr. ouron, urine) Presence of red blood cells in urine. Cf hemoglobinuria. See stone, setfast.

hematology Science of blood.

hematoma See blood blister.

hemiplegia (hemi- + Gr. plege, stroke) Paralysis of one side of body.

hemisphere (hemi- + Gr. sphaira, ball or globe) Half of spherical organ. **cerebral h.** See brain.

hemlock (Conium maculatum) poisoning Occurs if the plant, which contains an alkaloid, is eaten, though this is unlikely except if food is scarce. Symptoms: dilated pupils, weakness, staggering. Consciousness is lost just before death. Treatment: purgatives, tannic acid and stimulants, eg strychnine or atropine.

hemoconcentration Condition in which proportion of blood cells to plasma is greater than normal, ie above 50%. Occurs, normally, after exercise and excitement; abnormally in dehydration, qv. See hematocrit.

hemodynamic Study of blood circulation.

hemoglobin Oxygen-carrying pigment of red blood cells formed in bone marrow. Consists of protein, globin combined with iron-containing pigment. Average **h.** in blood is 14gms./100ml.; decreases in anemia and hemolytic diseases.

hemoglobinometer (hemoglobin + Gr. metron, measure) Instrument for measuring concentration of hemoglobin in blood.

hemoglobinuria (hemoglobin + Gr. ouron, urine + -ia) Presence of free hemoglobin in urine. Cf hematocyturia, setfast, hemolytic jaundice.

hemolysin (hemo- + Gr. lysis, dissolution) Naturally occurring substance which destroys red blood cells, causing hemolysis, eg in rare cases mare produces **h.** against red cells of her fetus. When foal is born it absorbs mare's **h.** from the first milk (colostrum) and suffers hemolytic jaundice, qv.

hemolysis Liberation of hemoglobin from red cells. Caused by the chemical hemolysin, by freezing, heating or contact with water. See hemolytic jaundice, jaundice. Cf beta **h.**

hemolytic Of hemolysis.

hemolytic jaundice Disease of newborn foal caused by reaction between antibodies in dam's colostrum and foal's red cells. A few fetal red cells cross into mare's blood stream and in rare instances, because of an inherited difference, they cause mare to produce antibodies; these are concentrated in the colostrum which foal swallows during its first feed; antibodies are absorbed through stomach lining into foal's blood stream and destroy its red cells. Condition is result of inherited blood groups. Fetus is not affected until it is born because antibodies do not cross placenta. Symptoms vary. Acute cases develop within 36 hours of birth and jaundice is severe. Urine turns red and breathing and heart rate increase, especially on exertion. Foal dies in a matter of hours, unless treated. Other cases may not develop for 2–4 days and jaundice, although marked, does not cause severe symptoms until just before death. Diagnosis: on examination of blood. Red cell count is below 3 million/cu.mm., hemoglobin below 7gms./100ml. and hematocrit below 20%. Treatment: transfuse compatible blood to replace lost red cells. Prevention: mare's blood or colostrum can be tested and affected mare diagnosed in last two weeks of pregnancy. Foal should be muzzled in the first 24–36 hours and fed donor colostrum and artificial milk. (See plate 34.) After 24 hours antibodies in mare's milk can no longer be absorbed by foal's stomach and it is then safe to allow foal to suck from its dam. Once mare has been affected, she is more liable to suffer condition in other pregnancies.

hemophilia (hemo- + Gr. philein, to love) Disease characterised by inherited defect in blood cells. Rare, but reported in closely related Thoroughbreds due to deficiency in coagulation factor 8. Probably sex-linked defect associated with sex chromosome X; **h.** carried by fillies and occurs only in colts. Symptoms: blood blisters in skin forming without apparent reason or on slightest knock. See chromosome, coagulation.

hemopoiesis (hemo- + Gr. poiesis, formation) Forming of red blood cells in special tissues such as bone marrow. See red blood cell.

hemorrhage (hemo- + Gr. rhegnynai, to burst forth; syn. bleeding) Escape of blood normally contained in blood vessels, ie veins, arteries and capillaries. Occurs if these are broken by trauma, increased fragility of walls and/or increased blood pressure. **H.** may be external, eg in wound, or internal, eg in ulceration or rupture of a vessel. (See birth **h.**) Blood may be from artery, vein or capillary. That from an artery is usually bright red and gushes out under pulsating pressure; from a vein it is darker and emerges in a steady flow. **H.** is stopped by natural mechanism of clotting (coagulation, qv) and can be helped by direct or indirect pressure (see tourniquet). **petechial h.** See bleeder, petechia.

hemosiderin (hemo- + Gr. sideros, iron) Form in which iron is stored.

hemostasis (hemo- + Gr. stasis, halt) The stopping of bleeding.

hemostatic (hemo- + Gr. statikos, standing) Substance or drug that stops bleeding.

heparin Substance, formed by liver, which prevents blood clotting. Used as anticoagulant when collecting blood samples. See blood tests.

hepatic Of the liver.

hepatitis Inflamed liver caused by bacterial or viral infection, poisonous chemicals and certain plant toxins such as ragwort. **serum h.** Highly fatal toxic disease of liver. Follows use of antiserum and characterised by jaundice, nervous signs, staggering and death. Thought to be due to virus or allergic reaction. See swamp fever; abortion, viral; tuberculosis; cirrhosis.

herbicide poisoning May occur if horse allowed to graze next to field sprayed with **h.** (weed killer). Symptoms: loss of appetite, loss of weight, depression, muscular weakness. Post-mortem findings: inflamed alimentary tract, changes in liver and kidney and sometimes congestion of lungs.

hereditary (L. hereditas) Inheritance. Established **h.** conditions include parrot jaw, coat colouring. Suspected **h.** tendencies: navicular disease, temperament, cryptorchidism. See rig, Welsh Mountain pony.

hermaphrodite (Gr. hermaphroditos) Individual with male and female tissue in sex organs. See intersex.

hernia (L.) Protrusion of abdominal (or other) contents (gut, organs, omentum) through containing walls. May be inherited, congenital or caused by trauma. Consists of opening (ring) and pouch (sac) lined with peritoneum. **diaphragmatic h.** When abdominal contents pass through abnormal openings in diaphragm. **scrotal h.** When abdominal contents enter scrotum through inguinal canal. **strangulated h.** When contents of any type of **h.** are squeezed by opening causing pain and death if not relieved. **umbilical h.** When muscular ring (through which vessels pass to umbilical cord in fetus) does not close after birth. Soft external swelling develops at age 4–6 weeks. This can easily be reduced by pressing contents of sac back into abdomen. Cf umbilical abscess. Treatment: surgery to remove pouch and close ring. Essential for strangulated and diaphragmatic types though umbilical **h.** often disappears unaided by yearling stage.

herpes See equine herpesvirus.

hexachlorethane Colourless crystals with smell of camphor but almost tasteless. Used to treat liver fluke in cattle and sheep. Infections uncommon in horses and drug not specifically recommended for them.

hexachlorophane White powder with slight smell of phenol. Used to treat liver fluke in cattle and sheep but not specifically recommended for horses.

hexamine Colourless odourless crystals, which taste first sweet then bitter. Given by mouth to acidify urine, in treatment of cystitis and infections of urinary tract. Dose: 4–8gms.

Hg Chemical symbol for mercury.

Hibitane Trade name. See chlorhexidine hydrochloride.

Highland pony (colloq. Garron) Largest of British mountain and moorland types. Those on mainland up to 14.2 hands; on Scottish islands smaller. Rhum Island ponies are probably oldest established. Extremely strong breed used for pony trekking and carrying stags. Colours: black, brown, grey, dun and chestnut with flaxen mane and tail. Sometimes have black dorsal stripe. Assn: **H.** Pony Soc., c/o J. McIldowie, Dunblane, Perthshire.

hilus (L., a small thing) Part of organ where vessels and nerves enter, eg on ovary, kidney.

hip joint Ball and socket joint formed by head of femur and acetabulum of pelvis. Joint is characterised by absence of external ligaments but contains round ligament, a short strong band attached to rim of acetabulum and notch in head of femur. **h.j., dislocation of** Uncommon and can occur only if round ligament is ruptured. Symptoms include deformed angle of leg so that toe and stifle turn out and hock turns in. Treatment: anaesthetise, manipulate back into position, rest horse.

hippiatra Ancient Gr. for veterinary surgeon. **hippiatry** Veterinary medicine. Greeks based words on hippus (horse), showing their main veterinary interest was in the horse.

hippo- (Gr. hippos, horse) Combining form meaning relationship to horse.

hippomane (Gr., horse madness; syn. pad) Brown, yellowish, white or greenish rubber-like structure in allantoic (placental) fluid; found only in horse family. Develops in first 4 months of pregnancy and grows to form flat, oval, or rectangular object about 10 by 5cm., 1½cm. thick; made up of cells and salts; has no known biological function; traditionally believed to have mysterious powers. Often found on floor/ground after mare has foaled.

hippus (ancient Gr.) Horse, as in Eohippus. See evolution.

histamine Substance produced from amino-acid histidine when living tissues are damaged. Causes capillaries to dilate and become more permeable and water passes from blood into surrounding tissues, eg injection beneath skin causes a weal of oedema. **H.** also causes smooth muscle in uterus and lungs to contract and is released in anaphylactic reactions and allergies, eg during attack of asthma and broken wind it causes small air tubes to constrict.

histological Of histology, eg **h. section** Small sample of tissue, usually mounted on slide, for studying under microscope.

histology (Gr. histo-, tissue + -logy) Detailed study of normal and abnormal (pathological) anatomy.

Histoplasma farciminosum Fungus which causes epizootic lymphangitis, qv. (Used to be called Cryptococcus or Blastomyces.)

Hobday (after Sir Frederick **H.**, FRCVS; syns. laryngeal ventriculectomy, ventricle stripping) Operation to relieve roaring/whistling caused by paralysed muscles controlling vocal and arytenoid cartilage of voice box (larynx). Uusually performed under general anaesthesia, less commonly under sedation and local anaesthesia. Larynx is opened and a burr (round instrument covered with spikes) used to strip mucous membrane from inside cups formed by vocal cords. Part of cord may be removed. In healing, cords are pulled back against larynx walls so they no longer obstruct air passage. Horse is then mute. Operation can be modified and arytenoid cartilage pulled to one side by a ligature (prosthesis). See wind.

hock Joint in hindleg between gaskin (second thigh) and cannon bone, equivalent to human ankle. **capped h.** Soft swelling over point of **h.**, containing fluid in sac (bursa, qv) caused by bruising. Does not usually impair action.

holocrine (holo- + Gr. krinein, to separate) Type of gland in which the entire secreting cell forms secreted matter of gland, eg sebaceous gland, qv. See gland.

Holstein German horse used for driving and riding, particularly hunting. Similar to Hanoverian but with little Thoroughbred blood. Believed to date back to 13th century and to have been improved by imported Yorkshire Coach horses (similar to Cleveland Bay but now virtually extinct). Most often brown.

homatropine hydrobromide Colourless crystalline odourless powder. Used in eye-drop solutions to dilate pupil. See mydriatic.

homeostasis (homeo- + Gr. stasis, standing) Tendency to remain stable, eg blood levels of salts, sugar and protein.

homidium bromide Dark-purple bitter-tasting crystalline powder without smell. Used to treat Trypanosoma congolense infection. Intramuscular injection may cause local swelling. Dose: 10mg./kg. body wt.

hoof (L. ungula) Horny casing of foot, qv.

Hoppengarten cough See influenza.

hormonal Of a hormone.

hormone (Gr. hormaein, to set in motion, spur on) Chemical substance produced by gland or body organ and which travels in blood or lymph stream to a distant part, on which it has an effect, eg follicle stimulating hormone (FSH) secreted by pituitary gland in head, causes follicle to grow in ovary. **adrenocortical h.** One produced by part of adrenal cortex. **adreno-cortico-trophic h.** One from anterior pituitary gland which acts on adrenal cortex. **anterior pituitary h.** Secreted by anterior lobe of pituitary gland. See gland, pituitary, sex **h.**'s, adrenaline, cortisol, oestrogen, follicle stimulating hormone, insulin, luteinising hormone, oxytocin, progesterone, prostaglandin, testosterone, thyroxine.

horn (L. cornu) (1) Anatomical description for **h.**-shaped part, eg **h.** of uterus. (2) Hard cells which form hoof. See foot.

horse See Equus and various breeds. Cf pony. **h. fly** See tabanid fly. **H. and Mule Assn of America,** 407 So. Dearborn St, Chicago, Illinois (Zip no: 60605). **h. sickness** See African horse sickness, Crofton weed. **h. tails** (equisetum) Plant found on damp land which causes symptoms similar to bracken poisoning, qv.

host (L. hospes) Animal which harbours or nourishes a parasite, eg horse is **h.** of redworm.

hot-blooded Colloq. for any high-spirited horse, usually of Oriental origin, eg Thoroughbred. Cf cold-blooded.

hotting up Colloq. for signs of 1st stage labour. See birth.

Hucul Type of Konik, qv.

humane With feelings befitting man, ie merciful. **h. killer/killing** See euthanasia.

humerus Long bone between shoulder joint and elbow joint (one either side of chest).

humour/humor (L., a liquid) Term meaning oedematous swelling in body, particularly legs. See oedema.

Hungarian Shagya Hardy horse similar to Arab and sometimes termed type of half-bred Arab, but usually without dished face. Originated from Hungarian mares (similar to Przewalskis) crossed with Arab stallion named Shagya. Now used for riding and driving. About 14.2 hands, most often grey.

hunter Type rather than breed, the only essential being that it can stand a day's hunting. Divided into three groups for show purposes—heavy-weight to carry 14st. 7lb. or over, middle-weight 13st.–14st. 7lb., light-weight under 13st. Assn: **H.** Improvement and National Light Horse Breeding Soc., 8 Market Square, Westerham, Kent (Westerham 63867).

hyaline (Gr. hyalos, glass) Glassy, transparent as in h. membrane of lungs of newborn foals suffering from convulsions. See neonatal maladjustment syndrome.

hydrated aluminium silicate See clay.

hydrocephalus (hydro-, from Gr. hydor, water + kephale, head) Abnormal accumulation of fluid in head. May be congenital or acquired. In either case, due to interference with drainage of cerebro-spinal fluid. Rare in horses.

hydrochlorothiazide (trade names: Direma, Vetidrex) White crystalline odourless powder with slightly bitter taste. Increases excretion of sodium in urine; used as diuretic to treat oedema. Dose: 100–250mg. IM once a day.

hydrocortisone (trade names: Cortisol, Cortril, Ef-Cortelan, Hydrocortistab, HydroCortisyl, Hydrocortone) White crystalline odourless powder with bitter taste. Has general actions and uses of a corticosteroid, qv. Dose: locally as ointment, or 2.5–10mg./kg. body wt. IM, daily in divided doses. See allergy, inflammation, corticosteroids, cortisone.

Hydrocortistab Trade name. See hydrocortisone.

HydroCortisyl Trade name. See hydrocortisone.

Hydrocortone Trade name. See hydrocortisone.

hydrogen peroxide solution Colourless odourless liquid with slightly acid taste; also known as 20 vol. **h.p.** indicating volumes of oxygen obtained from one volume of solution; used as antiseptic and deodorant, to wash wounds, especially of feet because these are most likely to be contaminated with anaerobic bacteria such as cause lockjaw. Bleaches hair and other coloured organic matter.

hydropericardium Accumulation of fluid in pericardium (sac surrounding heart). Present in septicemia, qv. See oedema.

hydrophobia (hydro- + Gr. phobos, fear) Fear of water, as in sign of rabies.

hydrops amnii (L., Gr.) Abnormal accumulation of fluid in membranes surrounding fetus.

hydrothorax Accumulation of fluid in pleural cavities, ie surrounding lungs. Caused by heart failure and septicemia.

hydroxy-methyl progesterone Long-acting progesterone, qv.

hygroma Swelling, usually in bursa, eg on front surface of knee joint. Caused by a kick, falling on knees, hitting fence or, rarely, individual that kneels, cow-like, when getting up. Treatment: remove cause, eg if horse paws at manger, feed should be put on ground. Drain fluid, inject corticosteroids, apply elastic bandages. Long-standing injury may need surgery.

hyoid (Gr. hyocides, u-shaped) Bone between vertical parts of lower jaw. Supports root of tongue, throat and voice box and is attached to skull by rods of cartilage. Sometimes fractured by trauma, causing difficult swallowing.

hyper- (Gr. hyper, above) Prefix meaning above or in excess.

hypercalcemia (hyper- + calcium + Gr. haima, blood) Excess calcium in blood; above 11–15gms./100ml. blood serum.

hypercapnia (hyper- + Gr. kapnos, smoke) Excess of carbon dioxide in blood; normal: 40mm.Hg pressure in arterial blood.

hyperemia (hyper- + Gr. haima, blood) Excess blood in a part. See hemorrhage, inflammation.

hyperextension Over-extension of limb or joint. See stay apparatus.

hyperflexion Overflexion, as in **h.** of limb. See contracted tendon.

hyperglycemia (hyper- + Gr. glykys, sweet + haima, blood) Abnormally high level of sugar content in blood. Normal level: 60–140mg./100ml. blood. Cf hypoglycemia.

hyperimmune serum Solution of antibodies prepared from horse that has been vaccinated to produce extremely high levels of antibody in blood stream. Serum is then taken and put into another individual to protect against infection, eg tetanus antitoxin, the antidote of lockjaw.

hyperkalemia Excess potassium in blood. Cf hypokalemia.

hyperparathyroidism Increased amount of hormone (parathormone) secreted by parathyroid glands; causes removal of calcium from bones, raising calcium level in blood. **primary h.** Caused by tumour of glands, but never reported to have occurred in horses. **secondary h.** Caused by low levels of calcium in blood as a result of (1) low calcium or high phosphate diet, (2) failure to absorb calcium from intestine, (3) pregnancy and lactation, (4) rickets (qv). Severe cases may cause loss of bone, which is replaced by fibrous tissue (osteitis fibrosa). See calcium and phosphorus, bone.

hyperphosphatemia Excessive phosphates in blood. Normal level: 3–6gms./100ml. blood serum.

hyperplasia (hyper- + Gr. plasis, formation) Abnormal multiplication of normal cells.

hypersalivation Excessive salivation. See choke, grass sickness.

hyperthermia Raised temperature. See temperature.

hyperthyroidism (syn. ex-ophthalmic goitre) Over-activity of thyroid gland and excessive uptake of iodine from blood. Too much thyroid stimulating hormone (TSH) is produced and gland becomes enlarged and fibrous with an excess of colloid.

hypertrophy (hyper- + Gr. trophe, nutrition) Excessive growth of organ or part, eg **h.** of heart muscle due to disease or increased work.

hyperventilation Increased exchange of air in lungs due to deeper or faster breathing.

hypo- (Gr. hypo, under) Prefix meaning below, beneath, under or deficient.

hypocalcemia (hypo- + calcium + Gr. haima, blood) Abnormally low levels of blood calcium.

hypochromia (hypo- + Gr. chroma, colour) Decrease in hemoglobin content of red blood cells.

Hypoderma Genus of warble fly, qv.

hypodermic injection Administration of drug beneath skin, through a needle.

hypoflexion of limbs Condition in which there is too little flexion in muscles and tendons supporting legs. Affects newborn foals; cause unknown. Pastern bone descends so that fetlock is close to, or on, ground. Usually occurs in all 4 legs. Treatment: bandage joints to give support and, possibly, give antibiotics. Cf hyperflexion.

hypogammaglobulinemia Abnormally low levels of gammaglobulin in blood. See immunity.

hypoglycemia (hypo- + Gr. glykys, sweet + haima, blood) Abnormally little glucose in blood. Occurs in newborn foals which are weak and ill-nourished; not usually associated with convulsions, as would be case in adult horses. Cf hyperglycemia.

hypokalemia Abnormally low level of potassium in blood. Often occurs in chronic diarrhoea.

hypoplasia (hypo- + Gr. plasis, formation) Incomplete or faulty development.

218

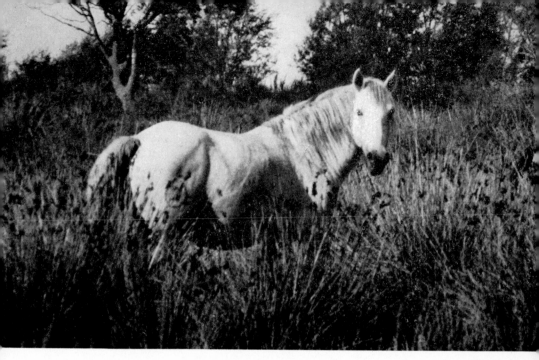

23   A pony in its natural surroundings, the marshy Camargue district of southern France.
See *Camargue, feral*

24   Donkey (Equus asinus) with the typical dark shoulder stripe

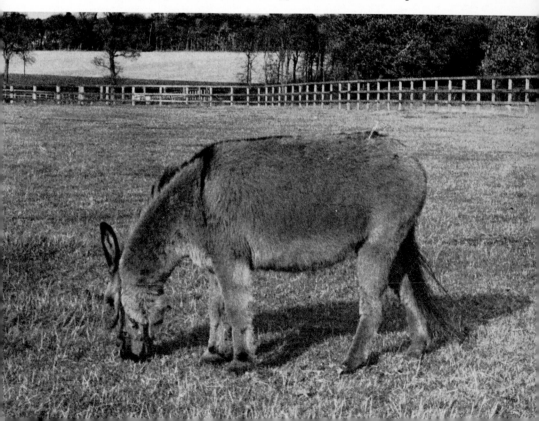

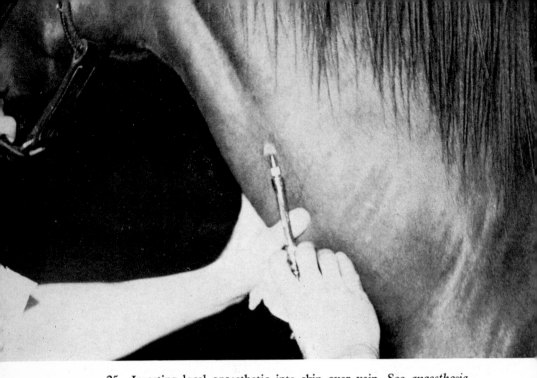

25 Inserting local anaesthetic into skin over vein. See *anaesthesia*

26 Internal parasites of the horse: l to r: 2 seatworms, 2 tapeworms, many small redworms, 3 large redworms, 3 redworm larvae, 2 botfly larvae; below: immature whiteworm

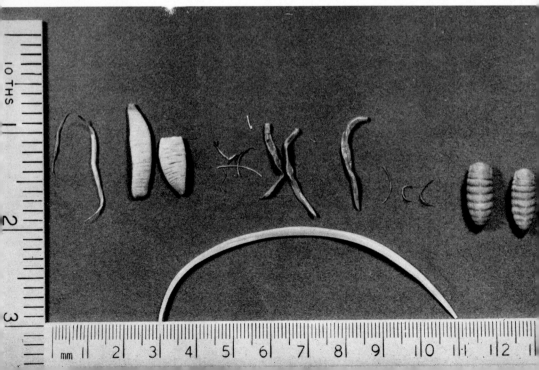

hyposodonty Having long teeth. Sign of old age. Noted in study of equine evolution, to determine length and type of teeth and therefore type of food eaten and period when fossilised remains lived. Cf brachydonty. See evolution.

hypothermia (hypo- + Gr. therme, heat + -ia) Temperature below normal, ie 38°C. (100.4°F.). See temperature, neonatal maladjustment syndrome.

hypothyroidism Any condition caused by inactivity of thyroid gland, when its uptake of iodine from blood is negligible.

hypothysectomy Operation (usually experimental) on pituitary gland. Either dissection of gland or severance of its nerve supply.

hypotonia Reduced activity or tone, eg of muscle in wasting or congenital condition.

hypoventilation Reduced amount of air exchange in lungs as a result of shallow or slow rate of breathing.

hypoxemia Low level of oxygen in blood; usually measured in pressure; normal 80–100mm.Hg. See anoxemia.

hypoxia Low oxygen content. See anoxia.

hysterectomy (hystero- + Gr. ektome, excision) Surgical removal of uterus. Rare in mares.

I

I Chemical symbol for iodine, qv.

Iceland/ic Pony developed from Norwegian and Irish ponies taken to I. by first settlers. Extremely hardy with shaggy dun coat and usually about 12.2 hands. Now used for riding or as pack pony but at one time settlers ate ponies' flesh and enjoyed encouraging stallions to fight.

ichthyosis Condition in which skin becomes dry and rough as a result of excessive growth (hypertrophy) of horny layer. Cf dry coat.

ICSH See interstitial cell stimulating hormone.

icteric Of jaundice.

icterus (L., Gr. ikteros) Yellow discoloration of skin, tissues and organs. See jaundice.

idiopathic Of unknown cause.

idiosyncrasy (idio- + Gr. synkrasis, mixture) Habit peculiar to an individual; his unusual susceptibility to some drug, protein or substance. See allergy.

ileocaecal Of ileum and caecum, particularly **i.** opening into caecum, at which impaction may lodge or ulcer form. **i. valve** Projection of mucous membrane; prevents food passing from caecum to ileum. See colic.

ileum End part of small intestine opening into caecum. See alimentary canal.

ileus (L., Gr. eileos, from eilein, to roll up) Obstructed intestines due to lack of movement. **meconium i.** Stoppage due to first dung. See meconium retention. **paralytic i.** Paralysis of gut. See colic.

iliac thrombosis (syns. thrombosis of posterior aorta or iliac arteries) Blood clot (see thrombus) which decreases blood supply to hindlegs. May be caused by disease of artery, redworm larvae damaging artery, or by infection; most common in geldings, following castration. Symptoms: lameness (claudication), painful spasm of muscles if exercised, sweating, anxiety. Affected leg will be cooler than opposite one and veins stand out less. No satisfactory treatment apart from rest.

ilium One of 3 bones comprising pelvis (see ischium and pubis); consists of a wing, broad flat part to which gluteal muscles are attached, and shaft joined to ischium. Tuber coxae (point or angle of hip) and tuber sacrale (croup) are part of ilial wing.

Ilotycin Trade name. See erythromycin.

IM Abbr. for intramuscular/ly, qv.

imbalance Lack of balance. Colloq. fluid **i.** See fluid balance.

immaturity Lack of maturity or development. Applied to whole or part of animal. **i. of behaviour** During period of learning. See behaviour. **i. of newborn** Foal which is weak, undersized and undernourished, born after 325 days' gestation (300–25 days usually termed premature). **sexual i.** Not having reached full sexual powers, before puberty. See maturity. **i. of skeleton** Before growth of bone has stopped. All bones have stopped growing by age 5 years but individual bones stop at various ages, eg cannon at about 12 months; forearm (radius) 24 months. Growth occurs at ends of bones (epiphyses). See growth plate.

Immobilon/Revivon Trade name.See etorphine hydrochloride.

immune (L. immunis, safe) Protected against particular disease, eg by vaccination.

immunity (L. immunitas) Reaction between an infecting organism (bacteria, virus or fungus) and the body. Individual resistant to infection said to possess **i.** (opp. susceptibility). **I.** may be natural or acquired; active or passive. **acquired i.** Reaction of the body following vaccination or contact with infection. **breed i.** Some breeds are more resistant to infection than others. **inherent i.** Inherited **i. natural i.** Body's resistance without external stimulation, eg skin, mucous membranes, secretions produced by cells and acidity of secretions all provide barriers to invasion by bacteria. **passive i.** Transference of **i.** by innoculation with serum from one immune individual to a susceptible one. See vaccine, antiserum. **species i.** Certain diseases such as tuberculosis, anthrax, rabies are common to most species, but many diseases are species specific, eg human diphtheria does not affect horses.

immunology Science of immunity.

impaction See colic.

Imperacin Trade name. See oxytetracycline.

implant Drug in tablet or other solid form for inserting beneath skin. Prepared so that drug leaves site at a steady rate over weeks or months. Most often used to give oestrogen and progesterone in treating infertility.

impotence (L. in, not + potentin, power) Lack of sexual power; in stallion lack of sexual drive (libido), ie mounting behaviour, pelvic thrust, erection of penis or ejaculation. **temporary i.** May occur if horse is ill or inexperienced. See behaviour.

Improved Bigourdan See Bigourdan.

impulse Wave of energy passing along nerves, muscle etc. See heart i., nervous i.

incidence (L. incidere, to occur) Rate of occurrence, eg number of cases suffering from specific disease.

incision Cut or wound as made by surgeon's scalpel. See surgery.

incisor (L. incidere, to cut into) Front tooth. See teeth.

inclusion body Minute structure in cytoplasm or nucleus of cell, often containing virus, eg negri **i.b.**'s are found in cytoplasm of nerve cells in rabies; Cowdray A **i.b.**'s found in nuclei of lung and liver in herpes-virus I and adenovirus infections.

incompetence See aortic semilunar valve.

incontinent (L. incontinentia) Unable to control urination or defecation. See enuresis.

inco-ordination (L. in, not + co-ordination) Uncontrolled movement. See cerebellar degeneration, encephalomyelitis, lockjaw, meningitis, wobbler syndrome, segmental myelitis.

incubation (L. incubatio) Act of hatching. In laboratory, process by which virus or bacteria is innoculated into special substances known as media. Germ then grows after being incubated at certain temperature (usually 38°C.). **i. period** Time between infection and appearance of symptoms, eg glanders: 1–3 months or more, influenza: 1–5 days, lockjaw: 5–15 days, strangles: 4–8 days.

indigestion Literally failure to digest, ie poor digestion. See colic.

Indigofera dominii Australian plant poisonous to horses. See birdsville disease.

inductothermy Form of heat treatment. See physiotherapy.

infarct (L. *infarctus*) Death of tissue due to obstructed blood circulation. Occurs in small intestine due to lodging of blood clot that has broken away from aneurism (qv) caused by redworm infection. See colic, redworm.

infection Non-specific condition caused by bacteria, fungus, virus. Fever, dullness and disturbed functions in particular organs are diagnostic, eg lungs (pneumonia), kidneys (nephritis) and liver (hepatitis). **local i.** That in, eg abscess, metritis (inflamed uterus). Type of **i.** can be diagnosed by examining white blood cell count and differential; bacterial **i.** causes marked increase in total white blood cells and/or an increase in polymorphonuclear leucocytes; viral **i.** causes increase in lymphocytes, although some viruses, eg arteritis, cause a reduction in white cell count and a depression of lymphocytes; parasitic **i.** is characterised by an increase in eosinophils. (See blood tests.) If there is a discharge, or if fluid or tissue can be obtained by needle puncture or biopsy, the **i.** can be identified by laboratory growth and analysis.

infectious Disease spread by infection. **i. equine anemia** See swamp fever. **i. equine bronchitis/cough** See influenza. **i. equine encephalomyelitis** See encephalomyelitis.

infective arthritis See joint-ill.

infertility (L. *in*, not + *fertilis*, fruitful) Inability to conceive. In mare, may be due to fault in genital organs, eg underdeveloped ovaries, or more commonly infection of uterus. In stallion may be due to immature behaviour which inhibits ejaculation or to poor-quality semen. Term relative to definition, eg mare said to be infertile because she does not conceive in given period; serious **i.** is when mare fails to breed in 2 or more consecutive stud seasons; stallion fails to achieve conception in about 60% of 40 mares (or fewer) under reasonable conditions of stud management. Treatment: hormones, antibiotics, good management.

inflammation Tissue reaction to injury. Symptoms: redness, heat (due to more blood vessels in area opening up), swelling (due to vessels becoming more permeable, so fluid passes into tissue spaces) and pain (due to stretched nerve endings). Blood vessels release white blood cells, antibacterial and antitoxic materials which clump bacteria together. White cells (phagocytes) invade area and, with amoeboid action, remove dead cells. Treatment: assist and control i. by applying heat (to draw blood to part) then cold (to draw it away). Phenylbutazone and cortisone reduce pain and swelling, antibiotics counteract any infection. See physiotherapy, oedema.

inflammatory Characterised by inflammation.

influenza (syns. flu, infectious equine bronchitis, Newmarket cough, Hoppengarten cough, infectious equine cough) Highly infectious disease caused by myxo-virus, 2 main types known: A/equi 1 (Prague strain) and A/equi 2 (Miami strain). Symptoms: fever: 39°–41°C. (102.2°–105.8°F.), watery nasal discharge, persistent hacking cough, shivering, loss of appetite, inflamed throat. Signs are present for about 48 hours although some horses cough for several weeks after apparent recovery. Secondary bacterial infection is uncommon. Diagnosis: on symptoms and increasing level of antibodies in blood between acute and convalescent stage. Culture of the virus may be possible from nasal washings. See blood (serological tests), virus. **i. vaccines** See Duvaxyn 1 E, Fluvac-Equine, Grippequin, Prevac, Prevac T.

infrared Energy rays of between 7,700 and 120,000 angstroms. Used for heating, often in foaling boxes.

inhalant Drug or substance which is breathed in, eg benzoin for colds or infected sinus. Not recommended for horses.

inheritance Characters passed from parent to offspring. See hereditary.

inject To use needle or catheter to put solution (eg of drug) into muscle, vein or connective tissue beneath skin. **injected mucous membrane** See mucous membrane.

injection (L. injectio) Act of forcing liquid into cavity or part of body. **hypodermic i.** One below skin; usually with syringe and needle. **intradermal i.** One into substance of skin. See also intravenous, intramuscular, subcutaneous.

injury (from L. in, not + jus, right) Colloq. for sprain, wound, damage inflicted by force.

inoculate Colloq. to vaccinate. To introduce serum vaccines or infectious materials or vaccines into body; to implant micro-organisms on to culture media in laboratory.

insect Member of class Insecta, which belongs to phylum Arthropoda, qv. Typical **i.** body has head, thorax and abdomen, three pairs of walking legs and one or two pairs of wings; parasites such as fly and louse have lost both pairs of wings. Those important in equine medicine: subclass Apterygota (order Phthiraptera)—louse, qv; order Siphonaptera —see flea; order Diptera—see bot, tabanid fly, warble fly.

insecticide (L. insectum, insect + caedere, to kill) Substance or drug which destroys insects, used, eg in control of African horse-sickness, qv. **i. poisoning** Symptoms: overactivity of gut causing salivation, abdominal pain, diarrhoea, possibly vomiting; muscle twitching, weight-loss and death from respiratory failure.

insemination (L. inseminatus, sown) Act of introducing semen into vagina or uterus. **artificial i.** By mechanical process or apparatus. **natural i.** By coitus. See artificial insemination, behaviour.

insertion (L. from in, into + serere, to join) Point where muscle is attached to bone.

inspiration (L. inspirare from spirare, to breathe) Act of drawing air into lungs. If accompanied by roaring/whistling or rattling noise, wind unsoundness likely. See wind.

insufficiency (L. insufficientia) Inadequate, low levels, reduced function. **cardiac i.** Abnormal pumping of heart.

insufflation (L. in, into + sufflatio, a blowing up) Act of blowing powder, gas or air into cavity, eg **i.** of lungs in artificial respiration, qv.

interfering (syn. speedy cutting) Action in which horse strikes part of inside of one leg with inside of foot or shoe of opposite leg. Point of impact may be from coronary band to knee (carpus) of foreleg or up to hock of hindleg.

interferon Protein formed by cells when stimulated by virus. Capable of conferring infection-resistance on other cells in same animal, or in another individual given **i.** May be natural or synthetic.

intersex Individual with some anatomical characteristics of opposite sex, so that diagnosis of sex is confused. May have: (1) some reproductive organs of both sexes; (2) female and male sex chromosomes in same cells or in two different lines of cells; (3) inherited material (ie

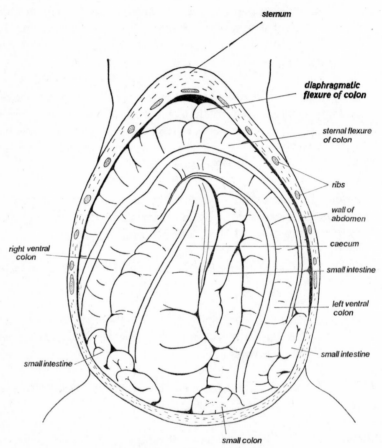

sternum

diaphragmatic
flexure of colon

sternal flexure
of colon

ribs

wall of
abdomen

caecum

small intestine

left ventral
colon

right ventral
colon

small intestine

small intestine

small colon

20   Intestines seen from below

that in spermatozoa (or ova) of different sexuality to that in body cells. **true i.** (syn. hermaphrodite) One with gonads of both sexes, either a separate ovary and testis or combined into an ova-testis (pseudo-hermaphrodite has gonads of only one sex but has reproductive organs with some characteristics of opposite sex; individual may be classed as male or female depending on gonad present, eg male has large female external genitalia but possesses testis). **free-martin** Sterile female with male characteristics. Condition common in cattle twins, but not reported in horses. See chromosome.

interstitial cell stimulating hormone (ICSH of stallion same as FSH of mare) Produced by anterior lobe of pituitary gland; one of pituitary-gonadotrophin group of hormones. Acts on interstitial cells (qv) or testes causing them to produce male sex hormone testosterone, qv.

intestines (L. intestinus, inward, internal, Gr. enteron) Colloq. for whole of alimentary canal, qv.

intra-articular In or into a joint, as in **i.-a.** injection.

intradermal injection One into skin. Used in tuberculin and mallein tests.

intramammary Into mammary gland. **i. injection** Forcing of drug, usually antibiotic, through teat canal. Used to treat mastitis. May cause pain (mare's canal narrower than cow's).

intramuscular/ly (IM) Injecting drug into muscle; usually neck, hind-quarters or brisket.

intranatal During birth.

intraocular (intra- + L. oculus, eye) In the eye.

intraperitoneal In the peritoneal cavity.

intratracheal Into trachea (windpipe). See tube.

intra-uterine injection (syn. irrigation) Putting drugs, usually suspended in water, into uterus via a catheter inserted through cervix. Used to treat infection. See metritis.

Intraval sodium Trade name. See thiopentone sodium.

intravenous/ly (IV) Injecting drug into blood stream via needle or catheter in vein, usually the jugular. Vein is raised by pressing it on heart side of site to be injected.

intubation (L. in, into + tuba, tube) Act of inserting a tube. See tube, anaesthesia.

intussusception (L. intus, within + suscipere, to receive) Telescoping of one part of intestine into immediately adjacent part causing blockage. See colic.

in utero (L.) In uterus, eg exported **i.u.,** before birth.

in vitro In test tube, or laboratory; as in action of antibiotic against bacteria **i.v.**

in vivo In living body, eg action of antibiotic against bacteria **i.v.**

involuntary muscle See smooth muscle.

involution (L. from in, into + volvere, to roll) Changed or decreased tissue or organ. See uterus, involution of.

iodine (chemical symbol: I) Blue-black plates with metallic lustre, distinct penetrating odour and acrid taste. Used in solution, externally, to treat ringworm or to blister, qv. I_{131} Test dose of radio-active **i.** IV. Its course in body can be followed with a geiger counter and amount circulating measured in blood plasma. Used to test activity of thyroid gland, qv.

ion (Gr. ion, going) An atom with a positive (cation) or negative (anion) charge of electricity.

iridocyclitis (irido- + Gr. kuklos, circle + -itis) Inflamed iris and ciliary body of eye. See eye, diseases of: moon blindness.

iris Part of eye, qv.

Irish Hobby Pony of middle ages, around 14 hands. Believed to have had ambling gait and to have originated from Spanish Jennet, qv.

iritis Inflamed iris. See eye, diseases of.

iron poisoning Excessive **i.** is toxic. Symptoms: diarrhoea, drowsiness, shock and coma. Treatment: give milk of magnesia, milk of lime and treat for shock, qv.

irradiation (L. in, into + radiare, to emit rays) See radiation.

ischemia (Gr. ischein, to suppress + haima, blood) Deficiency of blood to a part, eg to hindleg in iliac thrombosis, qv.

ischium One of 3 bones comprising pelvis (see ilium and pubis). Forms back of pelvic floor (front is pubis). See pelvis.

isotonic Fluid in equal concentration with another, eg 0.9% sodium chloride (salt) is **i.** with fluid concentration of body cells. This means such a fluid can be injected without water from tissues draining towards site and without damaging cells; if applied to eye will not smart.

Istin Trade name. See danthron.

Italian See Neapolitan.

IV Abbr. for intravenous/ly, qv.

J

jack Male ass, qv.

janet Female mule, qv.

jaundice (Fr. jaunisse, from jaune, yellow; syn. icterus) Condition in which too much bile pigment circulates in blood and is deposited in tissues and organs. Yellow colour can then be seen in mucous membranes of mouth, eye and vagina. Due to: (1) excessive breakdown of red blood cells, liberating large quantities of hemoglobin from which bile pigment is formed—as in hemolytic disease of newborn foals, swamp fever; (2) damaged liver which cannot excrete hemoglobin brought to it as a result of normal destruction of red cells—as in poisoning with ragwort, chloroform, lead, arsenic, copper, phosphorus, carbon tetrachloride or infection with bacteria or virus; (3) obstructed bile ducts leading from liver, so that pigment seeps back into blood instead of being excreted into gut—as in whiteworm infection, impacted colic or growth. See hepatitis, hemolytic jaundice, colic, poisons, hemolysis, hemoglobin.

jaw One of 2 bony structures in head, bearing teeth. **lower j.** Formed by mandibular bones and carrying lower incisor and molar teeth. **parrot j.** See parrot jaw. **upper j.** Formed by maxillary bones and carrying upper incisor and molar teeth. See also skull.

Jennet See Spanish Jennet.

jenny Female ass.

Jockey Club See Thoroughbred, veterinary rules.

joint (syn. articulation) Union of 2 or more bones capped by cartilage or other tissue. **synarthrodial j.** Bones united by fibrous tissue, bone or cartilage; no movement or joint cavity, eg skull bones, bones of pelvis. **diarthrodial j.** Bones united by a capsule, with surfaces in a cavity containing fluid and having movement. **J.** usually has smooth surfaces of dense bone or cartilage, **j.** capsule with fibrous outer covering and inner lining which secretes **j.**-oil (synovia). Ligaments may support **j.** by binding bones together. Movement of **j.** may be gliding, eg knee (carpus), angular, eg leg **j.**'s which flex and extend. Equine **j.**'s do not normally circumduct, adduct or abduct (these movements are typical of human arm). **amphiarthrodial j.** Bones directly united by cartilage and ligaments and with limited movement, eg **j.**'s between vertebrae. **j.-ill** (syns. infective arthritis, navel ill, pyemia) Erosion of joint surfaces caused by micro-organisms, Streptococci, Salmonella or E. coli. Found in foals up to 6 months and in older horses that have suffered a penetrating wound. Symptoms: painful swelling of **j.**'s especially knee, hock, stifle, hip and elbow, damaged surface either side of **j.** (probably causing lameness in later life), fever, anemia, white blood cell count above 10,000 per cu.mm., possibly abscess just inside navel. (Condition can be considered a local septicemia, qv.) Cause: in foal, organism may enter body through mouth or navel (umbilicus) and become established if immunity is low (eg due to lack of colostrum). Diagnosis: on symptoms and finding pus cells in synovial fluid. Treatment: lance and drain umbilical abscesses, inject antibiotics into joint; also small amount of cortisone or similar anti-inflammatory drug; disinfect to prevent

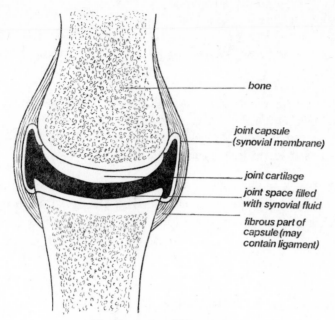

21 Knee, a gliding joint

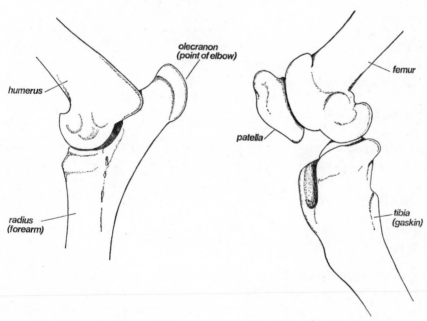

22 Elbow, a hinge joint   23 Stifle, a gliding joint

organism spreading to other foals. **j. mice** Particles of bone which break off and lie free in joint cavity. Caused by trauma or arthritis. May be responsible for lameness. Diagnosed on X-ray and should be surgically removed.

jugular (L. jugularis, jugulum, neck) Of neck, eg **j. vein** One of 2 major veins in front of body. Carry blood from head and neck and lie in furrow on either side of neck; convenient for intravenous injections and collecting blood for transfusions, laboratory analysis, etc.

Jutland Danish saddle horse developed from imported Cleveland Bays and improved with Thoroughbred blood. **J. Draught** Danish war horse of 12th century. Extinct in pure form.

K

K Chemical symbol for potassium.

kaolin (syn. China clay) White odourless tasteless powder. Given by mouth to absorb toxic substance (see poisoning) and form protective coating for mucous membranes. Dose: 50–200gms. Also used as poultice, qv.

Kathiawari Saddle horse named after peninsula on NW coast of India. Probably developed from Arab and Siwalik. Noted for in-turning ears, tips of which almost touch.

Kentucky Saddle horse See American Saddle horse.

keratin Special type of insoluble protein, which contains sulphur. Main constituent of outer layer of skin, hair and horn. See foot.

keratitis Inflamed cornea of eye. See eye, diseases of.

Kiang One of 2 sub-species of ass. Lives in Tibetan mountains, in small herds; is very shy and may be on verge of extinction. See ass.

kidney Organ which filters blood and forms urine, excreting waste products nitrogen, urea, acids and water. One either side of aorta in upper part of abdomen. Right k. shaped as playing-card heart; left k. bean-shaped. Each k. weighs about 700gms. (newborn foal about

170gms.); covered by thin fibrous capsule; consists of outer cortex containing glomeruli, qv, and inner medulla formed of collecting tubes which empty into central pelvis, drained by ureter which carries urine to bladder. **K.** functions by filtering unwanted products from blood which passes through capillaries in glomerulus in close contact with thin-walled tube (loop of Henle and collecting tubule) that carries filtered fluid. Further exchange of salts, acids and water by contact of tubes with blood vessels produces urine, which passes to ureter. **k., diseases of** (1) Infection causing abscess. See sleepy foal disease, septicemia of

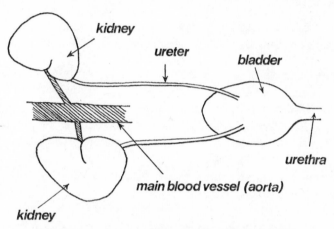

24   Kidneys, showing their relationship to bladder

newborn foal. (2) Degeneration caused by bacterial toxins and metallic poisons. (3) Damage caused by massive quantities of hemoglobin in severe setfast (qv). (4) Hemorrhage due to back injury. (5) Stones, rare but may collect in **k.** Any inflammation of **k.** cells is termed nephritis. Nephrosis is rare condition in which **k.** is waterlogged due to excess pressure if outflow of urine is blocked, eg by stone or congenital defect.

kilo- (Fr. from Gr. chilioi, thousand) Combining form used to indicate one thousand times, eg kilogram=1,000gms. See weights and measures.

Kimberley horse disease See crotalaria plants.

Kladruber Fast-disappearing Austrian/Bohemian breed, developed from Spanish Jennet. Named after place in Czechoslovakia where it is bred at Imperial Stud. An ancestor of Lippizzaner; used as carriage horse and characterised by roman nose, heavy, arched neck and high action. Breeders aim for either black or white horse of 17/18 hands. Smaller **K.** now being bred to produce dressage horse.

Klebsiella Genus of gram-negative micro-organisms (bacteria); with short rods and capsule, of tribe Escherichieae, family Enterobacteriaceae, order Eubacteriales. **K. pneumoniae** Cause of infected genital organs and spread by coitus. Occasionally responsible for abortion and septicemia of newborn, qv. Treatment: antibiotics, especially neomycin; sexual rest.

Klepper Strong, long-lived pony of Baltic regions of Estonia and Livonia. Often dun with black mane, tail and dorsal stripe.

Knabstrup Danish spotted horse (with leopard, snowflake or blanket markings) similar to Fredericksborg in all but colour. Pure form almost extinct in Denmark but colouring has been passed on to many circus horses (cf Appaloosa). Assn: British Spotted Horse Soc., c/o Miss J. Eddie, Nash End, Bisley, Stroud, Gloucestershire (Bisley 257).

knee Colloq. for carpal joint. True **k.** of horse is stifle. See carpal joint. **popped k.** See carpitis.

knock knees (syn. medial deviation of carpal joints) Condition of foal in which forelegs become concave or bowed. May straighten as foal grows. Severe cases sometimes helped by stapling, ie inserting metal staples on either side of growth plate, on inside of limb. This stops growth for limited period and allows outside of growth plate to develop.

knuckling (syns. straight in front, upright) (1) Condition of young horse in which forelegs are straight and fetlock joints permanently flexed. In severe cases animal may walk on front surface of fetlock joint. Cause is contracted flexor tendons; may be congenital or result of deficiency of calcium, phosphorus, vitamin A and/or D. Successful treatment possible only in mild cases. It consists of plaster casts and supporting bandages, correct diet and, sometimes, cutting of flexor tendons. (2) Action when horse stumbles. May result from fetlock joints which are too straight.

Konik (Polish, small horse) Polish pony; several types, one of which resembles Tarpan; others may have Arab blood. Some can change grey summer coat for white winter one.

L

lab. Abbr. laboratory.

labium (pl. labia) Fleshy border, eg l. of vulva.

laboratory (L. laboratorium, abbr. lab.) Place where investigatory tests are performed. See cross-matching, blood tests, dope test, filter, pregnancy tests.

labour Part of foaling process divided into 1st, 2nd, and 3rd stage l. See birth.

laburnum poisoning (plant Cytisus laburnum) May occur if horse eats any part of plant, especially flowers and seeds which contain alkaloid cytisine. Symptoms: excitement, inco-ordination, sweating, convulsions, coma and death from asphyxia. No specific treatment available, though anti-convulsant drugs may help.

labyrinth (Gr. labyrinthos) System of intercommunicating cavities or canals, eg in bone or internal ear. See bone, ear.

laceration (L. laceratio) Wound, tear in skin. See wound.

lacrimal (L. lacrimalis, lacrime, tear) Of tears. **l. duct** Conveys tears from eyelids to discharge them close to nostrils.

lactate (1) To secrete milk from mammary glands, qv. (2) Salt of lactic acid.

Lactobacillus Genus of micro-organism of tribe Lactobacilleae, family Lactobacillaceae, order Eubacteriales. Gram-positive anaerobic bacilli. **L. acidophilus** Bacteria present in large gut concerned in digestion. Used for re-seeding gut during diarrhoea. Foals 5gms. twice daily in feed or as small drench, adults 50gms. daily.

lactoglobulin Protein globulin in milk; normally passed by foal in urine during first 36 hours after birth.

lamella (L., dim. of lamina) Thin leaf or plate of bone.

lameness Disturbance in natural gait. Weight is unevenly distributed, in most cases so that horse can avoid as much pain as possible. **l., diagnosis of** Head and withers rise when painful foreleg meets ground; head is lowered as lame hindleg meets ground. Front limb lameness is best seen by watching head and withers; hindlimb lameness by watching horse as it moves away—point of hip on side of lame leg rises as leg meets ground. Stride of affected hindleg is shortened. **L.** is best seen at walk or trot when severe cases readily detected, but slight l. may require considerable experience. After identifying lame leg, find site of pain by (1) palpation (pressure by fingers or metal pincers over foot), (2) manipulation (flexing of joints and firm but forced retraction and extension of various parts of limb), (3) feeling for swellings and heat. Special techniques include radiography (X-ray), withdrawal and analysis of synovial fluid from joints, faradic stimulation of muscles (see physiotherapy) and nerve block, qv. **l., cause of** Painful inflammatory reaction in part of limb. Origin may be (1) traumatic, as in sprains, strains, (2) infection, especially abscess in foot, local or general lymphangitis, (3) entry of foreign body, eg nail, thorn, etc in foot or higher in leg. Inflammation may affect joint surfaces and their capsules (arthritis and capsulitis) or ligaments that support joint; tendons (tendonitis) or sheaths (tenosynovitis) through which they pass; the lining of bones (periostitis); bones themselves (osteitis); lamina of pedal bone (laminitis), muscles (myositis) and bursae between muscle or tendon and bone (bursitis). Inflammation always follows consistent pattern, ie escape of small quantities of blood and fluid, due to tearing of muscle, tendon, ligament, capsule, etc, followed by increased flow of blood to part, degree of swelling and pain. Fractures produce special inflammatory reaction resulting in formation of a callus, ie bridge of new bone uniting fractured parts. If fracture involves a major weight-bearing bone, eg cannon, femur or humerus, immobilisation of the ends may be impossible and healing cannot occur. In other bones, eg pastern, splint or sesamoid, union between fractured parts may be partial or complete. See carpitis, corn, curb, capped elbow, gravel, hock (capped) joint, navicular disease, osselet, ringbone, sand cracks, bucked shin, sidebone, bruised sole, spavin, bog spavin, splint, bowed tendons, windgall. **l., treatment of** Remove cause if possible, control and further the inflammatory process. Apply heat and cold alternately, massage, inject anti-inflammatory drugs. See physiotherapy. Rest is essential for most injuries although exercise may help muscle injuries.

laminae Velvety membrane or sheet containing fine leaf-like projections. **sensitive l.** Membrane lining pedal bone of foot and interlocking with insensitive l. (a similar membrane attached to hoof wall but unlike sensitive l. does not contain blood vessels). Together these structures bind hoof to bone. See laminitis, seedy toe, foot.

laminitis Inflamed sensitive laminae of hoof, characterised by heat and pain causing severe lameness. Usually present in more than one foot. Thought to be due to allergy (qv), to protein as a result of overfeeding with rich food or infection of uterus or disturbed alimentary canal. Exact way condition develops is not known, possibily due to effect of histamine on blood vessels in membrane (lamina) lining pedal bone. Most common in horses fed grain or on rich pasture. Symptoms: acute pain, sweating, increased heart rate and respiration, sometimes raised temperature; standing with feet bunched together under body with head low and back arched. Usually difficult to get horse to move and then gait is shuffling. Horses usually lie down and have difficulty getting up. There is marked heat and pain on pressure on the hoof. Disease often leads to separation of hoof wall from sensitive laminae, horn crumbles (see seedy toe) and pedal bone may drop through sole. (See plate 16.) Cases that recover develop concave hoof walls with horizontal ridges. Treatment: antihistamine, anti-inflammatory and pain relieving drugs, eg corticosteroids and phenylbutazone; reduced diet and forced exercise.

lampas Swelling and hardening of mucous membrane lining hard palate immediately behind upper incisors. Sometimes forms prominent, inflamed ridge but, contrary to popular belief, condition is not significant.

Lancefield classification Classification of hemolytic Streptococci into groups A to N, based on precipitin test. Those in group C important in equine diseases. See Streptococci.

Lanoxin Trade name. See digoxin.

laparo- (Gr. lapara, flank) Combining form meaning relationship to flank or abdomen.

laparotomy (laparo- + Gr. tome, a cutting) Surgical incision through flank or abdomen as in caesarian section, qv. **exploratory l.** Opening of

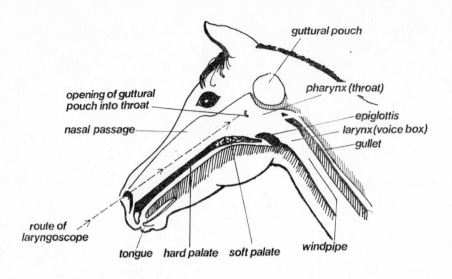

25 The way a laryngoscope is used to see voice box

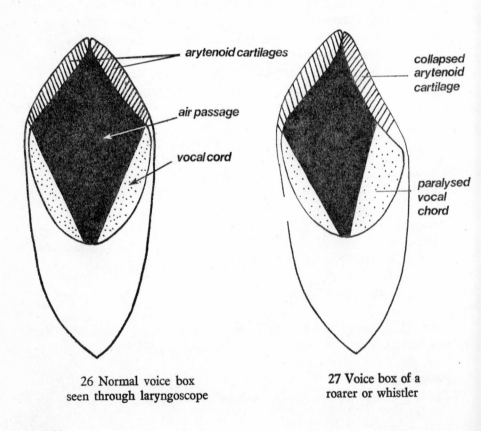

26 Normal voice box
seen through laryngoscope

27 Voice box of a
roarer or whistler

abdomen in colic or other condition to confirm diagnosis by direct examination of viscera.

Largactil Trade name. See chlorpromazine.

larva (pl. larvae) Young or immature stage in life history of insect or parasite, eg redworm l., whiteworm l. **migrating l.** Young parasite travelling through body.

laryngeal Of larynx (voice box). **l. paralysis** Condition when muscles controlling arytenoid cartilage and vocal cords of larynx are paralysed. Usually results in horse whistling/roaring. **l. prosthesis** Modification of Hobday operation, qv.

laryngismus (L., Gr. laryngismos, a whooping) Spasm of larynx.

laryngitis Inflamed larynx.

laryngoscope (laryngo- + Gr. skopein, to view) Flexible or straight tube containing lights and mirrors. Used by inserting into nostril, to get direct view of voice box (larynx).

laryngotomy (laryngo- + Gr. tome, a cutting) Surgical incision of larynx. See Hobday.

larynx See voice box.

Lasix Trade name. See frusemide.

lateral cartilages Cartilages partly fibrous tissue and partly hyaline cartilage. They are attached to wings of pedal bone and form bulbs of heel.

lateral gait See gait.

Latvian Heavy Russian horse developed from Zemaitukas, Oldenburg, Ardennes (Swedish) and Finnish draught. Have been used as heavy-weight hunters. **L. harness horse** Heavy-weight whose trotting ability is encouraged. Bred mainly on **L.** state farms.

laxative Mild purgative, eg liquid paraffin, glycerine.

lead (1) Term used in electrocardiography to describe position of recording tracing, eg **l. one** (I) in which electrodes are on left and right forelimbs, **l. two** (II) on right foreleg and left hindleg and **l. three** (III) on left foreleg and left hindleg. See electrocardiogram. (2) Chemical symbol Pb. Metallic element. **l. poisoning** Caused by chewing painted objects or grazing pasture near l. works. Metal is absorbed from alimentary tract and passes to liver. From here it is excreted back to gut in bile and, via kidneys, to urine and in lactating mares, to the milk. It is also taken up by bones, heart, lungs, muscle and brain. Symptoms: convulsions, staggering, muscular spasms, dullness, abdominal pain and constipation, followed by diarrhoea, weight-loss, swelling of limbs, gradual paralysis of hind legs, larynx and pharynx, causing shallow breathing or roaring. Tiny granules of l. sulphide may cause band of blue/black colour in gums. Diagnosis: on symptoms and l. in blood and feces. At post-mortem: typical smell on opening carcase, dirty grey/red muscles. Liver shows fatty degeneration. Poisoning is confirmed if there are more than 25 parts per million of l. in kidneys and 10 p.p.m. in liver. Treatment: give saline purgatives, soluble sulphates, sodium sulphate, magnesium sulphate by mouth; and calcium disodium versenate sub. cut.

lecithin (Gr. lekithos, yolk of egg) Acid containing phosphorus found in nerve tissue, semen, yolk of egg, bile and blood.

Ledercort veterinary Trade name. See triamcinolone.

leg A front or hindlimb, more usually termed foreleg, hindleg.

length Measurement of distance. **crown to rump l.** Measurement from head to rump of fetus, qv. See weights and measures.

lens Glass or transparent substance shaped to converge or scatter rays of light. See eye.

leptospirosis Acute disease characterised by increasing hemolytic anemia caused by Leptospira pomona and L. icterohemorrhagica. Symptoms: fever, fluctuating temperature, loss of appetite, depression, jaundice. Recovery may be followed by relapses. Diagnosis: upon hematological examination of blood. Treatment: inject penicillin and streptomycin. See also eye, diseases of: moon blindness.

lesion (L. laesio, laedere, to hurt) Pathological damage or abnormal condition of tissue, may be visible to naked eye (macroscopic) or only through microscope (microscopic).

leucocyte (from Gr. kytos, cell) See white blood cell.

leucocytosis Increased number of leucocytes in blood (normal level: 5–10,000 per cu.mm.). Indicates infection with micro-organisms or parasites.

leucopenia (leucocyte + Gr. penia, poverty) Condition when white cells in blood fall below 5,000 per cu.mm.; may be caused by infection with arteritis virus or radiation overdose. Cf leucocytosis.

levamisole hydrochloride (trade name: Nemicide) Liquid drug for treating lungworm and gastroenteritis caused by parasites.

levo- (L. laevus, left) Combining form meaning towards left (opp. dextro-).

libido Sexual drive. Increases in both sexes in natural breeding season, ie late spring and early summer. Can be artificially boosted with hormones, or lighting. See pituitary.

Lieberkühn glands (after German anatomist Johann L.) Glands in small intestine, producing digestive juice.

ligament Band of fibrous tissue connecting bones or supporting organs.

TABLE OF LIGAMENTS

Important l.'s are:

ligamentum nuchae	extends from poll to withers helps to support head
round l. of hip joint	secures head of femur to pelvis
broad l. of uterus	membrane suspending uterus from roof of abdomen
check l. superior and inferior	see stay apparatus (and for sesamoidean l.'s, suspensory l.)

ligation (L. ligatio) Application of ligature.

ligature (L. ligatura) Band, cord or fine thread for tying blood vessel. Cf stitch.

light Electromagnetic force having velocity of about 186,284 miles per second. See infrared, ultraviolet, pituitary gland.

lignocaine hydrochloride White crystalline powder with slightly bitter taste, followed by local numbness. Used in general anaesthesia, with adrenaline, and in ointment to lubricate catheters for insertion into bladder or other sensitive area.

Limousin Heavy, late-maturing French saddle horse; developed from English Thoroughbred. Now dying out.

lingula (pl. lingulae) Small, tongue-like structure, eg front part of cerebellum (see brain).

liniment Fluid preparation which has oily, soapy or alcoholic base, applied externally with friction.

linseed oil Oil from seeds of Linum usitatissimum. Yellowish-brown liquid with characteristic odour and bland taste. Used as laxative to treat impacted colic and occasionally tapeworms. Now largely replaced by other treatments. Dose: 0.25–1 litre. See danthron, colic.

lint (L. linteum from linum, flat) Absorbent dressing.

lipoma Fatty tumour. See growth.

Lippizzaner Proud-looking but tractable breed almost always grey, famous for dressage at Spanish Riding School, Vienna. Developed in Austria (stud founded 1580s) and later (1780s–World War II) at Babolna Stud near Bana, N Hungary. L. developed from Kladruber, N Italian horse and, later, Arab.

liquid paraffin Transparent colourless, odourless and tasteless oily liquid. Bland laxative used to soften and lubricate feces in treatment of meconium retention and colic. Dose: adult $\frac{1}{2}$–1 litre, foal about 200ml. By enema: 100–200ml. See meconium retention; colic.

liquorice Dry root of species Glycyrrhiza. Powdered l. is buff or yellow with characteristic odour and taste. Used to disguise taste of medicine. Dose: 30–60gms.

lithiasis Condition in which calculi form. See stones.

lithotomy (litho- + Gr. tome, a cutting) Surgical removal of stone from duct or organ. See stones.

Lithuanian heavy draught Horse bred on same lines as Latvian (qv). Believed to date from 1870 when Zhmud Horse Breeding Soc. was formed to cross this horse with Ardennes (Swedish).

litre Unit of capacity in metric system; volume occupied by 1kg. of pure water. See weights and measures.

liver (L. jecur, Gr. hepar) Largest gland in body capable of over 100 different functions; weighs about 5kg. in adult, lies in abdomen between diaphragm, stomach and intestines; divided into right, middle and left lobe. It is supplied by arteries, veins, nerves and lymph channels and has bile duct which carries bile to duodenum. (Horse has no gall-bladder) L. of newborn foal relatively large, with ratio to body wt. of 1:35 compared to 1:100 in adult. L. stores sugar in form of glycogen; converts amino-acids to protein; stores fat and vitamin A; transforms substances into simpler or more complex ones, thus protecting body against poisons; copes with drugs and synthesises carbohydrate and fat; forms blood proteins, albumin and globulin; regulates blood's concentration of fat, sugar, amino-acids and other nutrients and produces bile including bilirubin, waste product formed in breakdown of hemoglobin. L. made up of minute cells arranged in sheets, between which blood circulates freely. Between adjacent sheets are tiny canals into which bile is secreted; these join together to deliver bile to intestine in common bile duct. Each l. cell therefore has contact with blood on one side and bile canals on the other. Section of l. examined under microscope shows cells arranged in lobules which form columns radiating towards central vein. This receives blood that has passed between the sheets of l. cells and carries it to the great veins of the heart. l. biopsy See biopsy. l., **diseases of** See cirrhosis; jaundice; abortion, viral; swamp fever; tuberculosis; ragwort.

lobe (L. lobus, Gr. lobos) Defined portion of organ, eg anterior l. of pituitary.

local (L. localis) Of a restricted part of area, eg l. anaesthesia. See anaesthesia, nerve block.

lochia (Gr. lochia) Chocolate-coloured discharge from uterus after foaling, composed of blood and uterine secretions. Exercise helps evacuation.

lockjaw (syn. tetanus) Horrific disease caused by Clostridium tetani, an anaerobic bacterium which lives in soil and body tissues away from oxygen (in abscesses, beneath scabs or in alimentary tract). Germ produces toxin which causes spasm of muscles (tetanic spasms). Symptoms: stiffness, rigid limbs and neck as flexor and extensor muscles contract at same time (spasm is brought on by noise or contact with skin), difficult jaw movement and swallowing, head thrust forward, ears pricked, tail raised and difficulty in getting up. Diagnosis: on signs of gradually increasing intensity, characteristic stance, spasm of 3rd eyelid when face is gently tapped with finger. Incubation period 5–21 days; foals particularly at risk in first 6 weeks because bacteria can enter through the umbilicus. Older animals may be infected through wounds, especially on legs, which become contaminated with soil and dung. Treatment: see mephenesin. Prevention: antitetanic serum gives immunity for about 30 days. Vaccination with tetanus toxoid provides lasting immunity but needs annual booster injection. See tetanus toxoid.

locomotion (L. locus, place, + movere, to move). Movement, as in walking.

locomotor Of locomotion.

Lorexane Trade name. See gamma benzene hexachloride.

lotion (L. lotio) Liquid used for washing. See wound.

louse (L. pediculus; pl. lice) Skin parasite of phylum Arthropoda, class Insecta, order Pthiroptera. Some suck blood (sucking l.). Others chew. (biting l.). They have small flat wingless bodies. Lice that live on horses: Damalinia equi (formerly known as Bovicola equi or

Trichodectes equi, found in Australia and belong to sub-order Mallophaga, biting lice); Haematopinus asini (sub-order Siphunculata, sucking lice and, common in UK, sub-order Anoplura). Eggs are laid on skin, hatch in 20 days and are killed by dry heat. Sucking lice cause irritation and loss of hair. Diagnosis is easy on warm days when the parasites are active, particularly around mane and tail. Treatment: see gamma benzene hexachloride.

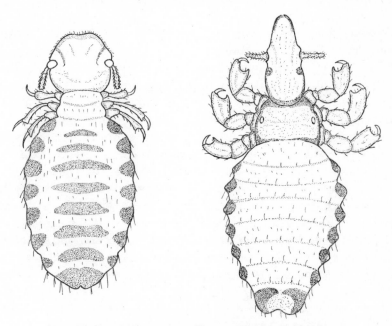

28 (*left*) Biting louse (Damalinia equi) and sucking louse (Haematopinus asini)

lucern (medicago sativa) poisoning Ingestion of plant can cause photo-sensitisation and liver disease associated with jaundice, dark-coloured urine and wasting. See poisons, liver.

lumbar Of the back. **l. vertebra** See skeleton, vertebrae.

lumen Cavity or channel inside a tube, eg l. of alimentary canal.

Lundy pony Hardy, thick-skinned animal which runs wild on **L.** island, in Bristol Channel. Thought to have developed from mainland's native ponies, particularly New Forest and Galloway.

lung (L. pulmo, Gr. pneumon) One of 2 breathing organs in chest. It brings air into close contact with blood stream for exchange of gases. As chest expands and contracts air is drawn down and up windpipe, into and out of l. Air passes through smaller tubes (bronchi and bronchioles) into many millions of minute air sacs (alveoli). Capillaries in alveolar walls expose blood for exchange of oxygen and carbon dioxide. L. is divided into apical, cardiac and diaphragmatic lobes. See broken wind, percussion, pneumonia.

lungworm Nematode parasite of the order Strongyloidea, family Metastrongylidae. Slender roundworm living in air passages of lungs where it lays eggs. These are coughed up and swallowed. L. is host-specific; type affecting horses and donkeys is Dictyocaulus arnfieldi, which has a direct life history and does not require intermediate host. Male is about 36mm. (1½ins.) long and female 60mm. (2½ins.). The swallowed eggs pass out in feces, where they hatch and are picked up by another host. The larvae bore through intestinal wall, to mesenteric lymph nodes, and enter lymph stream. Venous blood carries them to heart, through right ventricle, to lungs. Here they develop into adults and lay eggs, completing the cycle. They irritate and inflame bronchi (causing bronchitis, coughing and pneumonia) and the larvae cause diarrhoea. (Donkey can carry large numbers without showing symptoms, so should not graze with horses unless checked.) Treatment: see diethylcarbamazine citrate, levamisole hydrochloride.

Lusitano Attractive, lightly-built Portuguese breed, possibly descended from Minho. About 15 hands, often grey and frequently used in Portuguese bullfighting.

lutein (L. luteus, yellow) Hormone which causes formation of corpus luteum (yellow body) in ovary after ovulation.

luteinising hormone (LH) Hormone produced by anterior lobe of pituitary gland. Acts on ovaries of mare causing rupture of ripe follicle (ovulation); and on testes in colt stimulating them to produce male sex hormone testosterone.

Lutormone Trade name. See chorionic gonadotrophin.

lymph (L. lympha, water) Transparent, slightly yellow liquid present in lymphatic vessels. **l. gland** (syn. node) See lymphatic system.

lymphadenitis (lymph- + Gr. aden, gland + -itis) Inflamed lymph nodes. See gland.

lymphangitis (L. lympha, lymph; syn. Monday morning leg) Inflamed lymphatic vessels and usually lymph nodes (lymphadenitis). Characterised by hot, painful swellings beneath skin, especially in legs. Caused by infection, which enters through skin, injury to lymph channels which become blocked, or overloading of lymph stream due to excess feed. There is chronic inflammation of vessel walls and abscesses may develop, discharging serum. Fibrous tissue may form beneath skin, causing chronic thickening. Specific diseases in which l. occurs are glanders, epizootic l., ulcerative l. See separate headings, also lymph glands and plate 39.

lymphatic system System of thin-walled channels similar to veins, but without valves. Channels contain fluid consisting of water, protein, fat and small number of cells (lymphocytes). Channels start as blind-ended tubes in extremities, organs, muscles etc; by joining with others they form network, becoming larger nearer point where they enter blood stream close to heart. They drain tissue fluid and are essential part of body's fluid balance, transport system (see blood) and defence mechanism (see immunity, lymphocyte). **l. gland (node)** Structure at intervals in lymph channels. Acts as filter and contains large number of lymphocytes. Gland is responsible for producing protective substances (antibodies) and preventing microbes spreading through body. Becomes swollen and inflamed (lymphadenitis) and may be seat of abscess when infection occurs at point of body which they drain, eg pastern area may affect **l.g. in groin** (of hindleg) or axilla (foreleg). L.g.'s which can be felt if swollen: between branches of lower jaw (sub-maxillary), near ear (parotid), near throat (pharyngeal), in front of shoulder (pre-scapular) and inside thigh (femoral). Internally l.g.'s mostly affected by infection are those associated with drainage of lungs and intestine. See lymphangitis, sinusitis, strangles.

lysis (Gr., a losing, setting free) Destruction or decomposition of cells, eg hemolysis, l. of red blood cells.

M

μ (pronounced mew) Abbr. micron. See abbreviations, virus.

MA Abbr. Master of Arts.

magnesium carbonate White granular odourless tasteless powder. Heavy and light forms. Used as antacid in foals. Dose 2–12gms. **m. hydroxide** White odourless tasteless powder, used as antacid in foals. Dose: 2.5–5gms. **m. oxide** White odourless slightly alkaline-tasting powder, used in heavy and light forms as antacid. Dose: foals, 2–12gms. **m. sulphate** (syn. epsom salts) Colourless odourless crystals with salty taste. Used as purgative. Dose: 30–120gms. given with a lot of water. Unreliable action in horses. **m. trisilicate** White odourless tasteless powder. Used as absorbent and antacid to treat diarrhoea. Dose: foals, 1–6gms.

mal (Fr., L. malum, ill) Disease. **m. de caderas** Weakening disease causing staggering. Occurs in horses, mules, sheep, goats and cattle in S. America. Caused by Trypanosoma equinum and spread by tabanid and stable flies. **m. de coit** See dourine. **m. de zousfana** Algerian form of surra, qv.

maladjustment Failure to adapt to environment, as in **m.** of newborn foal (see neonatal maladjustment syndrome).

male Masculine sex, ie stallion, colt (colloq. horse). Castrated **m.** is a gelding, qv. **m. genital organs** Two testes, their ducts (vas deferentia), the urethra, penis and accessory glands (prostate, seminal vesicles and bulbo-urethral glands). **m. sexual behaviour** See behaviour.

malformation (L. malus, evil + formatio, a forming) Abnormal development. See cleft palate, conformation, parrot jaw.

malignant (L. malignans, acting maliciously) Disease or condition with tendency to become worse. **m. oedema** Acute infection of wounds caused by organisms of the soil, notably Clostridium septicum, Clostridium chauvei. Infection causes swellings (that contain air and froth which exudes from the wound), high fever, depression and death in 24–48 hours. Not common in horses. **m. tumour** Growth that spreads. See growth.

mallein/m. test (L. malleus, glanders) Extract of bacteria Loefflerella mallei used to diagnose glanders, qv. Types (1) 1ml. of dilute **m.** injected under skin, body temperature recorded every 3 hours between 12–24 hours. Positive reaction indicated by plaque round site of injection and rise of temperature to 39.5°C. (103.1°F.). (2) 0.1ml. of concentrated **m.** injected into lower eyelid. Positive reaction indicated by swelling 24–48 hours later.

Malleomyces mallei Syn. for causal organism of glanders, qv.

malnutrition Bad nutrition or feeding. See food.

malposition (L. malus, bad + positio, placement) Abnormal position of fetus. See dystocia.

Mammalia Division of vertebrate animals possessing hair and suckling their young; includes horse. See evolution.

mammary glands (syns. udder, bag) Two modified skin glands between mare's hindlegs on either side of mid-line. Each gland is a short flaccid cone consisting of a glandular mass or body and a teat (papilla) in which there are usually two small openings. Swell in last 4 weeks of pregnancy and may run milk (lactate) before birth of foal. Abortion or death of one twin may trigger off lactation. See birth, colostrum, plate 35.

Mangalarga Breed developed in Brazil, about 100 years ago, from an Alter stallion imported from Portugal. Later improved with Andalusian blood. **M.** is heavy variation of Criollo found throughout S America.

mange Infective skin condition caused by mites of order Acarina. **chorioptic m.** (syns. foot **m.**/itchy leg) Caused by Chorioptes equi, found in fetlock and pastern region; especially common on horses with long feathers, qv. Scabs appear, horse stamps its feet and rubs, scratches or bites affected region. Diagnosis: on parasites found in scab. Treatment: clip hairs from affected area and apply gamma benzene hexachloride. **demodectic m.** Scaly or pustular skin condition caused by Demodex folliculorum, a mite which lives in hair follicles or sebaceous glands of skin or in miebomiam glands of eye. Infection is spread by contact. Treat with gamma benzene hexachloride. **psoroptic m.** Caused by Psoroptes communis var. equi, mites which burrow into skin causing thick, heavy scabs. **sarcoptic m.** Caused by Sarcoptes scabiei var. equi. Mites enter skin, causing thickened areas where females lay eggs. These hatch in 25 days and larvae either stay in their burrows or make new ones at an angle. (Larvae moult and become nymphs which form further burrows.) Mites feed on tissue fluid and skin cells, causing small itchy red blisters. Hairs fall out leaving bald patches. Infection is by contact and infected bedding or grooming tools. **S.m.** is a notifiable disease (see veterinary rules). Diagnosis: on recovery and identification of mite. Treatment: see benzene hexachloride, gamma benzene hexachloride. Burn, or thoroughly disinfect, any contaminated material, such as bedding and grooming kit.

Manipur Pony bred in **M.** state of Assam. Reputed to date from 7th century, when used for polo. Probably has Mongolian and Arab blood (has Arab-like flared nostrils). About 12 hands.

mare hemorrhage See birth hemorrhage.

Marinol Trade name. See benzalkonium chloride solution.

marking Mark on horse. (1) Shape and/or position of white hairs in darker coat. (2) Arrangement of hairs, eg whorl. (3) Anatomical **m.**, eg prophet's thumb mark (see depression). **m.**'s include: blaze (down face, ie from between eyes to muzzle), hammer spots (dark spotting in brown coat, most common over quarters), sock (on pastern), star (centre of forehead), stocking (hock or knee down to hoof), flesh mark, wall eye, saddle or girth **m. m. certificate** (Thoroughbred) Paper containing diagrams of head, muzzle, left and right side of horse on which veterinarian draws horse's **m.**'s. Description of **m.**'s must be anatomically correct, eg white extending a third of the way up cannon; or flesh mark between nostrils, touching left one and entering right. Certificate must be sent to Weatherbys (see Thoroughbred) to register foal, name yearling etc. Also included in horse's passport.

marrow Red or yellow soft material in central cavity of long bones (cannon, radius, etc). Consists of fat, blood vessels, and blood-containing spaces (sinusoids). Red **m.** forms red blood cells (erthrocytes), a process known as erythropoiesis. Megaloblast is cell in wall of sinusoid which is forerunner of mature red cell; intermediate stages: early and late erythroblasts which possess nucleus and in which hemoglobin appears for first time, normoblast which contains full amount of hemoglobin, reticulocyte without nucleus and finally red cell. Horse **m.** can be obtained for diagnosis by inserting special needle into **m.** cavity at point of hip (see pelvis).

Martindale, The Extra Pharmacopoeia Book listing drugs, their actions and uses. Published by the Pharmaceutical Press. Cf British Veterinary Codex.

Marwari Indian war horse of middle ages, now saddle horse similar in ancestry and characteristics to Kathiawari, qv.

massage See physiotherapy.

mastitis Inflamed mammary glands or udder. Caused by infection, especially with Streptococcus. One or both glands become enlarged, firm and painful with cord-like swelling along abdomen as lymphatics become blocked. Diagnosis: on examination of milk for presence of pus cells and bacteria; condition must be distinguished from enlargements due to foal going off suck after weaning. Treatment: strip gland, insert ointment containing appropriate antibiotic such as penicillin and inject antibiotic.

masturbation (L. manus, hand + stuprare, to rape) Self manipulation of penis when horse rubs erect penis on underside of belly. Thought to have adverse effect on training programme and increase risk of unsuccessful coitus. Treatment: some horsemen advocate use of pollution ring, ie ring of material and/or rubber/metal fitted on to sheath. This causes slight pain if horse tries to draw (achieve penile erection).

Masuren Polish name for Trakehner horses, some of which were taken from East Prussians after World War II.

matching See blood tests, cross-matching.

mate To put mare and stallion together for coitus. See behaviour.

mater (lit. mother) Anatomical term for a protecting membrane. See dura **m.**, pia **m.**

materia medica Branch of medical science dealing with source, use and preparation of drugs. See British Veterinary Codex.

maternal (L. maternus, mater, mother) Of the mother, eg **m.** instincts (see behaviour), **m.** blood stream (see placenta).

mating (Ger. mat, companion) (1) Act of coitus or covering. (2) Selecting horses for breeding. See semen.

matrix Material surrounding cells, as in bone and cartilage.

mature (L. maturus) State of having reached full development.

maturity Age of attaining maximum development. **m. of bone** Indicates particular bone has completed its growth. **fetal m.** Length of gestation and ability of foal to live outside uterus. Between 300 and 325 days' gestation foal is premature, after that, immature until considered mature at 340 days. **skeletal m.** Shows all bones have stopped growing (at about 5 years). **sexual m.** Age of attaining capacity to breed. See puberty.

maxilla Irregularly-shaped bone that forms upper jaw. See skull.

maxillary sinus One of four pairs of air sinuses. Extends backwards to line in front of the eye. Floor is formed by bony plates surrounding last three cheek teeth. It is divided into front and back compartment and communicates with frontal sinus through a large oval opening. See skull.

MB, BS Abbr. Bachelor of Medicine and Science.

MCH Abbr. mean corpuscular hemoglobin, ie average hemoglobin content of a red blood cell. Measured in one thousandth of a microgram by dividing hemoglobin in grams per litre of blood by the number of red cells in millions per cubic mm. (normal range 12–18).

MCHC Abbr. mean corpuscular hemoglobin concentration, ie average hemoglobin concentration per cent expressed as amount of hemoglobin as a percentage of red cells ie hemoglobin in gm. per 100ml. blood divided by packed cell volume, × 100 (normal range 28–35%).

MCV Abbr. mean corpuscular volume (average volume of individual red blood cell) determined by packed cell volume divided by number of red cells in millions per cubic mm. × 10 and expressed in cubic microns (normal range 38–50 cμ).

mebendazole (trade name: Telmin) Drug similar to thiabendazole, qv.

Mecklenburg Heavy, German, warm-blooded saddle horse. Evolved from heavier, cold-blooded, military **M.**

meconium (L., Gr. mekonion) Feces stored in colon, caecum and rectum of fetus and usually expelled only after birth. Brown, black or green, hard or soft pellets, with slimy covering. Voided during first 3 days of life and followed by yellow milk dung. May be passed in utero due to asphyxia or illness. Foal is then born with coat saturated with **m.** and amniotic fluid stained brown. See birth, neonatal maladjustment syndrome. **m. retention** (syns. stoppage, ileus) Inability to void **m.** easily. Symptoms, in the first 3 days: rolling, straining, lying in awkward postures (head turned back, foreleg over head), refusing to suck, distended abdomen due to gas in intestine. Treatment: inject pain relieving drugs, give enema (qv) and liquid paraffin (200–300ml.) by stomach tube.

medicine (L. medicina) Drug or remedy; science of healing. **clinical m.** Applied in practice rather than in laboratory or institute. **equine m.** That applied to horses. **experimental m.** Investigation of disease based on experiments. **forensic m.** That relating to legality. **preventive m.** That which prevents disease. **proprietary m.** Drug or remedy manufactured under a trade name (see manufacturers' list at back of dictionary). **veterinary m.** Science and treatment of animal diseases.

mega- (Gr. megas, big, great) Unit of measurement 1 million times basic unit, eg 1 mega of penicillin is 1 million times 1 unit.

Megimide Trade name. See bemegride sodium.

meiosis (Gr.) A halving of inherited material in sex cells (sperm and egg) so that new individual receives equal amount of material from each parent. Each cell in horse contains 64 chromosomes (diploid number); but each sex cell contains 32 chromosomes (haploid number). After fertilisation haploid number is restored in new individual (zygote). Cf mitosis.

melanin (Gr. melas, black) Dark pigment of skin, hair, growth or eye. Grey horses may have deposits of **m.** in skin, especially under tail, size of walnut.

melanoma See growth.

membrane Layer of tissue covering a surface or dividing a space. See also mucous **m.**

menaphthone sodium bisulphite (trade name: Vitavel K) White crystalline odourless powder: synthetic water-soluble vitamin K. Essential for coagulation of blood, antidote to dicoumarol and rat poisons.

Mendel's law (after Gregor Johann **M.**, 1822–84) Particular trait or characteristic passed to offspring from one or other parent by dominant or recessive unit of inheritance (gene), eg active temperament said to be more easily transmitted (dominant) than passive one. See behaviour, coat colouring, gene.

meningeal Of meninges.

meninges (Gr., sing. meninx, membrane) Three membranes enveloping brain and spinal cord, ie dura mater, arachnoid, pia mater.

meningitis (Gr. meninx, membrane + -itis) Inflamed outer lining of brain (meninges) caused by infection with bacteria, virus or protozoa. Symptoms: gross disturbance in behaviour, eg circling, convulsions, paralysis, loss of consciousness, pushing against objects. Usually associated with inflammation of brain itself. See encephalomyelitis, borna disease, dourine, septicemia, surra.

mephenesin (trade names: Myanesin, Tolseram) Drug, used in human medicine, which Australian workers have found useful to lessen spasms in, eg, lockjaw. Dose: up to 15gms. 3 times a day.

mephyramine maleate White bitter-tasting odourless powder. Antihistamine and local anaesthetic drug used in allergic conditions and laminitis, lymphangitis and pulmonary oedema. Dose: 10–30ml. of 5% solution IM.

mercuric iodide See red mercuric iodide.

mercury poisoning Caused by eating cereals treated with mercurial compounds to prevent fungal growth. Symptoms: gastroenteritis, diarrhoea, shock, collapse and death. Chronic cases may develop inflamed mouth and kidneys. Treatment: corticosteroids and saline IV.

merocrine (mero- + Gr. krinein, to separate) Partly secreting; gland in which cells remain intact and discharge secretion, as salivary and pancreatic glands. Cf apocrine, holocrine. See gland.

mesenteric (Gr. mesenterikos) Of the mesentery.

mesentery Membranous fold of peritoneum (qv) which suspends organs and alimentary canal from body wall.

mesoderm (meso- + Gr. derma, skin) Middle layer of 3 main layers (germ or germinal layers) of embryo, lies between ectoderm and endoderm; forms connective tissue, bone, cartilage, muscle, blood vessels, lymphatics, nervous tissue, epithelium of pleura, pericardium, peritoneum, kidney and sex organs. Cf ectoderm, endoderm.

metabolism (Gr. metaballein, to change) General body changes in normal life; process by which energy is made available to body; affected by hormone thyroxine, qv. Cf anabolism, catabolism.

metabolite Substance produced by metabolism.

metacarpal Of metacarpus. **m. bones** Those forming front cannon and splint bones; the third **m.b.** (cannon) is strong, long bone taking weight of limb; the second and fourth **m.b.'s** are thin, elongated bones. See splint.

metacarpus (meta- + Gr. karpos, wrist) Part of leg between carpus (knee) and phalanx (pastern), ie cannon bone.

metamorphosis (meta- + Gr. morphosis, a shaping, bringing into shape) Change of shape or structure, eg fatty **m.**, infiltration of fat into cells or tissues.

metaphysis (meta- + Gr. phyein, to grow) Wider part of extremity of shaft of long bone, adjacent to epiphysis. See growth plate, bone.

metastasis (meta- + Gr. stasis, stand; pl. metastases) Spread of disease from one part to another, ie from a primary to a secondary focus. Characteristic of malignant tumours (in which secondary growths form in organs and tissues as a result of spread by blood or lymph streams); in bacterial infection (causing secondary abscesses, eg foal with abscess at umbilicus and others in liver, muscles, etc). See growth, joint-ill.

metatarsal Of metatarsus. **m. bones** 3 bones; hind cannon and inner and outer splint bones.

metatarsus (meta- + Gr. tarsos, tarsus) Area between hock and fetlock joint in hindleg.

metazoan Organism belonging to phylum Metazoa. Has multicellular body and includes all animal life above single-cell protozoa.

methoxhexitone sodium (trade name: Brietal Sodium) Short-acting barbiturate used for anaesthesia. Lasts 3–8 minutes after injection into vein. Used to cast horse before inserting tube into windpipe to give gaseous anaesthetic. Dose: 5mg./kg. body wt. IV. See anaesthesia.

methylprednisolone acetate (trade name: Depo-Medrone) Type of cortisone, qv.

Metis trotter See Orlov.

metre (Gr. metron, measure) Basic unit of linear measurement in metric system equivalent to 39.37 inches. See weights and measures.

metriphonate (trade names: Trichlorphon, Dyvon) White crystalline powder with characteristic odour. Effective against wide range of external parasites. Used to treat warble fly, qv.

metritis (Gr. metra, womb + -itis) Inflamed inner lining of uterus, characterised by discharge from vagina and which, in severe cases, may collect on thighs and hocks. Caused by infection with bacteria, mainly Streptococcus, E. coli, Klebsiella pneumoniae, Staphylococcus, Pseudomonas aerogenes or by fungus. Predisposing causes include abnormal entry of air into genital tract due to poor conformation of vulva; the after-effects of pregnancy and birth, or dysfunction of hormonal glands. Treatment: infuse antibiotics into uterus and inject sub. cut., eliminate predisposing causes. See Caslick, endometritis.

mg. abbr. for milligram. See weights and measures.

micro- (Gr. mikros, small) (1) Combining form meaning small. (2) In measuring, indicates a millionth, eg microgram, a millionth of a gram.

microbe (micro- + Gr. bios, life) Minute living organism; micro-organism, eg bacteria, fungus, virus.

microbic Of microbe.

microbiology (micro- + Gr. bios, life + -logy) Science of micro-organisms, including bacteria, fungi, viruses.

Micrococcaceae Family of Schizomycetes (order Eubacteriales) consisting of spherical cells, eg Staphylococcus, qv.

micron Abbr. μ. Measurement of size 1 millionth of a metre, ie 1 thousandth of a millimetre.

micro-organism (syn. germ) Any microscopic living organism, usually a bacterium, fungus or virus and capable of causing infection. See bacteria, fungus, virus.

microscope (micro- + Gr. skopein, to view) Instrument containing system of lenses; gives enlarged image of extremely small objects and reveals details of histological structures. **electron m.** One in which an **e.** beam forms image on fluorescent screen. Used for magnification many times greater than light **m.** Instrument rare and expensive. **light m.** Usual type of **m.** which uses light.

microsphere Minute radio-active particle which can be injected into a vein or artery and monitored, with a geiger-counter, to measure spread of radio-activity, thereby indicating course of blood stream. See iodine I_{131}.

microwave Short, electromagnetic wave of high frequency. See **physiotherapy**.

micturate (L. micturire, to urinate) To urinate or (colloq.) stale. See behaviour, urine sample.

Mierzyn (Polish, medium) Native Polish pony similar to Konik.

migration (L. migratio) Movement as in passage of white cells through walls of blood vessels, or parasites as **m.** of redworm larvae. See inflammation, redworm.

milk (L. lac) Fluid secretion of mammary glands forming natural food for foal. Cf colostrum. **m. warts** (syn. equine cutaneous papillomatosis) Infectious disease of horses up to 3 years old. Numerous small warts appear on nose and lips; caused by virus, infectious only to horse family and with incubation period of about 2 months. **M.w.'s** usually self-limiting and disappear in 1–3 months (see also growth). May ulcerate and bleed or recur if removed surgically. Can be treated by chemical cautery with, eg silver nitrate or glacial acetic acid.

miller's disease Colloq. big head, qv.

milligram Unit of weight in metric system, one thousandth of gram. See weights and measures.

millimeter Unit of linear measurement of metric system, one thousandth of a metre. See weights and measures.

Minel Trade name. See phenothiazine.

mineralocorticoid One of several hormones secreted by adrenal cortex; affects mineral (electrolyte) balance of blood and tissues. See desoxy-corticosterone acetate (DOCA) and glucocorticoid.

Minho (syn. Garrano) Popular, old-established Portuguese pony which probably influenced Alter, Lusitano and Galiceno breeds.

Ministry of Agriculture See veterinary rules, veterinary surgeon.

miosis (Gr. meiosis, diminution) Excessive contraction of pupil. See eye.

mite Colloq. for tick (qv) and smaller relatives belonging to order Acarina, sub-order Trombidiformes (harvest **m.** and Demodex, qv) and Sarcoptiformes (see mange).

mitosis Division of body cell (1st stage or prophase). Forms 2 cells, each containing identical amount of inherited material, ie in horse 64 chromosomes (diploid number). Cf meiosis. Fast-growing tumours show many cells in process of **m.**

mitral Shaped like a mitre. **m. valve** (syn. bicuspid valve) Valve guarding entrance between 1st and 2nd chamber on left side of heart. Consists of two cusps anchored to the ventricle wall by fibrous bands. See also heart.

ml. Abbr. for millilitre. See weights and measures.

molar (L. moles, mass) Tooth adapted for grinding. See teeth.

molybdenum poisoning May occur if horse grazes on plants which have taken up **m.** from contaminated soil. Symptoms: persistent diarrhoea any time up to 6 weeks after leaving pasture, weight-loss, harsh staring coat and depigmentation of hair. Treatment: give copper sulphate daily. (More common in cattle than horses.)

Monday morning Time when ill-health often discovered or starts, especially in Thoroughbreds which have been rested on Sunday. **M.m. disease** See setfast. **M.m. leg** See lymphangitis.

Mongolian Old-established breed. Large number live semi-wild on poor land, others are bred at farms. Varies according to district but usually around 13 hands with heavy head and smallish eyes. Has influenced other breeds, particularly Burmese, Turkoman and Manipur. Many **M.** ponies exported to Korea, Tibet and especially China, where known as Griffins or Chinese ponies. May be origin of, or have bred with, Przewalski.

monocyte Large white cell with oval, pale nucleus. See white cell.

monorchid Individual with only one testis descended. See rig.

monovular Derived from a single ovum, eg identical twins, rare in horses. See twin.

moon blindness (syn. periodic ophthalmia) See eye, diseases of.

morbidity Ratio of healthy individuals to sick ones in a community, eg disease with high **m.** affects many individuals.

Morgan American breed developed from one stallion, Justin **M.**, foaled in Massachusetts in 1789. He may have been type of American Quarter horse or part Arab. Breed flourished and **M.** stud farm established.

Breed is general-purpose with quiet disposition and is often used in light harness. Was raced until ousted by faster, specially-bred trotter (the Standardbred) on which it had strong influence. Now bred mainly under US government supervision. Usually bay, brown, black or chestnut and around 14-15 hands. Assn: **M.** Horse Club, PO Box 2157, Bishop's Corner Branch, W Hartford, Connecticut (Zip no: 06117).

Morochuco/Morochuquo Angular type S American Criollo (qv) living in mountainous areas of Brazil and Peru.

mosaicism See chromosome.

mosquito Insect of family Culicidae. See gnat.

mould poisoning May occur if horse eats mouldy plants or hay. Symptoms: frequent urination, nervousness, inflamed mouth, excessive salivation, inco-ordination, paralysis, depression, weakness, jaundice and in severe cases, death from internal hemorrhages.

Mouleki Colloq. Turkoman, qv.

mount To get on to, used to describe stallion on mare at time of coitus. See behaviour, male sexual; artificial vagina.

mouth Opening into alimentary canal. Houses teeth, gums, tongue. **m. injuries of** (1) Abrasions, caused by bit of bridle. May affect gums and angle of lips. (2) Wounds of cheek caused by kick, barbed wire, etc. (3) Fracture of one or both branches of lower jaw (from kick). (4) Abscess in the roots of molar teeth. (5) Tearing of root (frenulum) of tongue by rough handling. Treatment depends on nature of injury. If from bit, horse should be rested; if wounds or fracture, surgery; if abrasions, astringent lotions.

MRCVS Abbr. Member of the Royal College of Veterinary Surgeons, qv.

mucin Chief constituent of mucus, produced by small glands in lining of air passages, alimentary tract, etc.

mucoid Resembling mucus.

262

mucosa See mucous membrane.

mucous membrane Thin layer of cells consisting of epithelium and mucous glands. Generally used to mean those **m.m.**'s most easily seen, eg of eyelid, mouth, gums, vagina. **injected m.m.** Membrane in which blood vessels stand out abnormally. Sign of infection. See cyanosis.

mucus Slimy secretion which lubricates mucous membranes; contains mucin, inorganic salts, cells. Produced in excess in inflammation of mucous membranes, eg catarrh.

mud fever (syns. rain scald, dermatophilosis, mycotic dermatitis, heel bug, aphis, greasy heel) Skin infection caused by Dermatophilus congolensis. All ages susceptible and may occur singly or in epidemic. Coronet, bulbs of heel and lower legs usually affected, though may also occur on back and flanks. Lesions are matted hair and thick scabs which leave red, moist area when removed. Diagnosis: on laboratory examination of smears from underside of scab. Treatment: apply chloramphenicol lotion. Cf. acne, ringworm.

mule Offspring of male ass and female horse. Female **m.** is a janet. **M.** is usually infertile. See chromosome, Horse & **M.** Assn of America.

mulomedicus Romans' first term for veterinary surgeon. Later equorum medicus, then veterinarius (from veterinae—literally, old hack).

multiparous Mare which has had 2 or more pregnancies.

munai-su Veterinary surgeon of Mesopotamian people. Distinguished from the medical and witch doctor as early as 1800 BC. If a **m.-s.**'s patient died, he had to pay owner more than quarter of the animal's value.

murmur See heart murmur.

muscle (syn. flesh) Collection of fibres with ability to contract and exert a force. 3 types: striped, smooth and cardiac (heart). Striped **m.** is voluntary and found in muscles of legs etc. Smooth **m.** is involuntary and found in alimentary canal, uterus, walls of arteries etc. Cardiac **m.** of heart is characterised by capacity to contract rhythmically. **m.'s and tendons, abnormal conditions of** (1) Rupture of strong tendon

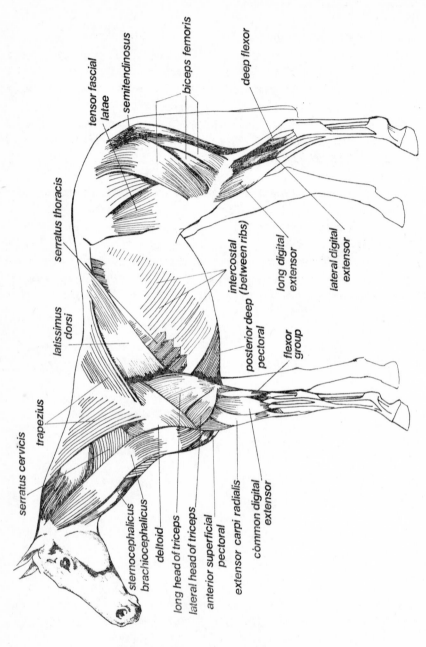

tensor fascial latae

semitendinosus

biceps femoris

deep flexor

serratus thoracis

intercostal (between ribs)

long digital extensor

lateral digital extensor

latissimus dorsi

posterior deep pectoral

flexor group

trapezius

serratus cervicis

sternocephalicus

brachiocephalicus

deltoid

long head of triceps

lateral head of triceps

anterior superficial pectoral

extensor carpi radialis

common digital extensor

29 The main muscles

264

(peroneus tertius) attached to back of femur and inserted on to cannon. It acts mechanically to flex hock when stifle joint is flexed. When ruptured, stifle flexes, but hock does not. Caused by overextension of hock joint. Symptoms: limpness below hock, as if fracture has occurred. Horse **can** bear weight and shows relatively little pain. When it walks there is a dimpling in Achilles tendon. Treatment: rest for several weeks. (2) Rupture of gastrocnemius **m.** Has its origin on back of femur and its insertion through a tendon to point of hock (tuber calcis). Its action is to extend hock and flex stifle joint. A small bursa lies on front of its insertion on front of hock and another is interposed between it and superficial flexor tendon. Symptoms: dropping of hock joint at an excessive angle. If on both sides, horse appears to be squatting and cannot straighten hind limbs. (3) Myositis. Inflamed **m.** due to strain, virus infection, setfast. (4) Ossifying myopathy. Laying down of scar tissue in **m.**, usually in hindquarters, or back of thigh, after injury. Adhesions limit action of **m.**'s and cause lameness. Often seen in American Quarter horse, qv. Symptoms: lameness, especially noticeable when walking; scar can be felt as an area of firmness. Treatment: remove fibrous lump surgically. (5) Tendonitis. Sprain of tendon, most common behind front cannon, ie deep and/or superficial flexor tendons.

TABLE OF MUSCLES

Part	Muscle	Action
lips and cheek	orbicularis oris	close eyelids
	levator nasolabialis	raise upper lip and nostril
	levator labii superioris proprius	raise upper lip
	zygomaticus	pull back angle of mouth
	incisivus superior	depress upper lip
	incisivus inferior	raise lower lip
	depressor labii inferioris	depress and pull back lower lip
	buccinator	flatten cheek

Table of muscles

Part	Muscle	Action
nostril	levator nasolabialis	
	dilatator naris lateralis	dilate nostrils
	transversus nasi	dilate nostrils
	lateralis nasi	dilate nostrils
eyelids	orbicularis oculi	close eyelids
	corrugator supercilii	raise upper lid
	malaris	depress lower lid
	levator palpebrae superioris	raise upper lid
lower jaw (mandible)	masseter	close mouth
	temporalis	close mouth
	pterygoideus medialis	close and move mouth from side to side
	pterygoideus lateralis	move jaw forward and from side to side
	occipito mandibularis	open mouth
	digastricus	open mouth and, when jaws are closed, to assist in swallowing
hyoid	mylo-hyoideus	raise floor of mouth, tongue and hyoid bone
	stylo-hyoideus	draw back tongue and raise larynx in act of swallowing

Part	Muscle	Action
	occipito-hyoideus	move hyoid bone during swallow
	genio-hyoideus	draw hyoid bone and tongue forward
	kerato-hyoideus	raise hyoid bone and larynx
	hyoideus transversus	raise root of tongue
neck	brachiocephalicus	move head and neck, and pull forward; sprain causes lameness
	sternocephalicus	move head and neck
	sterno-thyro-hyoideus	assist in swallowing and sucking movements
	omo-hyoideus	move hyoid bone and root of tongue
	scalenus	move neck and first rib
	cervicalis ascendens	extend neck
	rectus capitis ventralis major	flex or turn head
	rectus capitis ventralis minor	flex head
	rectus capitis lateralis	flex head
	longus colli	flex head
	intertransversales colli	turn neck to side

Table of muscles

Part	Muscle	Action
	splenius	extend neck or turn to side
	longissimus capitis et atlantis	extend neck or turn to side
	complexus	extend head and neck or turn to side
	multifidus cervicis	extend head and neck or turn to side
	obliquus capitis posterior	rotate head
	obliquus capitis anterior	extend head or turn to side
	rectus capitis dorsalis major	extend head
	rectus capitis dorsalis minor	extend head
back	longissimus cosarum	largest and longest muscle of body; extends back or turns to one side
	multifidus dorsi	extend back or turn to one side
	intertransversales lumborum	hold back rigid or turn to one side
	coccygeus	press tail down or turn to one side
	sacro-coccygeus dorsalis	raise tail and/or turn to side

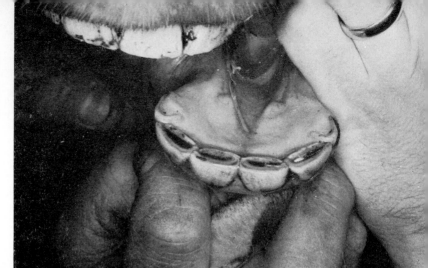

27 Lower jaw of four-month-old foal showing four front milk teeth in full wear and two others breaking through

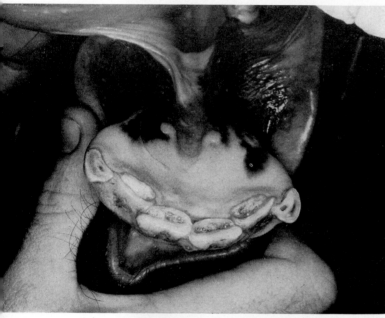

28 Lower jaw of three-year-old. The two middle teeth are in full wear, those on either side are coming through and the outermost milk teeth will be shed when the horse is four

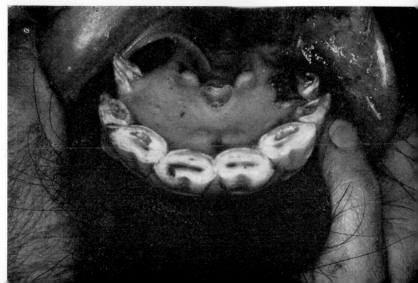

29 Lower jaw of a five-year-old, showing (left) a pointed canine tooth. The front teeth are all in full wear

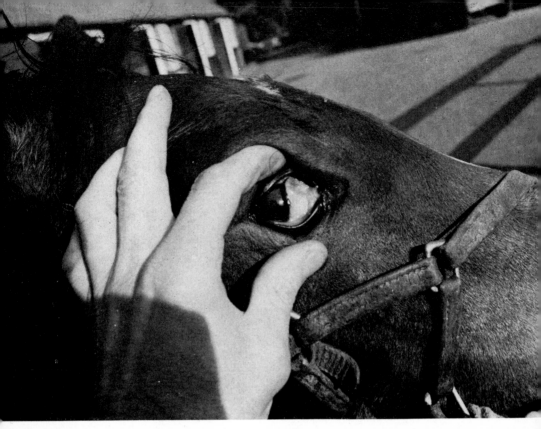

30 Spasm of the third eyelid, a symptom of lockjaw. See *eyelid*

31 A speculum, qv

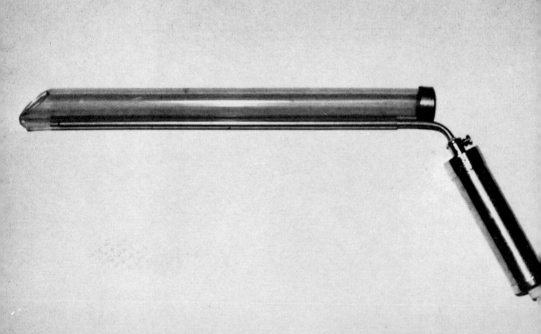

Part	Muscle	Action
	sacro-coccygeus lateralis	raise tail and/or turn to side
	sacro-coccygeus ventralis	press tail down
chest	serratus dorsalis anterior	assist in breathing (inspiration)
	serratus dorsalis posterior	assist in breathing (expiration)
	longissimus costarum	assist in breathing (expiration)
	levatores costarum	assist in breathing (inspiration)
	external intercostals	assist breathing
	internal intercostals	assist breathing
	retractor costae	move last rib
	rectus thoracis	assist breathing
	transverse thoracis	assist breathing (inspiration)
	diaphragm (qv)	principal muscle of breathing (inspiration)
abdomen	obliquus abdominis externus	compress abdominal cavity to assist in defecation, birth, breathing (expiration)
	obliquus abdominis internus	compress abdominal cavity to assist in defecation, birth, breathing (expiration)

Table of muscles

Part	Muscle	Action
	rectus abdominis	compress abdominal cavity to assist in defecation, birth, breathing (expiration)
	transversus abdominis	compress abdominal cavity to assist in defecation, birth, breathing (expiration)
	cremaster	pull up testicle from scrotum
forelimb (1) shoulder	trapezius	raise shoulder blade (scapula)
	rhomboideus	raise and pull shoulder blade forward
	latissimus dorsi	flex shoulder joint
	brachiocephalicus	extend shoulder and elbow joint; see m. of neck
	superficial pectoral	advance and adduct leg
	deep pectoral	pull limb back
	serratus ventralis	support chest between two shoulder blades
	deltoideus	flex shoulder joint and abduct leg
	supraspinatus	extend shoulder joint; bursa present between m. and shoulder joint
	infraspinatus	abduct leg

Part	Muscle	Action
	teres minor	flex shoulder joint and abduct leg
	subscapularis	adduct humerus bone
	teres major	flex shoulder joint and adduct leg
	coraco brachialis	flex shoulder joint and adduct leg
	capsularis	flex shoulder joint
(2) arm	biceps brachii	flex elbow joint, bursa present between tendon of biceps brachii and humerus bone
	brachialis	flex elbow joint
	tensor fasciae antibrachii	extend elbow joint
	triceps brachii (a) long head	extend elbow and flex shoulder joints
	(b) lateral head	extend elbow joint
	(c) medial head	extend elbow joint
	anconeus	extend elbow joint
(3) forearm	extensor carpi radialis	extend knee and flex elbow joints; tendon of m. possesses synovial sheath from 4″ above to middle of knee (see hygroma)

Part	Muscle	Action
	common digital extensor	extend toe and knee and flex elbow. Tendon of **m.** has sheath extending from above knee to upper part of cannon; and bursa between fetlock joint
	lateral digital extensor	extend toe and knee. **m.** possesses synovial sheath over knee and bursa at front of fetlock
	extensor carpi obliquus	extend knee joint. **m.** possesses synovial sheath over knee
	flexor carpi radialis	flex knee and extend elbow joints. **m.** posesses a synovial sheath from 3″ above knee to cannon
	flexor carpi ulnaris	flex knee and extend elbow joint
	ulnaris lateralis	flex knee and extend elbow joints
	superficial digital flexor	flex toe and extend elbow; tendon of **m.** possesses synovial sheathes extending from above knee to middle third of cannon; and between lower end of cannon to middle of second phalanx

Part	Muscle	Action
	superior check ligament	supports superficial flexor tendon above knee
	deep digital flexor	flex the toe and knee and extend the elbow; tendon of m. possesses synovial sheathes in common with superficial digital flexor, qv; bursa (navicular) placed between tendon and navicular bone behind pedal bone
	interosseus medius	see suspensory ligament
hindlimb		
(1) back	psoas minor	flex pelvis on back
	psoas major	flex hip joint and rotate thigh outwards
	iliacus	flex hip joint and rotate thigh outwards
	quadratus lumborum	flex pelvis on back
	tensor fasciae latae	flex hip and extend stifle joint
(2) hindquarters	gluteus superficialis	flex hip joint and abduct limb
	gluteus medius	extend hip joint, abduct limb; concerned in actions of rearing, kicking and galloping; bursa (trochanteric) placed between tendon of m. and trochanter of femur bone; see bursitis

275

Table of muscles

Part	Muscle	Action
	gluteus profundus	abduct thigh
(3) thigh	biceps femoris	extend limb as in rearing, kicking and galloping; bursa between m. and large and small trochanter
	semitendinosus	extend hip and hock joints
	semimembranosus	extend hip joint and adduct leg
	sartorius	flex hip joint and adduct leg
	gracilis	adduct leg
	pectineus	adduct leg and flex hip joint
	adductor	adduct limb and extend hip joint
	quadratos femoris	extend hip joint and adduct thigh
	obturator externus	adduct thigh
	obturator internus	rotate femur outward
	gemellus	rotate femur outward
	quadriceps femoris	extend stifle and flex hip joints
	(a) rectus femoris	

Part	Muscle	Action
	(b) vastus lateralis	
	(c) vastus medialis	
	(d) vastus intermedius	
(4) second thigh (gaskin)	long digital extensor	extend toe and flex hock
	lateral digital extensor	extend toe and flex hock
	peroneus tertius (entirely tendonous)	mechanically to flex hock when stifle is flexed
	tibialis anterior	flex the hock joints; bursa placed between tendon of m. and medial ligament of hock joint
	gastrocnemius	extend hock and flex stifle joints; bursa between tendon of m. and point of hock; tendon known as Achilles tendon
	superficial digital flexor	flex toe and extend hock; bursa placed under joint; tendon of m. behind hock
	deep digital flexor	flex toe and extend hock; synovial sheath round tendon of m. behind hock
	popliteus	flex stifle

Mustang (from Spanish Mestengo, stranger; syn. Bronco) Intelligent breed of great stamina, about 14 hands and often dun. Descended from first horses on American continent for thousands of years—those brought by Spaniards invading Mexico in early 1500s. American Indians stole or bargained for many of Spaniards' horses but were careless—or ignorant—about breeding and horses degenerated into today's Cayuse. Some **M.** horses roamed wild in America, becoming the legendary Wild West animals. (Term Bronco applied to roughest, wildest horses—hence Bronco-busting.) **In 1957 about 25 M.** mares and stallions were registered, which should prevent complete loss of **M.** blood.

MVB Abbr. Bachelor of Veterinary Medicine.

MVetMed/MVM Abbrs. Master of Veterinary Medicine.

MVSc Abbr. Master Veterinary Science (See veterinary surgeon.)

Myanesin Trade name. See mephenesin.

mycosis Any disease caused by a fungus, eg ringworm.

mycotic dermatitis See mud fever. **m. lymphangitis** See epizootic lymphangitis.

mydriasis Extreme dilation of pupil. See eye.

mydriatic Agent or drug which causes pupil of eye to dilate. Cf myotic.

Mylipen Trade name. See procaine penicillin.

myo-/my- (Gr. mys, muscle) Combining form meaning relationship to muscle.

myocarditis (myo- + Gr. kardia, heart) Inflamed heart muscle (myocardium). Occurs in bacterial infection, eg strangles, or viral infection with herpes, arteritis or influenza virus. Symptoms: reduced stamina and output of heart with rapid, irregular beat, abnormalities on electrocardiogram, collapse and sudden death. Diagnosis: on examination of electrocardiogram, qv. Post-mortem findings vary with stage of condition; if acute there are diseased cells in heart muscle, if of long standing, heart muscle may be interspersed with fibrous (scar) tissue. Treatment: eliminate infection, rest, give digitalis.

myometrium (myo- + Gr. metra, uterus) Smooth muscle lining uterus. Sensitive, especially during pregnancy, to hormone oxytocin, which causes it to contract. See biopsy, metritis.

myosin Protein of muscle.

myositis Inflamed muscle; caused by injury, sprain or infection. See blood blister, influenza, setfast.

myotic Agent or drug which causes pupil to contract. Cf mydriatic.

Mysoline Trade name. See primidone.

Myspamol Trade name. See proquamezine fumerate.

myxovirus Group of viruses including influenza. See virus.

N

nagana Disease of horses, camels, pigs, dogs and monkeys. Occurs in certain parts of Africa such as Abyssinia, Rhodesia and Mozambique. Caused by Trypanosoma brucei transmitted by tsetse fly, tabanid fly and stable fly. Trypanosomes live in blood and lymphatic systems breeding by longitudinal division. They are sucked in by a biting fly and develop in the insect's gut and salivary glands. When infected fly bites an animal, nodule develops at site. This becomes larger and trypanosomes multiply, causing fever and swollen lymph glands. A series of crises and remissions occurs (parasite is in blood only during active stages). Essential features of trypanosomiasis: intermittent fever; anemia, enlarged lymph glands, liver and spleen, progressive emaciation and sometimes drowsiness. Treatment: see diminazene aceturate, homidium bromide, quinapyramine salts and suramin.

Nandrolin Trade name. See nandrolone phenylpropionate.

nandrolone phenylpropionate (trade names: Durabolin, Nandrolin) Drug with actions similar to male sex hormone testosterone but not as potent. Causes body to retain nitrogen, phosphorus and calcium and helps build muscle and improve appetite. Used in wasting conditions; fractures, excess bone reaction after injury, eg splint. Dose: 200–400mg. injected once a week. Overdosage may cause temporarily smaller testes and virilisation in mares.

nasal Of nose. **n. cavity** Passage through length of skull, divided into right and left halves (by septum nasi). See wind, sinusitis. **n. passages** Air passages of head, divided by **n.** septum and ethmoid turbinate bones.

naso-lacrymal duct Tube between eye and nostril, through which tears drain. Enters nostril floor just inside entrance. May become blocked causing tears to overflow down face. See eye, diseases of.

natal (L. natus, birth) Of birth, qv.

Native Mexican Popular, versatile breed around 15 hands, based on Arab, Criollo or Spanish horses.

navel See umbilicus.

navicular disease (syns. navicular bursitis, bursitis, podotrochlearis) Inflamed bursa between deep flexor tendon and navicular bone. Bone and tendon develop adhesions which cause pain and lameness. Upright pasterns likely to increase concussion and make horses more susceptible to **n.d.** Symptoms: history of intermittent lameness which decreases on rest and after work (horse warms up), standing with affected toe pointed, shuffling gait, especially if both forefeet affected. Diagnosis: on symptoms, X-ray (navicular bone seen to have ragged edge and areas of rarefied bone) and nerve block. Treatment: inject bursa with corticosteroids. Only neurectomy (qv) will give permanent relief.

Neapolitan (syn. Italian) Horse developed around Naples, from Spanish stock in 16th and 17th centuries. Now extinct in true form, but said to have been long-lived, late-maturing and similar to Spanish Jennet, qv.

neck (1) Anatomical term meaning constricted portion, eg **n.** of uterus. (2) Part between head and thorax; differs according to breed, but ewe-**n.** (qv) usually considered a fault (see Turkoman). Sexually mature male develops thicker, more crested **n.** than gelding or female.

necrosis (Gr. nekrosis, deadness) Death of cells or groups of cells. **focal n.** That affecting liver of fetus infected with equine herpesvirus.

necrotic Affected by necrosis.

needle (L. acus) Instrument used for stitching wound. **hypodermic n.** Hollow tube used for injecting substances into skin, vein, muscle, etc.

Neftin Trade name. See furazolidine.

Nembutal Trade name. See pentobarbitone.

Neobiotic Trade name. See neomycin sulphate.

neomycin sulphate (trade names: Neobiotic, Neostat, Neo. Sulphentrin, Vonamycin) White or yellow-white odourless powder. Produced by Streptomyces fradiae; antibiotic poorly absorbed from alimentary tract and active against gram-negative and some gram-positive bacteria. Used in diarrhoea, joint-ill in foals (injected into joints with corticosteroids), in uterine infections and locally in dermatitis. Dose 100mg./ kg. body wt., daily in divided doses.

neonatal (neo + natus, born) Of newborn. **n. maladjustment syndrome** (syns. NMS, barker, wanderer, dummy, respiratory distress, convulsive foal) Condition of newborn foal characterised by grossly disturbed behaviour including convulsions, loss of suck reflex, muscle spasms, incessant chewing, wandering, coma, subnormal temperature, increased acidity of blood, low blood oxygen and abnormally high breathing rate sometimes accompanied by barking noise. Symptoms appear in first 24 hours. Cause is unknown but damaged brain, lungs and heart (due to pressure during birth) or disturbed fetal development is most likely. Treatment: good general nursing (see newborn foal), sedatives, anticonvulsant drugs, oxygen inhalation, intravenous sodium bicarbonate, corticosteroids and feeding by stomach tube. Foal may deteriorate and die or recover without apparent after-effects.

neonate Newly born, foal in first month or so of life.

neoplasm (neo- + Gr. plasma, formation) New and abnormal growth. See growth.

neoplastic Of tumour or growth.

Neostat Trade name. See neomycin sulphate.

neostygmine methylsulphate Colourless crystals or white powder with bitter taste and no smell; has action similar to physostigmine qv, counters enzymes that destroy acetyl choline and therefore promotes effects similar to parasympathetic (qv) nerve stimulation. Used in grass sickness; injection available in strength of 0.25%.

Neo. Sulphentrin Trade name. See neomycin sulphate.

nephritis (Gr. nephros, kidney, + -itis) Inflamed kidney caused by bacterial infection, toxins, poisons such as mercury, arsenic, oxalates and certain drugs. Diagnosed on finding protein in urine (proteinuria). See kidney, sleepy foal disease.

nephron (Gr. nephros, kidney + on, neuter ending) A unit of the kidney (qv) comprising glomerulus and collecting tubule.

nephrosis See kidney, diseases of.

nerve Colloq. for pathway which conveys messages to and from brain and spinal cord, controlling purposeful and automatic actions of body and its parts. See autonomic nervous system. **n. cell** (syn. neuron) Basic unit of nervous system; cell containing nucleus and one or more processes—dendrites (like branching of a tree) or axon (long, slender fibre). Axon carries nervous impulses which may be passed to other cells across junction known as synapse. See nervous system.

nerve block (syn. block) An injection of anaesthetic along course of **n.**, causing loss of sensation to area it supplies. Used to help stitching of wounds, minor surgery, or in diagnosis. **infra-orbital b.** Anaesthetic injected where **n.** enters or leaves infra-orbital canal of skull, ie 3cm. (approx. 1in.) below outer angle of eye and just below facial crest; or midway between nasal notch and front end of facial crest. Used for surgery of maxillary sinus, upper incisor and cheek teeth or nostrils and upper lip. **mandibular alveolar b.** One at entry to mandibular canal, on inside of lower jaw. Used for surgery of lower jaw, lower molars, incisors and lower lip. **supra-orbital b.** One blocking branch of 5th cranial **n.**, usually where it travels out of bony bridge over eye. Used in surgery of upper eyelid. **n.b. of legs** Used to diagnose lameness or repair wounds in area supplied by blocked **n.** (If pain is in foot, **n.** supplying foot is blocked and horse goes sound while anaesthetic lasts. If horse is still lame, the pain is above **n.b.**) (1) **median n.b.** At inside of elbow joint. Used with blocks of volar and musculocutaneous **n.** to diagnose lameness in knee joint (carpus) or for minor surgery. (2) **ulna n.b.** Anaesthetic injected 10cm. (approx 4ins.) above accessory carpal bone. Used for minor surgery of outside front of knee. (3) **musculocutaneous n.b.** One between distal ends of biceps and brachialis muscles. (See muscles, table of.) Used with blocks of median and ulna **n.**'s. (4) **tibial n.b.** About 10cm. (4ins.) above point of hock on inside of digital flexor muscle. Densensitises inside back of hock. (5) **volar and plantar n.b**'s Used to diagnose lameness or stitch wounds below knee or hock. Volar **n.**'s are branches of median **n.** Throughout cannon region, they lie either side of deep flexor tendon behind the artery and vein. Each volar **n.** divides into 3 branches at fetlock (on a level with sesamoid bones), 1 and 2 supply front of fetlock, pastern and coronary regions, the corium lateral cartilages and corono-pedal joint capsule, 3 the back (posterior) digital nerve, largest branch, supplies deeper structures of foot, including navicular bone. Plantar **n.**'s in hindlimb originate from tibial **n.** and are distributed in a similar way. Volar and plantar **n.**'s can be blocked high or low, eg wound across front of fetlock can be treated by injecting 5ml. of local anaesthetic over nerves on both sides of flexor tendons (volar or plantar **n.**'s). After about 15 minutes area is insensitive and wound can be cleaned and stitched. Area will remain insensitive for up to 1 hour (depending on type of anaesthetic). **posterior digital n.b.** Limited to diagnosis of navicular lameness. Anaesthetic is injected over **n.** in middle of pastern in groove between deep flexor tendon and the 1st phalanx (pastern bone).

TABLE OF NERVES

Cranial   12 pairs

Nerve		Function
I	olfactory	smell
II	optic	sight

Table of nerves

Nerve		Function
III	oculomotor	eye movement
IV	trochlear	eye movement
V	trigeminal	sensation eyelids, face, soft palate, mouth, gums, teeth, tongue
VI	abducens	eye movement
VII	facial	sense of taste, sensation of area round ear, movement of lips
VIII	acoustic	hearing and balance
IX	glosso pharyngeal	sensation and movement of soft palate and tongue
X	vagus	controls certain actions of larynx, heart and lungs
XI	spinal accessory	movement of neck muscles
XII	hypoglossal	movement of tongue
Spinal	42 pairs	

(a) 8 cervical (neck)
(b) 18 thoracic (chest)
(c) 6 lumbar (back)
(d) 5 sacral (croup)
(e) 5 coccygeal (tail)

(a) cervical nerves

1st
2nd
3rd   } supplies sensation to skin over ear, poll and neck; controls muscular movement in these areas
4th
5th

Nerve	Function
6th	sensation and movement to lower part of neck and front of shoulder; contributes to phrenic **n.**
7th ⎫ 8th ⎬	contribute to phrenic **n.** and brachial plexus
phrenic	movement of diaphragm
brachial plexus: formed from last 3 cervical and first 2 thoracic **n.**'s	sensation and movement of forelimb, braches include **median n.** **suprascapular n.** **brachial n.** **ulnar n.**

(b) thoracic nerves

1st to 18th	sensation of skin over chest and movement of muscles causing breathing motion of chest wall (rib cage)

(c) **lumbar nerves**

1st to 6th	muscle and skin of loins and croup
1st, 2nd, 3rd	sensation and movement of belly muscles, external genitalia
4th, 5th, 6th	forms lumbo-sacral plexus
lumbo-sacral plexus formed by 4th, 5th, 6th **l.n.**'s	supplies nerves giving sensation and control of movement to hind limb branches include **femoral n.** **obturator n.** **gluteal n.** **sciatic n.** **peroneal n.** **tibial n.**

Nerve	Function
(d) **sacral nerves**	
1st to 5th	sensation and movement to base of tail, perineum, anus, penis/vulva
(e) **coccygeal nerves**	
1st to 5th	sensation and movement of tail

nervous system Arrangement of nerve cells (qv) and their fibres (axons) which transmit nervous impulses from one part of body to another, in definite pathways through the spinal cord and/or brain. **central n.s.** (CNS) Concentration of nervous tissue in head and spinal cord. **peripheral n.s.** (PNS) part of **n.s.** outside CNS. **N.s.** is based on reflex arc in which two or more nerve cells (neurons) conduct nervous impulse from point of stimulation to structures of action, eg muscle acting to remove part away from needle. Most actions involve this type of stimulus and response, through nervous pathway which starts at a sensory cell (eg pain-sensitive cell in skin). Stimulus initiates nervous impulse (sensory) which passes along a nerve connected to CNS; this sparks off a further impulse (motor) that passes outwards to muscle. Nerve cells in CNS form pathways which intercept or control reflex arc by conducting messages up and down spinal cord. In this way the higher centres of nervous activity in brain are made aware of happenings in all parts of body, at a conscious or unconscious level: eg (1) horse that overcomes instinct to withdraw its leg from a painful stimulus exerts conscious or voluntary (and higher) control; (2) when horse increases its breathing rate at exercise, chest muscles are responding to nervous impulses started by body cells sensitive to changes in blood levels of oxygen and carbon dioxide; these impulses reach breathing centre of brain, which controls rhythmic rate and depth of breathing and alters rate and/or depth to compensate for changed gaseous concentration in blood.

nettle rash (urticaria) Form of allergic dermatitis caused by plant pollens or other protein antigens (see allergy). Weals develop on neck, flanks and quarters, varying from small spots to large areas. Hairs stand up and soft swelling beneath pits on pressure. Not usually painful but fluid may drain to dependent parts such as muzzle, abdomen or legs. Swelling of head is common in severe cases. Condition develops rapidly and usually disappears spontaneously, but can be controlled with antihistamine drugs, eg cortisone. See dog's mercury.

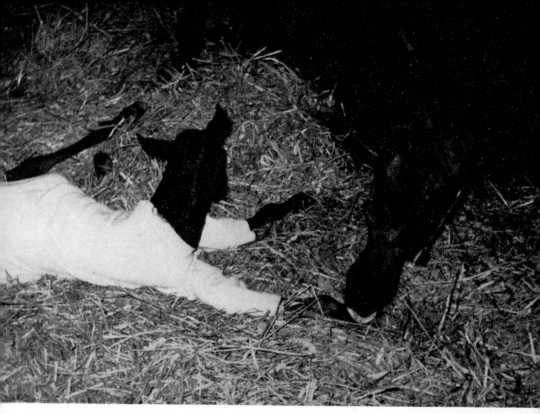

32 An old sweater can help a newborn foal keep warm. See *temperature, newborn foal*

33 Thoroughbred twins. One twin, in this case with the white markings, is usually larger than the other. See *twin*

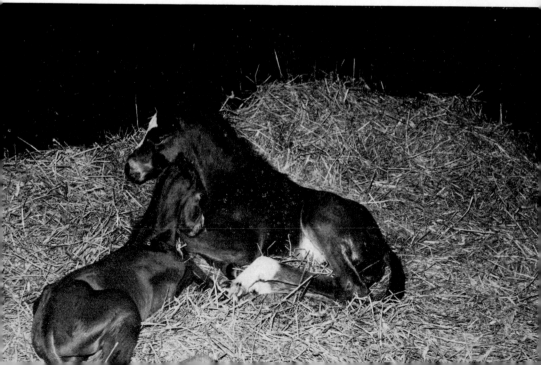

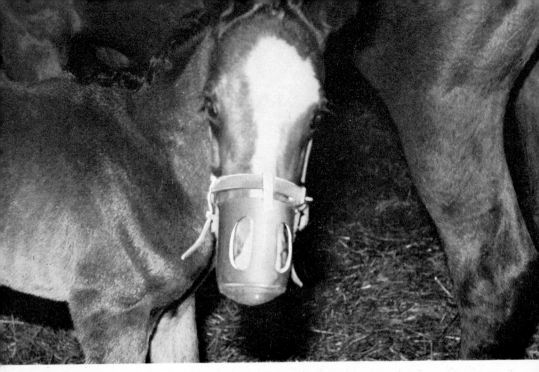

34 Foal muzzled to stop it sucking dam's milk. Practice prevents foal suffering from hemolytic jaundice, qv

35 Wet skin of mammary glands, showing foal has sucked recently

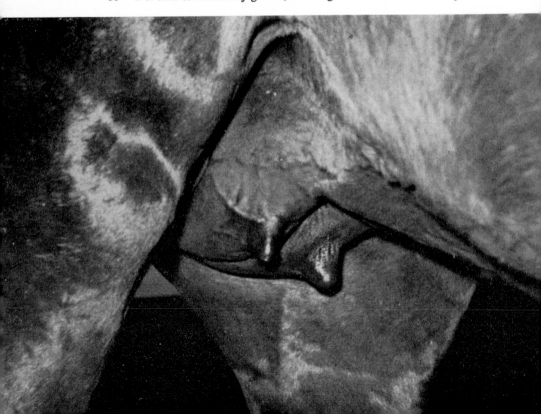

neural (L. neuralis, Gr. neuron, nerve) Of a nerve.

neurectomy Cutting of a nerve to abolish sense of pain (eg back (posterior) digital nerve at level of sesamoid bones). This removes sensation to navicular bone, allowing horse with navicular disease to go sound. Disadvantages are that loss of sensation removes protective reflexes and allows injury, may cause stumbling and shedding of hoof.

neuron (Gr. neuron, nerve) Nerve cell, qv.

neutralisation test Laboratory test for antibody/antigen reaction (qv) between toxin and antitoxin.

neutropenia (neutrophil + Gr. penia, poverty) Decrease in number of neutrophil white cells in blood. See blood.

neutrophilia Increase in number of neutrophil white cells in blood; sign of infection. See blood.

newborn Foal in first week of life. **n. foal, congenital abnormalities of:**

Condition	Synonyms	Predominant signs
patent bladder	ruptured bladder	straining; reduced urine flow, abdominal fluid (signs appear on 2nd or 3rd day)
hyperflexion of limbs	contracted tendons contracted forelimbs	knuckling over
hypoflexion of limbs		slack ligaments; reduced muscle tone
cleft palate hare lip		regurgitation of milk
parrot jaw	undershot jaw	
microphthalmia	button eyes	
umbilical urachal fistula	pervious urachus	wet cord stump
hernia		failure of umbilical and/or inguinal ring to close

n. foal, diseases of Groups: (1) Infective conditions characterised by fever, lethargy and weakened suck reflex. (2) Non-infective conditions characterised by gross disturbance in behaviour. (3) Congenital abnormalities. (4) Immunological conditions characterised by reaction between maternal and fetal tissues. See septicemia (group 1), neonatal maladjustment syndrome, prematurity, meconium retention (group 2), hemolytic jaundice (group 4). **n. foal immaturity** (syn. dysmaturity, lit. bad maturity) Foals born after 325 days' gestation, showing all appearances of prematurity, qv. **n. foal, nursing** (1) Restrain foal gently and help it stand. (2) Feed through stomach tube or by bottle. See food. (3) Raise surrounding temperature if foal's rectal temperature falls below 37.2°C. (approx. 99°F.). Use hot-air blowers, heated lamps, rugs, washable electric blankets. (See plate 32.) In severe cases stable temperature should rise to 26.6°C. (approx. 78°F.). (4) Remove meconium by enema and by giving liquid paraffin in food. (5) Place convulsive and comatosed foals on rugs or soft material to avoid damage to head. (6) Powder areas where bedsores are most likely, ie point of hip, outside of stifle and elbows. (7) Turn foal from side to side to help blood circulation.

New Forest pony Tough sure-footed breed that has roamed N.F. district of Hampshire for centuries (mentioned in Domesday Book, 1085). Able to eat acorns (see oak) without apparent harm. Attempts to improve breed include one by Queen Victoria, whose Arab stallion Zorah lived 8 years in forest. N.F. is now fairly static type and breeds true. Its natural home is densely populated compared with those of other mountain and moorland breeds and it is traffic-proof and popular child's pony when broken. Can be bought at sales in late summer. Usually about 14 hands and grey or brown, although any colour acceptable. Assn: **N.F.** Pony and Cattle Breeding Soc., c/o Miss D. Macnair, Beacon Corner, Burley, Ringwood, Hampshire (Burley 2272).

Newmarket cough See influenza.

nicotinamide White crystalline odourless powder with bitter taste. For actions and uses see nicotinic acid.

nicotinic acid White or creamy-white odourless acid-tasting crystals or powder; widely distributed in foodstuffs. It is classed a vitamin and, with nicotinamide, is part of enzyme system. Dose: 1–500mg. daily.

nictating membrane (syn. third eyelid) See eyelid.

nightshade poisoning Rare, as all members of family Henbane (deadly **n.** (syn. belladonna), thornapple, woody **n.**, garden **n.**, wild tobacco) unlikely to be eaten because they taste bitter. Symptoms: central nervous depression, salivation, inflamed gut with diarrhoea and colic.

nikethamide (trade name: Coramine) Colourless or yellow oily liquid or crystals, with slightly bitter taste. Used to increase frequency and depth of breathing; to counteract depressant effect of narcotics and anaesthesia; and to stimulate strength and regularity of heart. Dose: 2.5–6gms. IV, IM or sub. cut.

nitrate/nitrite poisoning Caused by eating artificial manures, plants and weeds which take up **n.**, eg oat, wheat and rye hay, barley, sugar beet. Symptoms: abdominal pain, diarrhoea, muscular weakness, inco-ordination, convulsions, difficult breathing, coma (seen as bluish mucous membranes) and death. Less severe cases may be listless and abort. Diagnosis: on symptoms and dark, chocolate-coloured blood. Treatment: methylene blue, 9mg./kg. body wt., as a 5% solution IV.

nitrofurantoin (trade name: Berkfurin E) Odourless yellow powder with bitter taste. Antibiotic used to treat respiratory infections (coughs, colds) in foals and adult horses; and in urinary or kidney infections but pH of urine must be below 8 as activity of drug greatly reduced by alkaline urine. 1st dose: 2gms./1000lb. followed by 1gm./1000lb. every 8 hours. Stop dosing if skin shows signs of allergy.

nitrofurazone (trade name: Furacin) Antibiotic used in infections of respiratory and urinary tracts. Has actions similar to nitrofurantoin, qv.

node (L. nodus, knot) Swelling. See gland.

Nonius Hungarian breed developed from Anglo-Norman stallion named **N.** Usually quiet-tempered and often dark bay. Two types: large— up to about 17 hands and used for agriculture; small—around 15.2 hands.

noradrenaline acid tartrate White crystalline odourless bitter-tasting powder; main substance released by medulla of adrenal gland when sympathetic nerves are stimulated. Causes rise in blood pressure. Less active than adrenaline, qv.

Noric See South German Cold Blood.

normochromic Having normal colour, eg normal hemoglobin content of red cells.

Northland Little-known Norwegian breed. About 13 hands, usually dark-coloured.

nose (L. nasus, Gr. rhis) Part of face beneath eye level and above muzzle; includes nostrils. **roman n.** Convex profile, eg in Kladruber.

nostrils (syn. nares) Entrances to air passages of head; skin and mucous membrane supported by ring of cartilage. **false n.** Blind sac in upper part of **n. true n.** Direct entrances to nasal cavity (air passage).

nucleus (L. dim. of nux, nut) Small body in cell, containing inherited material (chromosomes, genes) which controls cell function.

Numimbah horse sickness See crofton weed.

Nutrequin Trade name. Feed supplement containing vitamins, minerals, amino-acids.

nutrition See food.

Nymfalon Trade name. See chorionic gonadotrophin.

nystagmus (Gr. nystagmos, drowsiness, from nystazein, to nod) Involuntary rapid movement of eyeball. Occurs under anaesthesia or in brain damage or injury.

nystatin Yellow or light-brown powder with characteristic odour. Antibiotic active against wide range of fungi and yeasts. Poorly absorbed from alimentary canal. Used in dusting powder, cream or ointment to treat ringworm and other skin infections associated with fungi; also in uterine infection following fungal abortion.

O

oak poisoning (from common **o.**'s of Britain, Quercus robur and Q. petracea) Occurs if horse eats leaves or acorns (see New Forest pony). Symptoms, some days later: dullness, loss of appetite, constipation, sometimes followed by diarrhoea containing blood, excessive urination, pale mucous membranes and watery discharge from eyes. At post-mortem: inflamed gut and stomach. Treatment: give liquid paraffin.

obturator foramen Opening in floor of pelvis formed by ischium and pubis.

occipital puncture Colloq. for cisterna magna puncture, in which needle is inserted between occiput and first neck vertebra (atlas) to draw off cerebrospinal fluid for laboratory analysis.

occiput Area at base of skull formed by occipital bone. Projects above as poll.

oedema (syns. edema, filling, filled leg, plaque) Abnormal accumulation of fluid outside cells. It collects in spaces below skin, causing soft swellings that leave a pit on pressure. Due to: (1) more permeable blood vessels (ie they allow water and protein to pass freely), caused by toxins, allergy, infection; (2) abnormal decrease in protein in blood, eg in malnutrition or wasting diseases; (3) obstruction of blood returning to heart in veins; (4) heart disease causing increased blood pressure in veins; (5) kidney disease causing increased blood pressure and improper filtering of blood; (6) too much food, especially that high in protein; (7) inflammation from any cause, including sprain; (8) obstruction of lymph flow due to overloading of vessels, eg in **o.** of belly, close to udder at foaling time. **pulmonary o.** Fluid in lung due to capillaries damaged by toxins, allergy or circulatory failure. Common in virus infection and fatal neonatal maladjustment syndrome.

oesophagus (syns. esophagus, gullet) Muscular tube from throat to stomach (about 150cm. or 60ins.). Sited on left of lower part of neck. Extends through chest and diaphragm to open into stomach through a weak sphincter (ring of muscle), which prevents regurgitation of food except in rare cases, eg near to death, in grass sickness.

oestradiol Naturally-occurring oestrogen, qv.

Oestridae Family of insects belonging to sub-order Cyclorrhapha, containing bot, qv, and warble, qv.

oestriol Naturally-occurring oestrogen, qv.

oestrogen Hormone of steroid group. Natural **o.**'s include oestradiol, oestrone, oestriol, equilin, equilenin; secreted by ovary, placenta, adrenal cortex and testes. In mare, responsible for behaviour and changes in sex cycle (see oestrous cycle). **synthetic o.** See stilboestrol.

oestrone Naturally-occurring oestrogen, qv.

oestrous cycle (syn. estrous cycle) Sexual cycle of mare. Alternating periods of sexual activity, ie oestrus (when mare accepts stallion) and dioestrus (when she rejects him). Typical oestrus last 5 days, dioestrus 15 days. Cycle varies, being a regular 20 days probably only in spring and summer. It is controlled by pituitary glands through secretion of hormones FSH (follicle stimulating hormone) and LH (luteinising hormone). During oestrus, follicle develops in ovary, which ruptures, shedding egg into fallopian tube. Ovary secretes hormone oestrogen which causes oestrous behaviour and changes in genital tract including outpouring of mucus. Oestrus ends when egg is shed (ovulation) and a yellow body is formed (under influence of LH). Yellow body secretes progesterone which causes dioestrus and prepares uterus for fertilised egg which arrives from fallopian tube six days after fertilisation. If fertilisation does not occur, the yellow body ceases to function about the 15th day and thereby stimulates pituitary to produce more FSH and the cycle starts again. Life of yellow body is probably ended by prostaglandin secreted by uterus. Successful mating requires that stallion serves mare about 12 hours before ovulation, which usually occurs about 24 hours prior to end of oestrus.

oestrus State of being in heat, ie in an oestrous (receptive) state.

ointment (syn. unguentum) Semi-solid preparation for external use and with fatty base, such as lard, paraffin, lanolin.

Oldenburg Early-maturing German 'warm-blooded' breed of about 17 hands. Has influenced Lithuanian, Latvian and Friesian breeds and now has some Thoroughbred blood. Queen Elizabeth II has team of **O.** carriage horses. See cerebellar degeneration.

olecranon (Gr. olekranon) Bony point of elbow (ulna bone). See dropped elbow.

omentum (L., fat skin; pl. omenta) Fold, near stomach, of the membrane (peritoneum) lining abdomen.

Onager (Equus hemionus o.) One of 2 sub-species of Asiatic wild ass. Lives in herds in Afghanistan and Persia and was probably ass of the Bible. See ass.

opisthotonus Drawing back of head due to muscle spasms, as in brain injury. See bracken poisoning.

opium See powdered opium.

ophthalmoscope Instrument containing mirrors and light source. Used to see inside of eye and retina.

Opticorten Trade name. See dexamethasone.

Opticortenol-S Trade name. See dexamethasone.

Orbenin Trade name. See cloxacillin sodium.

ordinate Vertical line which, with abscissa (horizontal line), is used as reference on graph (in same way as lines of longitude/latitude on map).

Oribatid mite (colloq. beetle mite) Species of family Oribatidae belonging to class Arachnida (see Arthropod parasites). Small blind dark-coloured mite which lives in soil where it digests organic matter. It carries the intermediate form (cysticercus) of tapeworm, qv.

Oriental Literally: horse of the Orient, but widely used for any type of Eastern origin, eg Arabian, Turkish, Persian.

Orlov (after Count Alexis O.) Russian breed founded when Count O. crossed Arab stallion with Dutch mare in 1770s. Thoroughbred, Mecklenburg and Danish blood introduced and breed is renowned for Arab-like head and trotting ability. Up to 17 hands and sometimes termed O. trotter. Now, besides trotters, O. Rostopschiner is good saddle horse. A recent cross of Standardbred and O. has resulted in O. Standardbred sometimes known as Metis trotter which may be faster than O. trotter.

osselet (syn. arthritis of fetlock joint) Inflamed joint, joint capsule and insertion of lateral digital extensor tendon on front of pastern bone. Most common in two- and three-year-olds due to concussion, conformation of pastern and tearing of joint capsule and associated structures. Symptoms: distended front of fetlock because new bone (exostosis) has formed and joint produces too much synovia, pain on pressure or flexion of joint. Lesion usually develops gradually, eventually causing lameness. Diagnosis: on X-ray examination and symptoms. Treatment: rest, irradiation, corticosteroid injections, cold applications.

osteitis/ostitis Inflamed bone. Most common cause is fracture, qv.

osteoarthropathy Any disease of joints, bones. **hypertrophic pulmonary o.** Disease characterised by forming of new, irregular bone on surface of leg bones. Often occurs with some form of lung disease, eg infection, and each leg is affected. Symptoms include cough and difficult breathing. Cause: unknown, no known treatment.

osteodystrophia fibrosa See big head.

osteomyelitis Infection of bone marrow tissue and neighbouring bone. May occur after compound fracture (see fracture) or if site of surgery is infected. Symptoms: forming of cavities which discharge pus, pain, swelling, lameness and in severe cases, fever. Diagnosis: on symptoms, X-ray examination and an increasing white blood cell count (leucocytosis).

osteoporosis Abnormal rarefaction of bone. See big head.

osteosis Bone decay. May result from kick causing small piece of bone (sequestrum, qv) to fracture or break off, detached from blood supply. Abscess usually develops.

ovary One of pair of female glands; typically bean-shaped, varying from 4cm.–8cm. (2ins.–4ins.) long and weighing about 18gms. (3oz.). It is attached to broad ligament suspending uterus and enclosed in a capsule with an opening (ovulation fossa) through which egg passes at ovulation. **O.** consists of network of fibrous tissue in which numerous fluid sacs (follicles) develop; in each follicle is an egg. Follicle grows and eventually ruptures (ovulates) shedding egg into fallopian tube. Bleeding occurs into cavity of ruptured follicle and a yellow body (corpus luteum) is formed. See oestrous cycle, plate 37.

over-reaching Action in which hindfoot steps on heel of the forefoot on same side. Fault lessened by careful shoeing. Cf cross-firing, forging. See gait.

oviduct See fallopian tube.

ovulation The shedding of an ovum. See follicle stimulating hormone.

ovum (L.; pl. ova; syn. egg) Female gamete containing hereditary material. At birth, ovary contains about 30,000 ova; after sexual maturity they develop in graafian follicles; during heat periods one or two are released (ovulation) to enter fallopian tube for fertilisation. **O.** is one of the largest cells of body, 120–180 thousandths of a millimeter (or 120–180μ). It contains mass of cytoplasm surrounded by cell membrane (vitelline membrane) and a thick, transparent membrane (zona pellucida). During development chromosome numbers are reduced by half to haploid number (see chromosome). Egg survives only about 12–24 hours after ovulation unless fertilised. Unfertilised egg stays in fallopian tube and slowly disintegrates, but fertilised egg passes into uterus.

oxallic and malonic acids (trade name: Venagmin) Drug used to treat nosebleeds, uterine bleeding, purpura hemorrhagica. Dose: 3cc.

Oxazine Trade name. See piperazine salts.

oxygen Colourless odourless gas, given by inhalation, (1) with anaesthetic gases during anaesthesia, (2) to newborn foals suffering from low blood oxygen, and (3) to resuscitate foals that fail to breathe immediately after birth. See neonatal maladjustment syndrome.

oxyphenbutazone Chemical excreted in urine if horse is given phenylbutazone, qv. Synthetic o. (trade name: Tanderil) can also be given in conditions likely to benefit from phenylbutazone. See veterinary rules.

oxytetracycline hydrochloride/dihydrate (trade names: Terramycin, Imperacin) Yellow odourless bitter-tasting crystalline powder. Antibiotic with actions and uses similar to tetracycline hydrochloride, qv. Dose: 25–50mg./kg. body wt. by mouth and 3mg./kg. body wt. IV.

oxytocin (trade name: Pitocin) Hormone formed by posterior lobe of pituitary gland. Causes contraction of uterus, completion of 3rd stage labour, running of milk before and during birth and possibly the let-down of milk when foal is sucking.

Oxytocin S. injection Trade name. Solution of synthetic oxytocin. Used after foaling to restrict uterine bleeding. Dose: 10–40 units IM and 2.5–10 units IV. See birth.

P

P Abbr. for phosphorus.

pace See gait.

pacemaker, cardiac Sino-atrial (SA) node from which impulse causing heart beat originates. See heart impulse.

pachy- (Gr. pachys, thick, clotted) Combining form meaning thick.

pachyderma (pachy- + Gr. derma, skin) Abnormal thickening of skin, qv. Inexplicable condition in which horse loses hair over large parts of body and skin becomes thick, dry and scaly.

Pahlavan Form of Anglo-Arab, currently being established in Persia from English Thoroughbred, Arab and Plateau Persian.

pain (L. poena, dolor, Gr. algos, odyne) Sensation produced by stimulation of specialised nerve-endings; most plentiful in skin and membrane (eg peritoneum) lining body, body cavities, joints, etc. Symptoms: sweating, pawing ground, anxious expression, possibly rolling (see meconium retention, colic, plates 8–10) or lameness. **p.-killing drugs** Buscopan, pethidine, phenylbutazone.

Paint Horse developed in last few decades from American Quarter horse and Thoroughbred. Popular for its patchy colouring, which is similar to Pinto, qv.

palate Partition separating mouth and nasal cavities. Divided into hard **p.** (in front) and soft **p.** behind. Foals sometimes born with opening in, or complete lack of, **p.** (cleft **p.**). See soft palate.

Palomino Original golden horse of the West; colour rather than breed. Societies promoting **P.** allow all shades of gold, from pale blond to almost chestnut. Mane and tail should be cream and only markings allowed are white, on legs and face. Many foals born with blue eyes which darken with maturity—blue eyes not accepted in adult. Pinto, draught, albino and pony blood barred, otherwise any breed can be used to produce **P.** colouring. Probably of Spanish origin with Arab and Barb blood. May take name from Spaniard Juan de **P.**, who was given a **P.** by Hernan Cortes (conqueror of Mexico). Assns: **P.** Horse Breeders of America, c/o PO Box 249, Mineral Wells, Texas (Zip no: 76067); **P.** Horse Assn, PO Box 446, Chatsworth, California (Zip no: 91311); British **P.** Soc., c/o Mrs **P.** Howell, Kingsettle Stud, Cholderton, Salisbury, Wiltshire (Cholderton 273). Cf Haflinger, Highland, coat colouring.

palpation (L. palpatio) Act of feeling with hand, eg **p.** of foal's abdomen to detect tympany or fluid. **p. of ovaries** See rectal examination.

palpebra Eyelid, qv.

pan- (Gr. pan, all) Prefix meaning all.

pancreas Digestive gland in abdomen. It secretes substances which pass through duct to duodenum and help digest food. Also secretes hormone (insulin) which is absorbed into blood stream and controls level of blood sugar.

pancreatic (L. pancreaticus) of pancreas.

pancreatitis Inflamed pancreas.

Pange Popular cross between native Baltic mares and trotter stallion.

pannus (L., a piece of cloth) Ulcerative condition of cornea of eye or joint surface in which it becomes invaded with blood vessels.

papilla Anatomical term meaning small, nipple-shaped projection or elevation, eg teats of mammary glands.

papillae Pl. of papilla.

papilloma See growth.

papillomatosis Syn. milk warts, qv.

para- (Gr. para, beyond) Prefix meaning beside.

paracentesis (para- +Gr. kentesis, puncture) Surgical puncture of cavity to draw off fluid, eg from abdomen (**p.** abdomenis) of newborn foal with ruptured bladder. See bladder, rupture of.

paraffin See liquid paraffin.

Parafilaria multipapillosa Little-known worm parasite, about 4cm. long, found in tissue beneath areas of raised skin, usually on shoulders and hindquarters. Life-cycle not fully documented. Cf filaria, see Budyonovsky.

paralysis (para- + Gr. lyein, to loosen) Loss of use of a part due to injury or disease of nerve or brain. **facial p.** Common condition caused by injured facial nerve as it rounds back of lower jaw. Symptoms: drooping of upper eyelid and ear, nostrils and lips pulled to one side, drooping of lower lip. Usually occurs on one side; if on both (bilateral), it is more serious. Treatment: feed with soft mashes or, if severe, by stomach tube. Partial recovery may occur but horse may be left with permanent disability. **obturator p.** May occur after fracture of pelvis or at foaling. Symptoms: inability to move hindlimb due to paralysis of muscles obturator externus, pectineus adductor and gracilis. **pudic nerve p.** Infection or fractured pelvis injures nerve supplying retractor muscles of penis, so that it hangs limply from sheath. **radial p.** See dropped elbow. **supra scapula nerve p.** (syn. sweeny) Symptoms: wasting of muscles on shoulder, possibly lameness. Wasting is usually permanent but some recovery of muscle function is usual. Treatment: inject corticosteroids immediately after injury, use faradic stimulation. **tail p.** Tail root hangs limp and is not raised during defecating or staling; anus and surrounding skin may also be paralysed. Caused by fractured sacrum or injured tail (coccygeal) vertebrae. See Hobday, wobbler syndrome, stringhalt, wind, physiotherapy, corticosteroids, muscle.

parameter (para- + Gr. metron, measure) Measurement.

300

parasite (Gr. parasitos) Animal living on or in another and at host's expense. Those which affect horses: **external** (ectoparasites)—tick, qv, harvest mite, qv, mites causing sarcoptic mange, chorioptic mange, psoroptic mange, and demodectic mange (all see mange), louse, qv; **internal** (endoparasites)—tapeworm, qv, fluke, qv, redworm, qv, lungworm, qv, stomach worm, qv, whiteworm, qv, seatworm, qv, filiaria, qv, Parafilaria multipapillosa, qv, warble fly maggot (see warble fly), botfly maggot (see bot), Babesia (see biliary fever). See plate 26.

parasitic (Gr. parasitikos) Of, or caused by, parasite. **p. mange** Colloq. for sarcoptic mange. Notifiable disease. See mange, sarcoptic; veterinary rules.

parasiticide (L. parasitus, parasite + caedere, to kill) Drug or chemical used externally to destroy parasites on skin.

parasitology (Gr. parasitos, parasite + -logy) Science of parasites and parasitism.

parasympathetic nervous system Part of the autonomic nervous system, qv. Nerves which originate from brain and spinal cord. **p. nerve-endings** Supply blood vessels, glands, intestines and eye.

parasympathomimetic Agent or drug which mimics action of parasympathetic nerve, eg carbachol.

parathyroid (1) Beside thyroid gland. (2) One of 4 small glands, near thyroid, which control metabolism of calcium and phosphorus.

paravertebral Beside vertebral column. Used in connection with anaesthesia.

paresis (Gr. paresis, relaxation) Slight paralysis. See paralysis, wobbler syndrome.

paries Anatomical term meaning wall.

parietal (L. parietalis) Of a cavity.

parotid (para- + Gr. ous, ear) Situated near ear, eg **p.** gland.

parotitis Inflamed parotid gland.

parrot jaw (syn. undershot jaw) Short lower jaw. Inherited condition, results in overgrown front teeth and end molars, due to lack of wear from teeth in opposite jaw. Older horses may suffer malnutrition.

pars Anatomical term meaning division or portion of area, organ or structure.

parturient Of birth, qv.

parturition (L. parturitio) Act of foaling. See birth.

Paso Fino (Sp., fine step; syn. Chongo) Tough but attractive and gentle pony established on island of Puerto Rico, off S America, about 400 years ago. Descended from Spanish horses; now being exported to US. Has natural gaits similar to Peruvian Paso, qv.

passage Channel for moving from one place to another. **birth p.** See birth.

passport Document necessary for Thoroughbred in training travelling abroad. Contains marking certificate (qv), vaccination papers etc. Issued by Weatherby's. See Thoroughbred, veterinary rules.

pastern Part of leg between fetlock and coronet, formed by 1st phalanx. See ringbone. **split p.** Colloq. for fracture of 1st phalanx. Crack may start at any point and extend in any direction (but is rarely entire length of bone) or bone may be in small fragments (comminuted fracture). Causes acute lameness. Horse may pull up sound and go lame on way home or may be lame during exercise; usually sweats and shows distress. Diagnosis: on signs and X-ray (see plate 41). Treatment: rest in box on peat moss or woodshavings for 2–3 months then exercise gently 2–3 months. Bandage or plaster cast support may be necessary and if pieces of bone are separated, fix with internal screws. Complete recovery is usual unless arthritis of fetlock or corono-pedal joint sets in. **p. joint** Formed by 1st and 2nd phalangeal bones (pastern and coronary bones). Joint capsule bulges when distended by excess synovia at coronary band.

pasteurellosis Disease caused by infection with pasteurella bacteria. Uncommon in horses but may cause acute fever and infectious disease of respiratory tract, usually during long sea or road journey.

patella Large sesamoid bone articulating with femur and forming part of stifle joint. **upward fixation of p.** Locking of hindleg. Symptoms: hindleg locks briefly when extended, sometimes with repeated catching of **p.** when walking. Cause: poor conformation of central (medial) ridge (trochlea) of femur. Condition my be inherited or caused by loss of condition and muscular unfitness; often affects both hindlegs. Treatment: relieve pain by pushing **p.** to inside and down. Medial **p.** ligament can be cut to produce permanent cure.

patent (L. patens, open) Open. See ductus arteriosus. **p. bladder** See bladder, rupture of.

patho- (Gr. pathos, disease) Combining form meaning relationship to disease.

pathogen (patho- + Gr. gennan, to produce) Disease-producing microorganism, ie bacterium, fungus, virus.

pathogenesis Way that disease process develops in body.

pathogenic Resulting in disease.

pathognomonic (patho- + Gr. gnomonikos, fit to give judgement) Characteristic of a certain disease, eg spasm of third eyelid in lockjaw, qv.

pathognomy (patho- + Gr. gnome, a means of knowing) Science of signs and symptoms of disease.

pathologist Expert in pathology. See post-mortem.

pathology Science of disease as it affects body structures, tissues and organs.

pattern Design, arrangement, behaviour. **behavioural p.** Sequence of actions when horse reacts to external stimuli and to environment. See behaviour.

pCO₂ (PCO₂) Symbol for carbon dioxide gas partial pressure (tension). Usually measured in millimetres of mercury. It represents pressure exerted by CO_2 in a space (eg lungs) or fluid (eg blood). It is partial if other gases (eg oxygen) are present; and together they form a total pressure which is usually atmospheric.

PCV or p.c.v. Abbr. packed cell volume. See hematocrit.

pedal (L. pedalis/pes, foot) Of the foot. **p. bone** (pronounced peedal, syn. 3rd phalanx) Bone inside hoof. See foot. **p. osteitis/ostitis** Inflamed **p.** bone causing pain and lameness. Diagnosis: on X-ray examination. Treatment: rest, shoeing with pad underneath sole, possibly **neurectomy**. Outlook: unfavourable.

pediculosis Infested with lice. See louse.

peduncle Stem-like part, eg base of some warts.

pelvis Group of bones forming ring with sacrum (croup area of spine) above; ilia at sides and pubic and ischial bones, below. Cup-like area of ischium fits around head of femur, forming hip joint. Bones form area

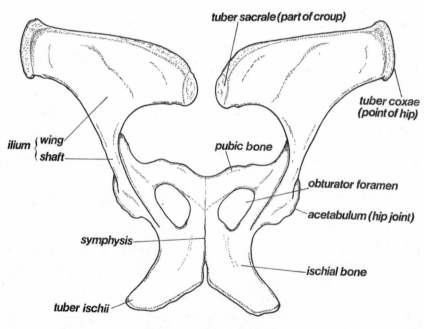

30 Pelvis, seen from above

of attachment for muscles and ligaments which control movement of back and hindlegs. Pelvic ring/girdle houses rectum, vagina and urethra in the mare; accessory glands and part of urethra in the stallion. Its diameter is about 24cm. (approx 9½ins.) in the mare and 18cm. (approx 7ins.) in stallion. **p., fracture of** Relatively common, particularly shaft of ilium. Caused by trauma, eg in fall or during galloping. Symptoms depend on site of fracture; tuber coxae—moderate lameness with point of hip on fractured side flatter than normal; shaft—severe lameness with refusal to take weight on affected leg; symphysis—severe lameness affecting both hindlegs. Diagnosis: on physical signs and on rectal palpation which detects grating of bones (crepitation). Treatment: rest 3–6 months on peat moss bedding. Slings may be necessary in severe cases. **renal p.** Funnel-shaped cavity in kidney at kidney duct (ureter).

Penavlon Trade name. See benzylpenicillin.

Penbritin Trade name. See ampicillin.

penicillin Powerful antibiotic. See benzamine **p.**, benzylpenicillin and procaine **p.**

penicillinase Enzyme-like substance which reacts against penicillin; produced by certain bacteria, eg Staphylococcus.

Penidural Trade name. See benzamine penicillin and procaine penicillin.

penis Male organ of coitus composed mainly of erectile tissue with common duct for semen and urine and with one end free, in prepuce, ending in glans penis. The whole is similar to human **p.** (rather than bull's **p.**) and has to become engorged with blood to make it erect. (See behaviour.) At rest it is entirely enclosed in sheath (lubricated by smegma). See plate 1.

pentobarbitone sodium (trade name: Nembutal) White odourless slightly bitter-tasting granules or crystals. Short-acting barbiturate with a more rapid effect than phenobarbitone, qv. Used as anticonvulsant in newborn foals and anaesthetic during surgery on young foals. Dose: 20–35mg./kg. body wt. See anaesthetic, neonatal maladjustment syndrome.

H.H.—T

Pentothal Trade name. See thiopentone sodium.

pepsin (L. pepsinum, from Gr. pepsis, digestion) Enzyme of gastric (stomach) juice which acts on proteins of food converting them into simpler substances. See digestion.

peracute (L. peracutus) Excessively acute, eg a disease.

Percheron Draught breed developed in La Perche district of France about 100 years ago. Now popular in many countries. Has very heavy body on short, comparatively feather-less legs. May be up to 17 hands and black or grey only. Assn: British P. Soc., c/o A. E. Vyse, Owen Webb House, Gresham Road, Cambridge (Cambridge 56778).

percussion (L. percussio) Act of striking part with short sharp blow to sound part beneath. **p. of chest** Can distinguish between hollow and solid part of lung. Two fingers are placed between each rib in rotation and lightly tapped with two fingers of opposite hand. With slack wrists this produces resonant sound where there is air in lung beneath. Chalk line can be drawn joining points where resonance becomes a dullness. Horse is then trotted and procedure repeated. In broken wind (emphysema) new chalk line will be well behind first one. Chalk marks on healthy horse will not move back as far. P. can identify consolidated (airless) areas of lung in pneumonia.

periarteritis (peri- + Gr. arteria, artery + -itis) Inflamed external coat of artery and surrounding tissues.

periarticular (peri- + L. articulus, joint) Around a joint, eg p. tissue refers to structures outside joint capsule.

pericarditis (pericardium + -itis) Inflamed membranous sac (pericardium) surrounding heart. Caused by infection with Streptococcus equi, Streptococcus pyogenes, and other bacteria or, in newborn foal, by injury during birth; often accompanied by septicemia, pneumonia or pleurisy. Symptoms: pain, shallow fast breathing, fever, increased heart rate. Diagnosis: on hearing grating or rubbing in heart area. Treatment: rest, antibiotics. See ausculation, birth, heart.

pericardium (L. peri- + Gr. kardia, heart) Fibrous sac which surrounds heart and is joined to membrane (epicardium) lining outside of heart.

perinatal (peri- + L. natus, birth) Occurring shortly before or immediately after birth. **p. mortality** Death from about 2 weeks before birth is due, to 1 week afterwards.

perineal Of the perineum.

perineum (Gr. perineos) Area between anus and scrotum/vulva.

periodic ophthalmia See eye, diseases of: moon blindness.

periosteum Special tissue which covers all bones of body and has bone-forming capacity. See periostitis.

periostitis Inflamed membrane (periosteum) lining surface of bone: caused by sprain, blow or infection. Symptoms: pain, swelling and heat. See ringbone, osselet, bone, bucked shin, spavin.

Perissodactyla (Gr. perissos, odd + daktylos, finger) Order of ungulates having odd number of toes on each foot. Includes horse (now one-toed). See evolution. Opp. Artiodactyla.

peristalsis (peri- + Gr. stalsis, contraction) Movements of alimentary canal which propel food along muscular wall. See alimentary canal, borborygmus, colic.

peristaltic Of peristalsis.

peritoneal Of the peritoneum.

peritoneum (L., G. peritonaion from per, around + teinein, to stretch) Smooth, glistening membrane lining abdomen and its contents; helps one part of gut slide easily on another.

peritonitis Inflamed peritoneum, qv. Caused by infection with bacteria, migrating redworm larvae, clot (thrombus) blocking arteries which supply gut, foreign bodies penetrating gut wall. Symptoms: fever, reluctance to move, grunting, looking round at flanks, raised white blood cell count (as condition progresses, count usually falls). **P.** may cause portions of intestine to stick together or to abdominal wall. Treatment: antibiotics and corticosteroids while primary cause is identified. See adhesion, blood tests.

per rectum Through rectum, as in administration of drugs by enema, or examination **p.r.**

Persian Originally a typical Oriental breed—beautiful and high spirited. Said to have descended from Tarpan, to have been known many years BC and to be ancestor of Arab. No longer a distinct breed.

perspiration See sweat.

Peruvian Paso Horse loved for its lateral gaits which, although smart and high-stepping, give wonderfully smooth ride. Inherent gaits are pace, marching paso and normal paso although undisciplined horse may break into trot or canter. Gaits may have caused tendency towards long pasterns, long hindlegs, sometimes with sickle hocks, and flexible leg and spinal joints. Thought to have descended fom Andalusians used by Spanish cavalry to conquer Peru. Later there was probably Arab influence and **P.P.** is now exported, particularly to US, where breed is popular in California and Arizona. Cf Paso Fino. See gait.

pervious urachus Condition when urine drips from umbilical stump of newborn foal. Happens if urachus (duct between bladder and placenta) does not close immediately after birth. Condition may be cured by antibiotics, but surgery necessary if it persists.

pessary (L. pessarium) Cone-shaped tablet of antibiotic or other drug for inserting into uterus. Used after difficult foaling or to treat infection. See infertility.

petechia (L.; pl. petechiae) Abnormal, round spot of blood under mucous membrane. Cf ecchymosis. See purpura hemorrhagica.

pethidine/p. hydrochloride Odourless colourless crystals or white crystalline powder with bitter taste. Relieves pain from smooth muscle, eg of alimentary canal. Effects last 3–4 hours; used in colic, meconium retention and with tranquillisers to sedate. Dose: 3–5mg./kg. body wt. IM.

Pfeifferella mallei Name formerly given to causal organism of glanders (qv).

PG See prostaglandin.

PGF₂ alpha Prostaglandin (qv) of uterus.

pH Symbol for measurement of alkalinity/acidity of body fluids: pH 7 is neutral; above 7 alkaline and below 7 acid. Normal pH of blood: about 7.40.

phago- (Gr. phagein, to eat) Combining form meaning eating or ingestion.

phagocyte Cell that devours and destroys (amoeba-like) micro-organisms or other cells and foreign particles. May be fixed, eg cell of reticuloendothelial system (qv) or free, eg white blood cell.

phagocytosis Process of phagocyte (qv) action.

phalangeal bones The first, second and third phalanx (or pastern, coronary and pedal bone) forming extremity of leg. See foot.

phalanges Pl. of phalanx.

phalanx (Gr. a line of soldiers; pl. phalanges) One of 3 bones below fetlock joint.

pharmacopeia (pharmaco + Gr. poiein, to make) See Veterinary Codex.

pharyngeal (L. pharyngeus) Of the pharynx (throat).

pharyngitis Inflamed pharynx. See strangles, influenza, virus, tongue swallowing.

PhD Abbr. Doctor of Philosophy. Degree entitles holder to title, Doctor.

phenacetin Fine white odourless and slightly bitter-tasting crystalline powder. Reduces temperature and relieves pain. Now rarely used in horses. Dose: 8–15gms.

phenamidine isethionate White odourless powder or crystals with slightly bitter taste. Used to treat biliary fever and other Babesia infections, particularly B. caballi, although controls Nuttalia equi. Dose: (1 usually adequate) 4% solution diluted with equal sodium chloride, 0.03ml./kg. body wt. sub. cut.

Phenergan Trade name. See promethazine hydrochloride.

phenobarbitone White odourless slightly bitter-tasting powder. Barbiturate drug with effect varying from mild sedation to full anaesthesia, depending on dosage and route of administration. **p. poisoning** Treat with artificial respiration and bemegride, picrotoxin, or nikethamide. See pentobarbitone, thiopentone.

phenol Colourless or faintly pink needle-shaped crystals with characteristic odour. Potent bactericide, but because it tends to penetrate skin, mucous memberanes and other tissues, its use as antiseptic has declined. See disinfectant.

Phenosan Trade name. See phenothiazine.

phenothiazine (trade names: Agrazine; Cooper's liquid **p.**, Minel, Phenosan; Phenovis; PTZ) Green or greyish-green tasteless crystalline powder with characteristic odour. Anthelmintic used against strongyles (redworm). In effective against tapeworm or whiteworms. Altered and excreted in dung and urine as harmless substance which, when exposed to air, may turn red. Variety of treatments—in single doses of 10–30gms. according to weight, age and condition. At this dose, drug will remove nearly all small strongyles and Strongylus vulgaris. Removal of S. vulgaris, S. equinus and S. edentatus is enhanced by piperazine. Worm control programmes include 1–2gms. daily for 3 weeks in every month, 5gms. weekly or 15gms. monthly. Many years' use may encourage development of resistant strains. Drug well tolerated by most animals, but may cause anemia, jaundice and photosensitisation, qv. **p. poisoning** Causes enlarged kidneys, liver and spleen. Foals should not be treated under 3 months old. Pregnant mares seem unharmed by drug.

phenotype (Gr. phainein, to show, + typos, type) Characters of an animal; result of its inherited material (genes) but not necessarily transmitted to progeny. Cf genotype.

Phenovis Trade name. See phenothiazine.

phenylbutazone (syn. bute; trade names: Butazolidin, Buta-Leucotropin) Fine creamy-white crystalline odourless powder with slightly bitter taste. Used to treat painful conditions including arthritis, torn muscle and wounds, splint, ringbone, bucked shin. Response to p. varies greatly;

if no improvement in 3–7 days it should be stopped. If successful, withdrawal of **p.** may allow reappearance of symptoms. Dose: 1–2gms. daily. (Excreted from body as oxyphenbutazone.) See veterinary rules.

phenytoin (trade name: Epanutin) White odourless powder made into solution to control convulsions, especially in foal (see neonatal maladjustment syndrome). Dose (foal): 5–10mg./kg. body wt. IM or IV, followed by maintenance doses 1–5mg./kg. every 2–4 hours for 12 hours, then every 6 or 12 hours depending on severity of convulsions.

pheromone Substance or hormone secreted by one animal and which alters behaviour of another, eg **p.** in mare's urine, when she is in oestrus, excites stallion, who exhibits flehmen posture, qv.

phonocardiogram (phono- + Gr. kardia, heart + gramma, a writing) Graph of heart sounds using instrument known as phonocardiograph connected to microphone placed on chest.

phosphorus (abbr. **P.**) (1) See calcium and **p.** (2) Can cause poisoning (sources: rat poisons and organophosphorus drugs). Symptoms: those of irritant poisons, ie abdominal pain, relief, then more pain, jaundice and nervous symptoms followed by convulsions, coma and death. Postmortem findings include inflamed mucous membranes of stomach and intestines, fatty degeneration of liver, jaundice and a smell of **p.** on opening abdomen. Diagnosis: chemical analysis of gut contents. Treatment: reduce shock with corticosteroids, heart stimulants and intravenous glucose.

photosensitisation Sunlight sensitivity. Occurs in unpigmented areas, eg white heels, face markings. Symptoms: inflamed skin and, especially on face, sores which ooze serum. Allergy or drugs (eg phenothiazine) may predispose to **p.**

phrenic (L. phrenicus, Gr. phren, mind) (1) Of the mind. (2) Of the diaphragm, eg **p.** nerve.

phthalylsulphathiazole White or yellowish-white odourless crystals or powder, with slightly bitter taste. A sulphonamide (qv) drug. Not absorbed from alimentary canal and used to treat diarrhoea in foals. Dose: 0.1–0.15gms./kg. body wt. See sulphanilamide.

phylum (L., Gr. phylon, race) Main division of animal or vegetable kingdom. Horses belong to **p.** Chordata which includes fish, birds, reptiles, amphibians and mammals. See evolution.

physiology Science of living organism and its parts.

physiotherapist Person specialising in physiotherapy.

physiotherapy (physio + Gr. therapeia, cure) Diagnosis and treatment using agents such as light, heat, cold. **cold therapy** Popular treatment for sprains, particularly those of deep and superficial digital flexor tendons of forelegs. Cold water from a hosepipe is played over injured parts for up to half an hour twice a day. Cold-water bandages are used but need constant changing. Bandages soaked in cooling lotions, generally based on lead acetate and zinc sulphate solution, are also used. Horse can be stood in bucket or boot and cracked ice packed around leg, more ice being added as original melts. **heat therapy** Includes poultices, electrically-heated boots, short-wave diathermy, inductothermy and microwave diathermy. Poultices can be made from bran or linseed, kaolin, etc, but a heated boot is more effective. This fits leg from knee or hock to hoof. Heating elements cover inside and run from a 16-volt battery. Heat can be applied up to 20 minutes and temperature allowed to fall over next half hour. Boot can be quickly removed if horse is restless. Heat from boot or poultice does not penetrate deeply so high energy waves can be used. Horse should stand on rubber mat placed on dry floor. In short-wave diathermy a flexible piece of metal between two pieces of rubber forms a pad. A lead connects it to a generator and it is kept off skin by perforated felt pad. It has been calculated that temperature of muscle 5cm. (2ins.) below skin can be raised 5 or 6°F. Inductothermy is used to treat tendons, ligaments, muscles, splints and bucked shins. Output of machine has to be varied as horse is not consistent in amount of heat it can tolerate. Microwave diathermy units are portable, so horse can be treated in own stable. After diathermy and inductothermy, sprained flexor tendons still need approximately a year's rest before fast work. Ultrasonic therapy gives pulsated heat; one 'on' period to four 'off' periods. The micromassage produced is particularly useful in muscle injuries. Faradism produces rhythmical muscular contractions. Power is from dry batteries which eliminates risk from mains electricity and allows machine to be used anywhere. Electrical contact is through indifferent electrode pad. Skin over saddle area is wetted and a plastic sponge moistened in water laid across back just behind withers. A leather pad, fitted underneath with two plates, is strapped over sponge. The two metal plates are connected to a single plug to which one lead of machine is fitted. The mobile electrode consists of chain and two sponges in chamois leather, to which the second lead is attached. Area to be treated is again wetted and substance, eg tragacanth mucilage, used to maintain good contact. Useful to diagnose site of injury—when painful muscles are contracted, patient is restless or moves away from mobile pad. Treatment varies between 20–30 minutes; number of contractions between 100–130 a minute, daily or every other day. Swimming allows horse to exercise without strain on legs and whirlpool baths are used to jet warm water on to horse, sometimes with magnesium sulphate added. In whirlpool boots, cold or warm water is added until it covers knee. Air is forced through a number of holes in the boot at level of fetlock by means of a compressor. Temperature of the water rises during treatment so ice must be added when cold therapy is used. Massage and manipulation are difficult as horse is such a large patient. Reference: Hopes, Raymond, BVMS, MRCVS.

Physostab Trade name. See chorionic gonadotrophin.

physostigmine salicylate Alkaloid from calabar bean of W Africa. Colourless odourless crystals with slightly bitter taste. Produces effects similar to parasympathetic nerve stimulation by preventing destruction of acetyl choline. Causes increased peristalsis, diarrhoea, constricts finer air tubes. Large doses cause muscle twitching. Used in eye to reduce pressure and counteract action of atropine.

phytoferol See tocopheryl acetate.

pia mater (L., tender mother) Innermost of 3 membranes known as meninges and covering brain and spinal cord. Cf. dura mater.

pica See appetite, depraved.

picadex Similar to piperazine. See piperazine salts.

picrotoxin White or off-white crystalline odourless powder with very bitter taste. Powerful stimulant of brain, increases frequency and depth of respiration, raises blood pressure. Used to counteract barbiturate poisoning. Dose: 60mg. IV or IM.

piebald See coat colouring.

pilocarpine nitrate Alkaloid from leaves of Pilocarpus plant. Colourless or white crystals with faintly bitter taste; action similar to effects of parasympathetic nerves. See autonomic nervous system. Used in eye drops, or as injection to treat impacted colic, but should be used with caution. Dose: 60–200mg. sub. cut.

Pinto (from Spanish pintado, painted) Type with patchy colouring, popular with American Indians for its natural camouflage. Similarly marked horses were drawn on walls of Egyptian tombs 3,000 years ago. Piebald **P.** termed Overo, skewbald is Tobiano. Either may have blue eyes. Developed from wide range of types and recognised as breed in 1960s. Assn: **P.** Horse Assn of America, PO Box 3984, San Diego, California (Zip no: 92103). Cf Paint.

Pinzgauer Draught breed first developed in Pinzgau district of Austria; said to trace to Friesian, but now dying out. Usually roan with short, compact, feather-less legs. Often crossed with South German Cold Blood.

piperazine salts (adipate, citrate, hydrate, or phosphate; trade names: Citrazine, Coopane, Entacyl, Antepar, Antoban, Helmezine, Pipricide, Radiol, Silbeverm, Verocid, Oxazine) White crystalline or granular odourless powders with slightly acid taste. Anthelmintic effective against seatworm and whiteworm at all stages in gut; acts by paralysing worms. Dose: 220mg./kg. body wt. (adipate and citrate), 185mg./kg. body wt. (hydrate and phosphate), all by mouth or stomach tube. Wide safety margin in overdose.

Pipricide Trade name. See piperazine salts.

Pirevan Trade name. See quinuronium sulphate.

Piroplasma (L. pirum, pear +Gr. plasma, something formed) Former name for protozoan parasite found in red blood cells. Now called Babesia. See biliary fever.

piroplasmosis Former name for infection caused by Piroplasma. Now called babesiasis/babesiosis. See biliary fever.

pithing Destruction of brain and spinal cord by thrust of blunt instrument, usually after shooting. See euthanasia.

Pitocin Trade name. See oxytocin.

Pitressin Trade name. See vasopressin.

pituitary Endocrine (ductless) gland connected to base of brain. About 2.5 cm. (1 in.) long in adult, with two parts (lobes): anterior (front) and posterior (back). Controlled by (1) releasing factors from hypothalamus (part of brain) and (2) its own hormones, ie those it produces which work on distant glands. When these react by liberating another hormone, p. cuts down its own secretion. Activity increases with amount of light filtering through eyes (it produces more of the sex **p. injection** (trade name: Pituitrin) Clear colourless liquid with faint hormones, which is why horses are more sexually active in summer).

Produced by posterior lobe	Acts on
oxytocin	smooth muscle of uterus
antidiuretic hormone	kidney
prolactic hormone	mammary glands
Produced by anterior lobe (syn. conductor of orchestra)	**Acts on**
follicle stimulating hormone (FSH)	ovaries
luteinising hormone (LH)	ovaries
adreno-cortico-trophic hormone (ACTH)	adrenal gland
thyrotrophic hormone	thyroid gland
interstitial cell stimulating hormone (ICSH)	interstitial cells of testes (causing production of testosterone)

odour, obtained from posterior lobe of p. gland. Has actions similar to oxytocin, qv. Also raises blood pressure, reduces excretion of urine (an antidiuretic) and raises levels of blood sugar. Used to treat inertia of uterus during birth or involution of uterus afterwards (see uterus). Oxytocin is generally preferred.

Pituitrin Trade name. See pituitary injection.

placenta (L., a flat cake; syns. chorioallentois, allantochorion) Membrane or organ developed by fetus to nourish it and transport waste material by close contact with mare's uterus. Formed in first 15 days of fetal life by fusion of 2 embryonic membranes, the chorion and allantois. By day 90 it is attached (implanted) to uterine wall. There is insufficient room in uterus for 2 placentae and carrying twins is difficult for mare (usually stunted or aborted if conceived; see twin). Material passes from fetal to maternal blood stream via capillaries that lie close together. Gases and materials pass by diffusion or by selective action of cells. They must pass 6 layers: (1) maternal capillary wall, (2) subcutaneous tissue, (3) epithelium, qv; then similar layers in placenta, (4) epithelium, (5) connective tissue, (6) capillary wall. This separation of blood streams of fetus and mare makes equine **p.** epithelio-chorial type. (Compare with human **p.** (hemochorial) which erodes maternal uterus and leaves 3 layers.) Mare's uterus retains all its tissue and does not bleed or lose many cells when **p.** is removed, ie it is non-deciduate. **P.** communicates with fetus by blood vessels of umbilical cord. This also contains the urachus, a duct from bladder through which urine passes and is stored as allantoic fluid, qv. **P.** is about 10mm. thick and is thinnest at part adjacent to cervix. It ruptures, releasing allantoic fluid (breaking water) at start of 2nd stage labour. Diseases of **p.** include infection with bacteria, fungus and probably virus, causing inflammation, (placentitis). These cause abortion or interfere with growth and nourishment of fetus. In twins capillaries and larger blood vessels may fuse, allowing blood streams to mix. **P.** normally weighs 2–5kg. (5–12lb.) at full term; usually expelled (about 30 minutes) after foaling. See abortion, afterbirth, plate 6. Cf yolk sac **p.**

placental Of the placenta.

plantar Of sole of foot.

Plantation Walking horse See Tennessee.

plantigrade (L. planta, sole + -gradus, walking) Characterised by walking on full sole of foot, eg man. Cf digitigrade. See evolution.

plaque Patch or raised area. See nettle rash.

plasma (Gr., anything formed or moulded) Fluid part of blood in which cells are suspended. Distinguished from serum by presence of fibrinogen.

plaster of Paris Calcium sulphate reduced to fine powder by driving off most of water. Used to make casts and cover bandages to immobilise part, eg fractured leg.

plate (1) Lightweight shoe, normally aluminium and about 3oz. Fitted when Thoroughbred races. Cf shoe. (2) Colloq. for media on which bacteria are grown in laboratory, eg blood agar **p.** (3) Flat, thin layer, eg of bone. See growth **p.**

Plateau Persian Light but hardy type. Bred by tribesmen roaming from Persian Gulf to Zagros Mountains bordering on Iraq.

platelet Oval or round disc-like cell in blood, concerned in clotting. See coagulation, blood.

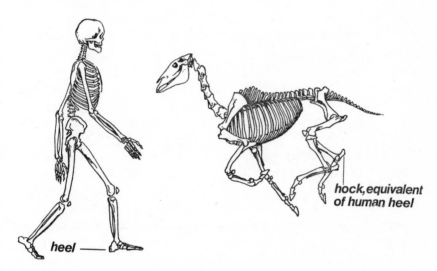

heel

hock, equivalent of human heel

31 The difference between plantigrade (walking on sole of foot) and digitigrade (raised on to the toes)

Platyhelminthes (platy- + Gr. helmins, worm) Phylum of flatworm including Cestoda and Trematoda. See tapeworm, fluke.

pleura (Gr. side, rib; pl. pleurae) Outer covering of lungs. It is moistened so that lungs can move and encloses potential cavity (pleural space).

pleural space Area around lungs.

pleurisy (Gr. pleuritis) Inflamed outer lining of lungs (pleura) caused by infection with bacteria or virus; usually associated with pneumonia and pericarditis. Symptoms are those of pneumonia, qv.

plexus (L., braid) Joining together of nerves. **brachial p.** See nerves, table of.

Pliohippus An ancestor of modern horses which lived in Pliocene period about 10 million years ago. See evolution.

PMS Trade name. See serum gonadotrophin.

PMSG Abbr. pregnant mare serum gonadotrophin, qv.

pneumonia (syn. pneumonitis) Inflamed lung tissue (as opposed to air tubes). Commonly associated with inflamed air tubes (bronchitis) and caused by infection with bacteria, virus, fungus, migrating parasitic larvae (see whiteworm, lungworm), inhalation of injurious particles or chemicals, allergic reaction. Symptoms: increased rate and depth of respiration, fever and coughing, especially in bronchitis and bronchiolitis (inflamed bronchioles). Abnormal sound, eg moist râle or high-pitched tone, may be heard on auscultation (qv) if bronchitis present. Areas of dullness can be detected if air sacs are obliterated by inflammatory reaction (see percussion). Treatment: antibiotics and/or removal of precipitating cause. **summer p.** Condition of foals under 6 months. Caused by Corynebacterium equi, organism inhaled or swallowed. Symptoms: abscesses in lymph glands and lung tissue, high temperature, distressed breathing, thick discharge from nostrils, areas of dullness and râles on auscultation of chest. There may be wasting and condition often fatal. The bacteria are sensitive to most antibiotics but these cannot help advanced cases because organisms are protected by thick-walled abscesses of creamy pus. **tuberculosis p.** Rare condition caused by Mycobacterium tuberculosis organism. Symptoms: increased cells in lung (not comparable with tuberculosis in humans). **virus p.** Caused by herpes and adeno viruses which inflame supporting tissues of alveoli and bronchioles. See also snotty nose.

pneumothorax Accumulation of air in pleural cavity as a result of injured chest wall.

pneumovagina Air abnormally present in vagina due to failure of vulva to seal entrance. See Caslick; uterus, infection of.

pO$_2$ (PO$_2$) Symbol for oxygen gas partial pressure (tension). Usually measured in millimetres of mercury. It represents pressure exerted by O$_2$ in a space (eg lungs) or fluid (eg 90–100mm. of mercury in arterial blood). It is partial if other gases (eg carbon dioxide) are present; and together they form total pressure which is usually atmospheric. See anoxia, neonatal maladjustment syndrome.

point of hock (syn. tuber calcis) See tarsal bones.

poisons Substances which harm body externally or internally and which can kill or interfere with function. Various amounts produce toxic effects; what is harmful in one circumstance may be harmless in another, eg food may be toxic if fed in excessive amounts or under unsuitable conditions. **inorganic p.'s** Lead, mercury, arsenic, phosphorus, salts. **organic p.'s** Carbon compounds, chloroform, carbon tetrachloride, ether, organic acids, alkaloids, glycosides, phytotoxins (see also rodenticide). Apart from substances which burn (strong acids and alkalis) most **p.'s** must be absorbed into blood to be toxic; they enter body by ingestion, inhalation, absorption through skin or injection. The liver detoxicates them and is therefore damaged or inflamed in most poisoining. Diagnosis: (1) diarrhoea, abdominal pain—due to metals and their salts (eg arsenic, copper, iron, strong acid or alkali, chlorates, phosphorus) and anthelmintics (eg carbon tetrachloride, phenol, turpentine); (2) convulsions—ammonium salts, lead, nitrate, phenol, opium, strychnine, ethylene glycol; (3) coma—bromide, carbon monoxide, zinc phosphide, barbiturate, anaesthetic, sedative, atrophine, phenol, turpentine; (4) muscular inco-ordination—ammonium salts, nitrate, lead, phenothiazine, nicotine, turpentine, oxylate; (5) dilation of pupils—atropine, hyacine, nicotine, aconite; (6) constriction of pupils—opium derivatives, physostigmine, pilocarpine; (7) distressed breathing—carbon monoxide, cyanide, nitrates, zinc phosphide, strychnine, yew, nitrite; (8) sensitisation—phenothiazine, dimadidium bromide, grasses, buckwheat; (9) blood in urine—chlorate, copper, kale, rape, bracken, lupin. See separate headings.

Polish Anglo-Arab Anglo-Arab widely and carefully bred in Poland. **P. Arab** Breed kept at a high standard by the Poles, a nation long renowned for horse breeding. Oldest Arab stud in Poland dates from 1500s and fresh stock has often been imported from Arabia. Arab studs in the USA have been founded with **P.** horses. See Arab. **P. Half-Bred** Type often produced Trackehnen blood.

poll Highest point of head, just behind ears. **p. evil** Infection of **p.** area (occipital bursa) with bacteria, often Brucella abortus. Painful swelling appears on one or both sides of neck just below **p.** Treatment: drain through needle and inject antibiotics. Surgery may be necessary in severe cases. See filaria, occiput.

pollution ring See masturbation.

polo pony Type rather than breed, term 'pony' being used loosely as animals used for polo may be up to 16 hands. Performance during the game, ie speed and agility, are only criteria. Many ponies have Thoroughbred blood or trace to Manipur (qv) ponies of Assam, where polo was popular in 7th century.

polycythemia (poly- + Gr. kytos, cell + haima, blood) Excess of red blood cells. See hemoconcentration.

polydipsia (poly- + Gr. dipsa, thirst) Excessive thirst and drinking. Associated with diarrhoea, excessive staling (polyuria) and diabetes mellitus. Follows saline medicine. See diarrhoea, behaviour.

polymixin(s) Antibiotic substances obtained from Bacillus polymyxa. **p.B sulphate** Used to treat uterine infection. Creamy, white powder which absorbs moisture and is effective against Proteus and Pseudomonas infections. Used locally, eg to irrigate uterus or in ointment to treat mastitis.

polymorph (abbr. polymorphoneuclear leucocyte) White blood cell, nucleus of which has several lobes. See blood tests, hematology (5).

polyp (Gr. polypous, a morbid outgrowth; syn. polypus) Growth from mucous membrane, occasionally found in nose or throat causing horse to make breathing noise (see wind). May also occur in bladder. See growth.

polypi Pl. of polyp.

polypropylene See wound.

polyuria (poly- + Gr. ouron, urine + -ia) Passage of large volume of urine, excessive staling.

pons (L., bridge) Tissue connecting two parts of an organ. See brain.

pony Any member of Equus caballus (qv) beneath 14.2 hands. Some breeds take **p.** (rather than horse) even if above 14.2, eg Camargue. **P.** seems more susceptible than horse to sweet-itch, laminitis. It rarely conceives twins, even when researchers try to induce them, cf Thoroughbred. Assns: National **P.** Soc., c/o Cmdr B. H. Brown, 85 Cliddesden Road, Basingstoke, Hampshire (Basingstoke 22906); Ponies of Britain Club, c/o Mrs G. Spooner, Brookside Farm, Ascot, Berkshire (Winkfield Row 2508); British Show **P.** Soc., c/o Capt. R. P. Grellis, Smale Farm, Wisborough Green, Sussex (Wisborough G. 279). See separate breeds, eg Dales, Dartmoor, Exmoor, Highland, New Forest, Welsh Mountain. **P. of the Americas** (syn. POA) Type developed in 1950s from Arab and American breeds, Appaloosa and Quarter horse. Up to about 13.2 hands. Sometimes has Appaloosa-type colouring.

popped knee See carpitis.

portal Of an entrance, eg to liver.

Portuguese Alter See Alter.

position (L. positio) Relationship of foal's spine to that of mare during delivery, eg **dorsal p.** Spine uppermost (normal). During last third of pregnancy fetus takes up **p.** upside down (head towards cervix) in uterus. Normally it revolves during 1st stage labour, so that it is born in dorsal **p. ventral p.** Foal upside down. Cf presentation, posture. See birth, dystocia.

posterior Anatomical for hind part or surface (opp. anterior).

post-mortem (L., after death) **p.-m. examination** (PME) Study of carcase to discover or confirm cause of death. Usual method is a mid-line (qv) incision to expose suspect areas and/or take tissue samples. These are put in preservative, eg formalin, for laboratory testing. **P.-m.e.** especially important on fetuses (to check for virus abortion), on sudden deaths and cases of suspected infectious disease. Usually required by underwriters if horse is insured.

postnatal Occurring after birth.

posture (L. postura) Alignment of foal's legs and neck during delivery or in utero, eg flexed or extended. Cf. position, presentation. See birth.

poultice (L. puls, pap; Gr. kataplasma; syn. cataplasm) Hot or cold substance applied to a part to alter its temperature or draw dirt, maggot or pus from area. See boil, physiotherapy, warble fly.

pound (L. pondus, weight) Unit of mass of avoirdupois system; contains 16 ounces; equivalent to 453.6gms. See weights and measures.

Pouseki Colloq. Turkoman, qv.

powdered opium Light-brown powder with strong characteristic odour and bitter taste. Obtained from capsules of Papaver somniferum. Actions and uses are those of morphine, qv. Dose: 3–8gms.

pox Skin eruptions which go through characteristic changes starting as small red spots and developing into blisters or vesicles. These burst leaving ulcer, on which scab forms, eventually falling off as condition subsides. May occur on skin or mucous membranes. See coital exanthema, acne.

precipitation Antigen/antibody reaction in which particles which clump together are smaller than those in agglutination reaction. Used in laboratory to test for presence of antitoxin in blood serum.

predispose To incline beforehand; action, fact or situation in body or environment which produces a tendency, eg cold draughts **p.** foal to infectious diarrhoea.

prednisolone (Trade names: Deltacortil, Deltastabl, Predsol-N) White or off-white crystalline odourless bitter-tasting powder. Actions similar to cortisone acetate, qv. Injected into and around joints. **p. acetate** (trade name: Delta-Ef-Cortelan) and **p. trimethylacetate** (trade name: Vecortenol) have similar uses.

Predsol-N Trade name. See prednisolone.

pregnancy State of being pregnant. **p. hormone** See progesterone. **p. tests/diagnosis** (1) Rectal palpation, ie put arm into rectum to feel fetus through wall. Usual 40 days after stallion's last service (and at intervals up to birth) but detection possible from 19th day. (2) Blood tests: measure PMSG (pregnant mare serum gonadotrophin). Reliable from day 45–100, either by mouse test or in test tube. Mouse test:

inject mare's blood into immature female mouse. Open mouse 48 hours later. Ovaries and uterus will be swollen and congested if mare is pregnant. (Similar to Aschheim-Zondek test using urine of human female.) Test tube method (immunological assay) by (a) hemagglutination inhibition or (b) agar gel diffusion. (3) Urine tests: detect oestrogens from day 150 to birth (cuboni test). (4) Ballottement: unreliable test in which clenched fist is pressed firmly against flank to feel fetus rise—and then fall when fist is retracted. (5) Ultrasonic: detection of fetal heart by placing probe of ultrasonic apparatus into mare's rectum. Used in research. May detect fetal pulse as early as 42 days' gestation and certainly from 3 months onwards.

pregnant (L. praegnans, with child; syn. gravid) Condition of having fetus in body after ovum has been fertilised by spermatazoon. Marked by interrupted oestrous cycle, calmer disposition (possibly), steady enlargement of abdomen, development of mammary glands. See also gestation. **p. mare's serum gonadotrophin** (PMSG) Mixture of follicle stimulating hormone (FSH) and luteinising hormone (LH) **in p.** mare from day 40–90. Can be measured in blood plasma (see blood tests) and given to mare as serum gonadotrophin, qv.

Pregnyl Trade name. See chorionic gonadotrophin.

premature (L. praematurus, early ripe) Birth of foal before it is mature, ie before 325 days' gestation. See birth, maturity.

prematurity Condition of weakness in foals born between 300–25 days' gestation. Symptoms: low weight, delay in standing for first time (over 2 hours after birth), reduced strength of suck and ability to maintain sucking position, emaciation, dehydration, tendency to suffer from diarrhoea and susceptibility to infection. Treatment: see newborn foal.

premium stallion One who travels to cover mares rather than staying at one stud. He stands in prearranged places in rotation so that mareowners know where he is. Stallion said to be at a **p.** of £x or x gns. System is common among English hunters, not among Thoroughbreds. French National Stud (Le Haras du Pin, Orne) runs **p.s.** service with Percherons and trotters. See veterinary rules (Ministry of Agriculture).

prepotent (L. praepotens) Having more power (than fellow parent) to transmit characteristics. See gene.

prepuce (syn. sheath) Double fold of skin which contains and covers non-erect penis. Contains glands which secrete smegma, qv.

presentation (L. praesentatio) The way foal is presented to birth passage; direction of spine. **anterior p.** Head first (normal). **posterior p.** Hindquarters first. **transverse p.** Lying across birth passage. Cf position, posture. See birth.

Prevac Trade name: influenza vaccine with aluminium hydroxide adjuvant. Prepared in W Germany.

Prevac T Trade name: influenza and tetanus vaccine combined. Safe in horses over 3 months old, including pregnant mares.

primidone (trade name: Mysoline) White crystalline odourless slightly bitter-tasting powder. Anticonvulsant used on newborn foals. Dose: 25–50mg./kg. body wt. See neonatal maladjustment syndrome.

primigravida (L. prima, first + gravida, pregnant) Individual pregnant for first time, ie maiden mare.

procaine hydrochloride Colourless odourless crystalline powder with slightly bitter taste, followed by local numbness. Acts as local anaesthetic. Effect increased when used with adrenaline to delay absorbtion. Used in solutions from 0.5–5% for operations such as removing of warts, stitching wounds, stitching vulva (Caslick). **p. penicillin** (trade names: Duracillin, Mylipen, Penidural) White crystalline powder. Antibiotic released slowly which forms a depot when injected. Dose: 0.5–10mg./kg. body wt. IM.

process (L. processus) (1) Prominence or projection, eg of bone. (2) Series of happenings, eg birth **p.**

progesterone (syn. pregnancy hormone) (1) Hormone secreted by ovaries, placenta and adrenal glands; prepares uterus to receive fertilised egg and necessary for implantation of fetus and maintenance of pregnancy; antagonistic towards oestrogen and associated with dioestrus (state of rejection). Together with oestrogen promotes growth of mammary gland, towards the end of pregnancy, and inhibits production of luteinising hormone and follicle stimulating hormone (see pituitary gland). (2) **synthetic p.** White odourless crystalline powder;

made into tablets for implanting into mares in an attempt to prevent abortion. Usual implant, 0.25–1gm., now thought to have little effect. See oestrous cycle. **P. implants** Trade name. See progesterone.

progestins Hormones secreted by yellow body (corpus luteum); 95% consist of progesterone, qv.

prognosis (Gr. prognosis, foreknowledge) Forecast of probable end of disease, ie prospect of recovery.

prolactin Female hormone produced by posterior lobe of pituitary gland. Acts on mammary glands causing them to develop and produce milk.

Prolan Trade name. See chorionic gonadotrophin.

prolapse (L. prolapsus from pro, before + labi, to fall) Passing outwards of part or organ through a natural opening or tear. **p. of uterus** See uterus, prolapse of.

promazine hydrochloride (trade name: Sparine) White crystalline odourless bitter-tasting powder. Has actions similar to chlorpromazine hydrochloride (qv) but less potent and toxic. Used as tranquilliser. Dose: 2.2–5.5mg./kg. body wt. IM or 1.1–3.3mg./kg. body wt. IV.

promethazine hydrochloride (trade name: Phenergan) White or cream-coloured odourless bitter-tasting powder. Antagonises histamine; has actions and uses similar to mepyramine maleate, qv. Dose. 5–20ml. of a 5% solution IM. See antihistamine.

prophase First stage in mitosis, qv.

prophet's thumb mark See depression.

prophylaxis (Gr. prophylassein, to keep guard before) Preventive treatment. See vaccine.

proprietary Medicine or drug marked under trade-mark, patent or copyright.

proquamezine fumarate (trade name: Myspamol) Drug with relaxant effect on smooth muscle and a mild tranquillising action. Used for relief of choke, colic, dystocia. Dose (39% solution) adult pony: 10–15ml., Thoroughbred: 10–20ml. IV. Can cause temporary staggering and prolonged lying down if injected too rapidly.

prostaglandin (PG) Natural hormone-like substance first described in 1930 by Lieb and Kurzrok. Isolated and named in 1934. Many types (in body tissues and fluids) which act on eg blood pressure, gut action, breathing, nervous system, inflammation. Inhibited by aspirin and anti-inflammatory drugs. **P.** secreted by uterus, PGF_2 alpha, causes yellow body (corpus luteum) to stop working, so that mare comes into season. Can be given to mare, by infusing 50–100μgm. to bring her into season.

prostate gland (Gr. prostates, one who stands before) Gland which stretches across neck of bladder, beginning of urethra and below rectum; consists of 2 lobes connected by an isthmus. It opens into urethra by about 20 ducts which convey a milky secretion with characteristic odour. Secretion acts like those of other accessory glands (seminal vesticles and bulbo-urethral glands), ie nourishing and forming fluid to carry spermatozoa.

prosthesis (Gr., a putting to) Replacement of a part by artificial substitute, as in modified Hobday operation.

protein (Gr. protos, first) Complex organic compound containing nitrogen; widely distributed in plants and animals; combination of amino-acids and their derivatives. **simple p.'s** Albumin, globulin, glutelin, alcohol-solubles, albuminoids, histones and protamines. **conjugated p.'s** Nucleoproteins, glycoproteins, phosphoproteins, hemoglobins, lecithoproteins, lipoproteins. **derived** p.'s Metaproteins, coagulated **p.'s,** proteoses, peptones and peptides, eg albumin, casein, legumin, fibrin. **P.** in blood consists of albumin and globulin in the ratio of about 0.8:1.0. Albumin maintains osmotic balance, ie it enables blood stream to retain fluid; globulin is made up of alpha 1, alpha 2 and beta 1, which are produced in liver and form part of hormones, bile pigment, mucus and blood clotting mechanism. Beta 2 and gamma globulins are formed from special cells lining blood spaces of liver and spleen and are part of antibody system of body. **p.-binding** Method of assaying levels of cortisone and other hormones in blood. See blood tests. **p. hydrolysate solution** (trade name: Protogest) Clear brown liquid with strong meaty taste. Product of digested first-class animal **p.** plus dextrose. Given to newborn foals suffering from malnutrition, dehydration or diarrhoea. Dose: 10ml./kg. body wt. every 4 hours.

proteinuria (protein + Gr. ouron, urine) Presence of protein in urine. Symptom of disease in kidneys or bladder. See nephritis, cystitis.

prothrombin (pro- + Gr. thrombos, clot + -in, chemical suffix) Glycoprotein present in blood plasma and converted to thrombin, also called coagulation factor II. See coagulation.

Protogest Trade name. See protein hydrolysate solution.

protoplasm Vital substance of living cells composed of proteins, carbohydrates and inorganic salts. See cell.

Protozoa Phylum of organisms with one-cell bodies, ie unicellular (cf metazoa). Life histories vary; parasitic species may be direct or indirect, with sexual or asexual multiplication. Members important in equine medicine include Trypanosoma brucei (see nagana), T. evansi (see surra), T. equinum (see mal de caderas), T. equiperdum (see dourine), Babesia equi and B. caballi (see biliary fever).

protozoan Organism belonging to phylum Protozoa.

protozoon (pl. protozoa) A single-cell organism.

proud flesh See wound.

proximal (L. proximus, next) Nearest (opp. distal).

PRQ Antiseptic Trade name. See benzalkonium chloride solution.

pruritus (L. from prurire, to itch) Condition characterised by itching or scratching. Symptom of skin infested with lice or mange mites. **anal p.** Itching caused by seatworm. See seatworm, mange, louse.

Przewalski (Equus przevalskii, after Russian explorer Col N. M. Przevalski) Wild horse, discovered in W Mongolia; virtually unapproachable by man. Looks like stocky, coarse pony, about 12 hands, with thick, dun-coloured coat, tufted tail and a mane which looks hogged and does not fall into a forelock. Head is large with small eyes and ears, and the hoofs horse-like rather than boxy. Pedigree book (published by Prague Zoo) records than on 1 Jan, 1972 there were 196 **P.** horses (85 stallions and 111 mares) in zoos around world and that 23 foals were born in 1971. It is unlikely any pure P.'s still roam wild. **P.** has 66 chromosomes, qv. See also Mongolian.

pseudo-glanders See epizootic lymphangitis.

Pseudomonas Group of bacteria one of which, **P.** pyocyanea, causes disease. Found in uterine and urinary infections. Gram-negative bacillus which responds to treatment with chloramphenicol and polymyxins.

pterygoid (Gr. pterygodes, like a wing) Shaped like a wing, eg shoulder blade (scapula).

ptosis (Gr. ptosis, fall) Drooping of upper eyelid caused by injured **third cranial** (oculomotor) nerve, by conjunctivitis or painful condition of eyeball. Usually affects only one eyelid. See eye; nerves, table of.

ptyalin (Gr. ptyalon, spittle) Enzyme in saliva, converts starch to maltose and dextrose.

PTZ Trade name. See phenothiazine.

puberty (L. pubertas) Age of full sexual powers, about 2 years in fillies, 3 in colts. Earlier in exceptional cases. See behaviour, male sexual.

pubic Of pubic bones. See pelvis.

pubis Smallest of 3 bones of pelvis (with ischium and ilium). Forms back part of pelvic floor and of obturator foramen; known as pelvic brim. See pelvis.

puff disease See dry coat.

pulmonary Of the lungs. **p. semilunar valve** 3 semilunar cusps forming valve guarding exit of right ventricle and entrance to **p.** artery. Prevents blood returning from artery to ventricle (see aortic semilunar valve).

pulp (L. pulpa, flesh) Soft tissue, eg **p.** of tooth (see teeth).

pulsation (L. pulsatio) Rhythmical beat. See pulse.

pulse (L. pulsus, stroke) Beat of artery coinciding with heart beat; felt by placing ends of fingers against artery, (1) on lower jaw, midway between angle of jaw and front teeth, or (2) on inside of foreleg, just in front of elbow. See heart rate. **p. rhythm** Normally regular but irregular in some heart conditions (atrial fibrillation, partial block, sinus arrhythmia). **p. quality** Refers to strength of beat. Strong in health, weak if heart is failing.

pupil (L. pupilla, girl) Opening at centre of iris of eye. See eye.

purgative (syn. cathartic) Drug which causes evacuation of intestinal contents (1) by increasing volume of non-absorbable matter, (2) by irritating intestine, increasing its movements (peristalsis), and (3) by direct stimulation of nerves (parasympathetic) supplying gut. **irritant p.** One that stimulates intestine. **p. overdose** Symptoms: severe diarrhoea, collapse and occasionally death. Treatment: give demulcent, eg kaolin. **saline p.** Acts by increasing fluid in gut.

purging See diarrhoea.

purpura hemorrhagica (L., purple) Acute non-contagious disease characterised by bleeding into mucous membranes and extensive soft swellings beneath skin. Usually follows acute infectious disease of upper respiratory tract, strangles, or stress of travelling. Cause: unknown. Damage to walls of small blood vessels results in plasma and blood leaking into surrounding tissues. Symptoms: face, muzzle or other parts of body develop extensive cold, painless swellings, which pit on pressure, mucous membranes of nose and mouth contain blood, temperature is unchanged, heart rate rises. Disease may last 1–2 weeks, majority of cases die from blood loss and secondary bacterial infection. Diagnosis: on symptoms (must be distinguished from equine viral arteritis, swamp fever and dourine). Examination of blood reveals fall in red cell count and hemoglobin level. Treatment: inject antihistamine and corticosteroid drugs. Give blood transfusions and calcium. Postmortem findings include hemorrhages (see petechia, ecchymosis) throughout body and congested organs and intestinal wall.

purulent (L. purulentus) Containing pus.

pus Inflammatory product consisting of cells, fluid and bacteria. See abscess.

put down Colloq. to destroy. See euthanasia.

pyemia (Gr. pyon, pus + haima, blood) Septicemia in which numerous abscesses occur in different parts of body. See joint-ill.

pyramidal disease See buttress foot.

pyrantel tartrate (trade name: Strongid) Drug used to treat redworm and whiteworm. Dose: 12.5mg./kg. body wt.

pyridoxine Component of vitamin B. See concentrated vitamin B solution.

Q

quadruped (quadri- + L. pes, foot) Four-footed animal, eg horse.

quarantine (Ital. quarantina) Period in which horse must be isolated, to avoid risk of spreading infectious disease. See veterinary rules (Thoroughbred Breeders' Assn).

quarter Part of wall of foot between heel and toe. See foot.

Quarter horse See American Quarter horse.

Queensland itch (syn. allergic dermatitis) Disease causing itchy skin and common in Australia. Sandfly bites cause allergy, producing lesions round tail, rump and on withers. Itching is intense and oozing sores develop. Treatment: antihistamine drugs and protection from bites by making stable insect-proof.

quid To chew grass or hay into mass (bolus) ready for swallowing, then drop it. May be result of injured throat or associated structures, neglected, overgrown teeth or partial paralysis of swallowing mechanism.

quinapyramine (chloride or sulphate; trade name: Antrycide) White, cream or pale-yellow odourless bitter-tasting powder. Active against Trypanosomes such as T. equinum (see mal de caderas). Dose: 4.4mg./kg. body wt. sub. cut. Overdose causes trembling, salivation, collapse; but recovery is usually swift. Local reactions common and dose should be divided and given at 2 or 3 sites.

quinidine sulphate White needle-like odourless bitter-tasting crystals. Slows heart rate. Used to treat atrial fibrillation (qv). Initial test dose of 5gms. given to detect idiosyncrasy, then 10gms. twice daily, increased to 3, 4 and 5 times on successive days until normal rhythm is re-established. Overdose causes diarrhoea and severe depressive illness leading to collapse and death.

quinsy (L. quinancia, sore throat) Abscess in throat. See strangles.

quinuronium sulphate (trade names: Acapron, Babesan, Pirevan) Odourless creamy-white to canary-yellow crystals with bitter taste. Used to treat biliary fever. Single injection will cure within 24 hours if disease is treated early. Signs of reaction, which may occur 10–15 minutes after injection: restlessness, muscular spasms, salivation and defecation. These may continue for a few hours, but are rarely serious and can be controlled with adrenaline or atropine. Because of risk of sensitisation, 2 weeks–3 months should be allowed before second treatment. Dose: 0.6–1mg./kg. body wt. sub. cut.

quittor Injury causing chronic inflammation of cartilage of pedal bone. Symptoms: pus-filled swelling, heat and pain around bulb of heel and coronary band. May cause lameness and hardening of cartilage, resulting in sidebones. Treatment: antibiotics and possibly surgical removal of damaged cartilage.

R

R. Abbr. for Roentgen. See radiation.

Ra Abbr. for radium, qv.

rabies (L. rabere, to rage) Fatal virus infection of central nervous system. Rare in horses but can affect any warm-blooded animal (including man). Symptoms: madness, biting other animals (which spreads the disease), chewing skin, fear of water, salivation, falling, rolling and eventually paralysis and death. Notifiable disease. See veterinary rules (Ministry of Agriculture), inclusion body.

rack See gaits.

rad Abbr. radiation absorbed dose. Measure of radiation, qv.

radial (L. radialis) of the radius. **r. paralysis** See dropped elbow.

radiation (L. radiatio; syn. irridation) Use of radio-active elements which emit rays. High-energy rays (eg X-ray) can penetrate skin and are used to diagnose broken bones (especially useful in hairline fractures, eg of pedal bone) and bony growths. Alpha, beta and gamma rays can be produced from radium (Ra) salts. Alpha rays have low penetrating power, beta rays slightly more and gamma rays are approx. same strength as X-rays. (Can be used to reduce inflammatory process, eg in arthritic joint, and treat skin diseases, by killing damaged or cancerous cells.) Ultraviolet rays have powerful germ-killing properties and are especially useful in diagnosing ringworm. International unit (IU) of **r.** is Roentgen (R.). 0–25 R. is unlikely to injure; more than 25 R. can cause burns and reduce red and white cells in blood (anemia and leukopenia); more than 400 R. can kill.

radio- (L. radius, spoke, ray) Combining form meaning relationship to radiation.

radio-active Having properties of radio-activity.

radiocarpal Of the radius and carpus, eg **r.** joint. See knee.

radiograph (radio- + Gr. graphein, to write) Photograph taken with X-ray equipment.

radio-iodine Radio-active isotope of iodine, usually I_{131} used in thyroid function test. See iodine.

radium (abbr. Ra after its radiant appearance) Rare metal. Its rays can be used in radiation, qv.

radius (L., spoke; pl. radii) Larger of 2 bones of forearm (cf ulna) between elbow joint (above) and knee, ie carpus (below). Lower end includes growth plate, qv.

radon Radio-active gas of radium. **r. seeds** Particles which emit gamma rays and can be put into plaster to treat cancerous or bony growths.

ragwort poisoning Occurs when pasture is scarce and horse eats **r.** (Senecio jacobaea, or other member of family: marsh **r.**, Oxford **r.**, groundsel). Plants should not be cut or pulled then left on pasture.

Symptoms: dullness, rapid pulse and breathing, weakness, constipation, jaundice and death in a few days or several weeks. Slow build-up of poison causes wasting, jaundiced mucous membranes, nervous symptoms charcterised by yawning, drowsiness and staggering. At post-mortem: enlarged, hardened (cirrhotic) liver, fluid in abdomen and lungs, spots of blood on small intestines, heart. Diagnosis: on liver biopsy and blood tests showing liver dysfunction. No known treatment available.

râle (Fr. râle, rattle) Abnormal harsh or soft breathing sound, depending on whether fluid is present in air passages. See auscultation, bronchitis, pneumonia. Cf rhonchus.

ramus Small structure given off by larger one. **r. of jaw** Branch of lower jaw.

RANA See animal nursing auxilliary.

rash Colloq. for spots on skin. See nettle rash, ringworm, acne, dermatitis.

rate Speed, frequency or measure of events. **basal metabolic r.** Amount of oxygen used by body at rest. **breathing (respiratory) r.** Number of breaths in 1 minute. **death r.** Number of deaths resulting from disease or particular circumstances. **erythrocyte sedimentation r.** (ESR) Time taken for red blood cells to settle when blood containing anticoagulant is allowed to stand. Expressed as percentage fall in a given time, usually 1 hour. Increased in infectious diseases, eg swamp fever; slowed in states of dehydration, eg diarrhoea. **fertility r.** Percentage of mares producing foals in any given stud season. **heart r.** Number of beats per minute. See breathing; blood tests, hematology (7); fertility; heart.

ratio Quantity of substance in relation to another. **A./G. (albumin/globulin) r.** Albumin to globulin in blood serum, normally approx. 2:1, reversed in liver disease to 0.5:1. **calcium/phosphorus r.** See calcium and phosphorus. **nutritive r.** That between protein, fats and carbohydrates in feed. See blood tests, food.

rat killer poisoning See rodent killer poisoning.

RCVS Abbr. Royal College of Veterinary Surgeons, qv.

reaction (re- + L. agere, to act) Response to physical or chemical stimulation. See behaviour, blood tests.

reagent Any material used in chemical or biological reaction.

receptor Sensory nerve-ending which responds to stimulus. See nerve cell.

recto-vaginal fistula Abnormal opening between rectum and vagina, caused by foreleg of foal puncturing vagina during delivery. See birth, hazards of; dystocia.

rectum Last part of large intestine. See alimentary canal.

recumbent Lying down. Horse rarely **r.** for long (see behaviour); if it is, sores may develop. See decubitus.

red blood cell (syns. erythrocyte, RBC) Cell of blood, 4–5μ diameter. Produced in bone marrow and unusual as it has no nucleus. Contains pigment (hemoglobin) and carries oxygen from lungs to all parts of body. See blood.

red mercuric oxide Scarlet odourless tasteless highly-irritant powder. Solution: **r.m.o.** dissolved in equal weight potassium iodide and water. 1% solution used repeatedly as mild counter-irritant. See blister.

redworm (syn, strongyle) Nematode parasite (roundworm) of order Strongyloidea, family Strongylidae. Several genera, viz.,

Strongylus vulgaris	14–16mm.
Strongylus equinus	6–35mm.
Strongylus edantatus	23–28mm.
Tridontophorus (4 species)	from 6–25mm.
Trichonema	4–17mm.
Posteriostomum and	
Gyalocephalus	

Lengths refer to males; females are smaller. All are parasites of large intestines (colon and caecum). Life history: female in intestine lays eggs which pass out with dung on to pasture; 1st larvae hatch, feed on bacteria and moult to become 2nd larvae; further moults lead to infective larvae. These are swallowed by new host. Inside host, habits differ by species, eg larvae of Trichonema enter wall of large intestine and develop inside nodules, then return to cavity of large intestine.

Larvae of S. equinus penetrate walls of caecum and colon and hibernate in nodules beneath peritoneum. After further development for about 11 days, 4th-stage larvae leave nodules and migrate to liver, where they stay 6–7 weeks. They return to intestine through pancreas and peritoneal cavity, where they develop further, then again travel to gut about 120 days after infection; larvae of S. edentatus cause nodules in mesentaries and wall of large intestine. Larvae of S. vulgaris enter blood vessels supplying small intestine and cause an aneurysm (qv) where the vessels branch from main aorta. S. vulgaris has longest life cycle, ingestion of larvae to appearance of adults in large intestines taking 6–12 months. **R.** damage can be divided into that caused by adults and that by migrating larvae. Adults suck blood from intestine walls and cause anemia, ulceration, hemorrhage, colic or diarrhoea. They can rupture intestines, especially in young horse, if present in large numbers. Larvae cause peritonitis, ulcerative enteritis, aneurysms, colic, liver disease, wasting and can migrate to heart, damaging valves. Treatment: workers are trying to perfect a vaccine, using irridated **r.** larvae; until this is available horses at grass should be wormed regularly (see dichlorvos, mebendazole, phenothiazine, pyrantel tartrate, thiabendazole). Larvae are infective only when on grass, so stabled horses not at risk unless allowed to graze contaminated pasture. See plate 26.

reflex (L. reflexus) Automatic nervous reaction to a stimulus at some point of body. **r. arc** See arc.

regurgitation (re- + L. gurgitare, to flood) Backward flow. **aortic r.**/ **mitral r.** Blood flows backwards against main stream due to faulty heart valves.

reproduction (L. re, again + productio, production) Process of conception, gestation and birth of foal. See behaviour, embryology, birth, Society for the Study of Animal Breeding.

resistance (L. resistentia) Horse's ability to withstand pathogenic microorganisms. Partly due to immunity, partly to natural defence mechanisms of body, eg white blood cells.

resonance (L. resonantia) The noise produced by percussion of a cavity. See percussion.

respiration See breath.

respiratory distress (syn. difficult breathing) See neonatal maladjustment syndrome.

reticulo-endothelial system Network of cells lining liver and bone marrow which engulf harmful substances. Cells are named phagocytes; their ingesting action, phagocytosis.

retro- Prefix meaning backward or behind, eg retropharyngeal, at back of pharynx.

Rhenish Draught horse from Rhine area of Germany. Usually about 16 hands, most often sorrel-coloured and with comparatively feather-less legs. Has own stud book.

rheumatism (L. rheumatismus, Gr. rheumatismos) Condition characterised by diseased connective tissue of body, especially muscles and joints. Not known to occur in horses. Cf arthritis.

rhinitis Inflamed mucous membranes of nose. See snotty nose, catarrh. Cf sinusitis.

rhinopneumonitis Virus now called equine herpesvirus I. See virus.

rhododendron poisoning Caused by eating r. (Ericaceae family). Symptoms: attempts to vomit, salivation, colic, shallow breathing, weakness, staggering, collapse and death after several days. Little, if any, evidence of inflammation at post-mortem. No specific treatment.

rhonchus (L., Gr. rhonchos, a snoring sound) Dry, coarse râle. See râle.

rhythm (L. rhythmus, Gr. rhythmos) Regular beat or recurrence. **gallop r.** Heart beat with accentuated extra sound, so that 3 sounds can be likened to noise of hoof beats at fast pace. Best heard after exercise. See heart sounds.

rib Long, curved bone. R.'s form walls of chest and are arranged in pairs. Each articulates with thoracic vertebra (above) and a cartilage attached to sternum (below). Most breeds have 18 pairs. Cf Arab.

riboflavine Orange-yellow crystalline powder with slight odour and bitter taste. Member of vitamin B group; forms part of enzyme system necessary for oxidation of carbohydrates, amino-acids and other pro-

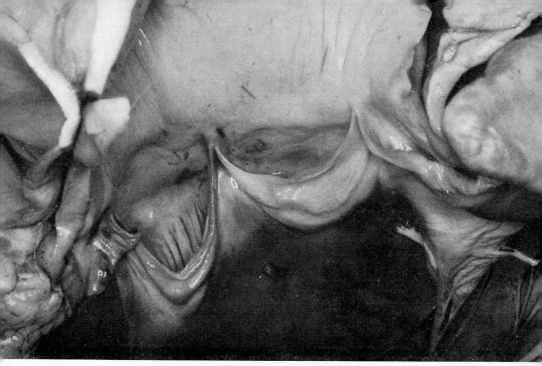

36   Aorta opened to show three cusps of semilunar valves guarding exit from left ventricle. See *aortic semilunar valve*

37   Ovary opened to show abnormal cysts. See *granulosa cell tumour*

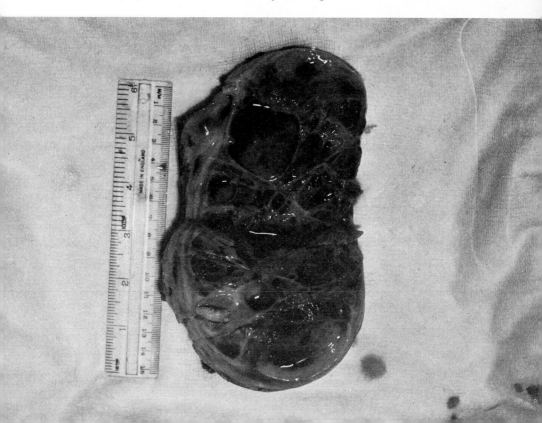

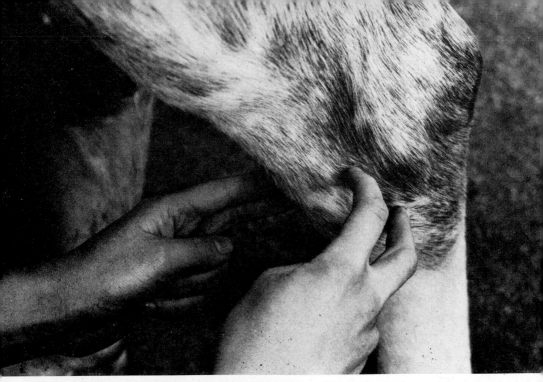

38 Feeling for bog spavin on inside and outside of hock. See *bog spavin*

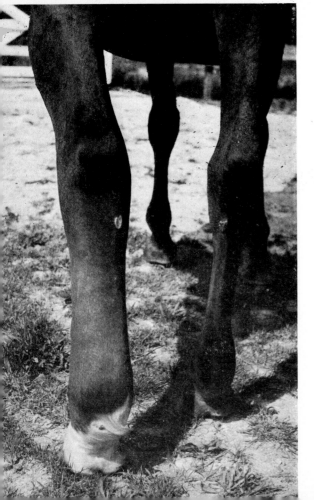

39 Swollen near-hind. See *lymphangitis, big leg*

ducts of metabolism. Important for red cell production and health of eye and capillaries. Storage organs: liver, heart, kidneys. Deficiency unlikely as **r.** widely distributed in foodstuffs. Moon blindness may be prevented, but not cured, by adding 40mg. per day to feed. See eye, diseases of: moon blindness.

rickets Disease of young horses characterised by lack of calcium in bones. Symptoms: stiffness, lameness, enlargement of growth plates (qv) resulting in firm, painful swellings on inside and outside of fetlock, knee and hock joints. In extreme cases—rare in horses—there may be bow-leggedness. Treatment: give vitamin D and correct any calcium/phosphorus imbalance. See calcium and phosphorus.

rig (syn. cryptorchid) Colloq. for state when one testis has not descended into scrotum; may be retained in inguinal canal (high testis) or in abdomen (intra-abdominal **r.**). Can also mean rarer state when neither testis has descended (double or bilateral **r.**). Condition may be inherited; likely to cause aggressive behaviour. Treatment: castrate under general anaesthesia, removing retained testis through flank. See Welsh Mountain pony.

rigidity (L. rigidus, stiff) Stiffness. See rigor mortis, neonatal maladjustment syndrome, convulsions, lockjaw.

rigor mortis (L.) Stiffening of body after death. Due to chemical changes shortening and hardening muscle tissues. Occurs 1–7 hours after death, varying with temperature (heat accelerates process, cold delays it) and cause of death (faster in conditions such as lockjaw). After a period of **r.m.** bacterial fermentation in tissues causes body to become limp.

ring Circular ridge in horn of hoof due to change of season, level of nutrition or laminitis, qv. See foot.

ringbone Growth of new bone (exostosis) on first, second or third phalanx due to inflamed bone lining (periostitis). Caused by trauma, underlying bone disease, nutritional deficiency or infection. **R.** classified as high (at lower end of 1st phalanx or upper end of 2nd); low (lower end of 2nd phalanx or top of 3rd); articular (involving joint surface of pastern or corono-pedal joint); or peri-articular (at distance from joint, not involving surface). Symptoms: pain, swelling and usually lameness. Diagnosis: on X-ray examination. Treatment: inject cortico-steroids, rest horse and, in extreme cases, cut nerve supply.

ringworm (syns. Dermatomycoses, mycotic dermatitis) Condition caused by fungal invasion of skin cells and hair fibres. (No type of worm is involved.) Occurs in all countries; more common in winter and where horses are stabled. Common causal organisms are: Trichophyton equinum, T. mentagrophytes, Microsporum gypseum and M. equinum. Spread by direct contact or infected bedding, saddlery, grooming kit, blankets or human clothing. Stables are difficult to disinfect because fungus spores can live for years. Fungi attack skin which oozes serum and forms scabs of matted hair. These peel off, leaving red, moist area. Infection spreads outwards and tends to form circles. These may amalgamate so that large areas are affected. Lesions are common on girth area, flanks and neck and tend to be deeper on young horses. Diagnosis: on examination of skin scrapings for fungus, which can be seen under microscope or grown on culture. Some fungal infections can be diagnosed by exposing skin or hairs to a fluorescent light (see radiation). Treatment: apply weak solution of iodine, salicylic acid or proprietary fungicide spray, ointment or lotion. Give griseofulvin by mouth. Control: **r.** not a health menace and has little economic consequence apart from Jockey Club ruling (Thoroughbreds) that affected horses must not go to race meetings.

roan See coat colouring.

roaring (syn. laryngeal paralysis) Abnormal noise made by horse breathing in. See wind, Hobday.

Roccal Trade name. See benzalkonium chloride solution.

rodent killer poisoning Rare condition when horse is affected by rodenticide. (1) ANTU (alphanaphthylthiourea), causes oedema of lungs and sac around heart. No treatment known. (2) Castrix, causes convulsions. (3) Fluoracetate, causes heart failure. (4) Red squill, causes convulsions and heart failure; chronic cases develop gastritis and enteritis. (5) Warfarin, interferes with production of prothrombin in liver and prolongs clotting time of blood. Symptoms: lameness due to hemorrhage, diarrhoea, often bloodstained, multiple hemorrhages throughout body. Treatment: give vitamin K, 5mg./kg. body wt.

rose Colloq. enlarged state of glans penis, qv.

roundworm Parasite of class Nematoda with six orders. Those important in equine medicine: Strongyloidea (redworm, qv, lungworm, qv, stomach worm, qv); Ascaroidea (whiteworm, qv); Filarioidea (filaria, qv); Spiruroidea (stomach worm).

Royal Animal Nursing Auxilliary (RANA) See animal nursing auxilliary. **R. College of Veterinary Surgeons** Opened 8 Apr. 1791 as Veterinary College of London. First professor of College and prime mover in its foundation was Lyons-born Benoit Vial (who used name Charles Vial de St Bel). First president of College (granted Royal charter 8 Mar. 1844): Hugh 2nd Duke of Northumberland. Addr.: 32 Belgrave Square, London SW1 (01 235 4971). See soundness, veterinary rules, veterinary surgeon. **R. Netherlands Draught horse** See Dutch Draught.

rubefacient (L. ruber, red + facere, to make) Drug or substance that increases blood flow to part. See blister.

running of milk Colloq. for premature secretion by mammary glands. Mare may run first milk (colostrum) as early as 3 weeks before foaling or if she aborts. See birth, colostrum, gland, oxytocin. **r. walk** See gait.

rupture Tear or break. See bladder, rupture of; cord, rupture of; birth.

Russ See Gotland.

Russian Saddle Syn. Orlov Rostopschiner, qv. **R. Steppe** Extremely tough type, either ewe-necked pony similar to Przewalski, or horse descended from English Thoroughbred crossed with Przewalski or Mongolian.

S

sac (L. saccus, Gr. sakkos) Pouch **allantoic s.** That part of placenta which contains fluid.

sacral (L. sacralis) Of the sacrum.

sacrum Single bone formed from 5 vertebrae fused together. It is triangular and forms joint with pelvis (sacro-iliac articulation). Articulation may be dislodged causing lameness. Spinal processes above form croup.

Saint John's wort (Hypericum species) Plant which causes photo-sensitisation (dermatitis over areas lacking pigment when exposed to light).

salicylate (aspirin) Pain relieving drug which may irritate intestinal lining causing hemorrhage and diarrhoea. Used to treat arthritis in preference to cortisone.

saline (L. sal, salt) Containing salt. **normal s.** 0.9% sodium chloride in water, ie approx. 1 teaspoonful to 600ml. (1 pint).

saliva (L.) Clear, alkaline fluid discharge into mouth by salivary glands. Contains a digestive enzyme and moistens food ready for swallowing.

salivation (L. salivatio) Increased saliva. **excess s.** Drooling of saliva due to colic, grass sickness, choke, foreign body in, or injury to, tongue, throat, teeth, gums and cheek. See ptyalin.

Salmonella Genus of aerobic gram-negative bacteria. Classified by serology for differing protein content, which is antigenically distinct. **S. abortivo-equina** (syn. S. abortus-equi) Organism causing abortion and septicemia. Once common but less so now. Causes abortion (in seventh or eighth month of pregnancy), retained placenta and infection of uterus (metritis). Foals develop septicemia (see septicemia of the new-born) and joint-ill (qv) during first few days of life. **S. enteritidis** Occasionally causes salmonellosis in horses. **S. typhimurium** Most common cause of salmonellosis (qv) in horses.

salmonellosis Disease of all animals often caused by Salmonella typhimurium. Causes acute enteritis or less typically joint-ill, qv. Symptoms: high fever, dullness, bloodstained diarrhoea and death, usually from 24–48 hours. May reach epidemic proportions on a farm. Spreads through pasture, feeding stuffs and drinking water contaminated with fecal material. Diagnosis: on recovery of organism from feces. At post-mortem there is extensive hemorrhage in wall of alimentary canal and enlarged lymph nodes. Treatment: sulphadimidine, chloramphenicol, nitrofurazone, neomycin.

salpingitis Inflamed fallopian tube, qv.

salt See sodium chloride, saline.

sandcrack (syn. toe, quarter or heel crack) Crack in wall of hoof from ground surface upwards; or starting at coronary band and extending downwards. Often several together. Caused by lack of foot care, injury to coronary band, weakening of wall from excessive drying. May result in lameness. Treatment: grove horn above or below crack and to either side; use shoe with clips to suport wall either side of crack.

sanguineous Of blood; bloody.

sarcoid (syn. equine sarcoid) Tumour on skin caused by virus. May appear on leg, head, shoulder, breast or flanks. Resembles simple wart at first but grows rapidly and ulcerates. On removal it tends to recur and may bleed. May be troublesome when mating if near genitalia, or when foal sucks if close to udder. Treatment: surgery, but radio-activity may be necessary to prevent recurrence. See growth.

Sardinian Pony of Italian island of Sardinia, about 13.2 hands. Roams free until broken for riding or driving.

scab Crust or hard covering of sore on skin. See ringworm, dermatitis.

Scandinavian breeds Include Fjord, Gudbrandsdal, Estonian or Smudish (Zmudzin) and Zemaitukas. See separate headings.

scapula See shoulder blade.

scar (Gr. eschara, scab on a wound caused by burning) Fibrous line in skin after healing of wound, qv.

Schleswig/er Heavy artillery or cart horse of German **S.** province.

scirrhus (Gr. skirrhos) Firm swelling of fibrous connective tissue. **s. cord** Infected spermatic cord, eg with Staphylococcus, after castration. Symptoms: swelling in region of wound, stiffness (due to pain). Treatment: surgical removal and antibiotics.

sclera (L., Gr. skleros, hard) White of eye; tough, outer covering of eyeball. See eye.

scleritis Inflamed sclera. See eye, diseases of.

343

sclerosing agent Substance which hardens tissues, eg sodium oleate, sodium morrhuate (used to treat fractured sesamoid bones). Other substances can be used to treat soft palate or abnormally distended (varicose) vein.

Scoline Trade name. See suxamethonium chloride.

scoliosis (Gr. skoliosis, curvation) Rare crooked spine in newborn foals. May be associated with limb deformities, but simple cases recover in few weeks.

Scottish breeds See Highland, Shetland.

scour See diarrhoea.

scrotal Of the scrotum. **s. hernia.** See hernia.

scrotum Fold of skin or sac containing testes (testicles).

seatworm (syn. Oxyuris equi) Nematode (roundworm parasite) of order Ascaroidea, family Oxyuridae, which lives in caecum and colon. Male 9–12mm. (just under ½in.) long, female 40–150mm. (approx. 1½in.–6in.). Life cycle: female passes to anus, where she lays eggs, which stick to skin; larvae develop in eggs, which then drop off host and are later eaten with food or drink. After further development larvae grow into adults, completing the cycle. They may irritate anus, causing horse to rub against objects. Treatment: see piperazine salts. See plate 26.

sebaceous (L. sebaceus) Secreting greasy substance, eg **s. gland** Gland in skin which secretes oily matter. Overactive **s.g.**'s may cause seborrhea, qv.

seborrhea (L. sebum, suet + Gr. rhoia, flow) Excessive discharge of grease from glands (sebaceous) of skin; may develop into infection. Most common in heels (see mud fever). Treatment: ensure clean bedding, wash area and apply astringent lotion.

second thigh See gaskin.

secretion (L. secretionem) A gland's production of substances such as hormone, digestive fluid.

sedative Drug which lessens activity of brain, reducing excitement, eg barbiturate.

sedimentation Deposit of particles on standing (settling out) or by use of centrifugal (spinning down) machine. See blood tests.

seed Colloq. for spermatozoa, qv.

seedy toe Separation of sensitive and insensitive laminae of foot. Follows chronic laminitis or infection. Horn becomes brittle and crumbles, leaving a gap between wall of hoof and pedal bone. Diagnosed by hollow sound when horn is tapped with metal object, confirmed by cutting away lower wall and exposing black tract and by X-ray examination. Cf sandcrack.

segmental myelitis Nervous disease characterised by hindleg inco-ordination, crossing over (qv). Cause: inflamed segments of spinal cord. Horse usually deteriorates until euthanasia is necessary.

selenium poisoning (syns. blind staggers, alkali disease) Important in N America and W Canada. Has been reported in Ireland. Source: s. content of soil and certain plants, eg astragulas (vetch), stanleya (prince's bloom), oonopsis (golden weed) and xylorrhiza (woody aster). These contain 2–6,000 parts per million of s., but horses usually avoid them unless food is scarce. Symptoms are acute, sub-acute or chronic. Acute poisoning—death occurs within a few hours, preceded by rapid and weak pulse, difficult breathing, bloat and colic. Post-mortem findings are hemorrhages and serum in abdominal cavity (ascites). Sub-acute poisoning (blind staggers)—weight-loss, staring coat, listlessness, staggering, impaired sight, abdominal pain, salivation and inability to swallow, finally paralysis and death. At post-mortem: chronic degeneration in all organs, particularly liver. Chronic poisoning (alkali disease)—loss of hair from mane and tail, rough coat, dullness, emaciation, anemia and depraved appetite. Rings appear on hoof and in severe cases there may be complete separation and shedding of hoof. No known treatment.

semen (L., seed) Thick, whitish secretion of stallion's testes and accessory sex glands. An average ejaculate of semen:

volume of **s.**	40–120ml.
number of sperm	100–150 million per cu.mm.
abnormal sperm (coiled tails and protoplasmic drops)	about 16%
pH (acidity/alkalinity)	about 7.330 pH units

seminal plasma	
specific gravity	**1.012**
ergothioneine	7.6mg./100ml.
citric acid	26mg./100ml.
fructose	15mg./100ml.
phosphorus	17mg./100ml.
lactic acid	12mg./100ml.
urea	3mg./100ml

It has been estimated that a minimum 500 million sperm per ejaculate are necessary for fertilisation and that the average content is 4–18 billion (American billion, ie 1,000 million).

semilunar valves See aortic **s.v.**, pulmonary **s.v.**

seminal vesicles Two long sacs lying either side of top of bladder and opening by ducts into urethra. 15–20cm. (6–8ins.) long in stallion but much shorter in gelding. They form part of accessory glands and provide nourishing fluid in which spermatozoa travel at ejaculation.

sense/sensation (L. sensus, sentire, thought, to think) Feeling conveyed by (afferent) nerves, eg of warmth, cold, pain. See arc.

sensitisation State of body or cells induced by specific substance. See allergy, anaphylaxis, immunity, photosensitisation.

sepsis (Gr. sepsis, decay) Bad or decayed. **puerperal s.** Occurs after foaling due to septic material absorbed from uterus and birth passage.

septicemia (septic + Gr. haima, blood + -ia) Presence of bacteria in blood. **s. of the newborn** Includes conditions such as sleepy foal disease, joint-ill, pneumonia, diarrhoea and meningitis, ie bacterial infections caused by Streptococci, Staphylococci, E. coli, Actinobacillus equuli (bacterium viscosum equi, shigella equirulis), Klebsiella pneumoniae. Similar conditions may be caused by virus, qv. Symptoms vary with main site of infection, eg if brain, it causes convulsions; if infected joints, lameness and painful swellings; if alimentary tract, diarrhoea; if lungs, rapid breathing. Characteristic signs are fever, gradual loss of suck reflex and strength to approach mare, inability to stand unaided, coma and convulsions. Dehydration (shown in sinking of eyeballs into sockets) is especially associated with diarrhoea and affected foals exude aromatic smell. Signs first show between birth and 3 days, although joint-ill may appear up to third month (see joint-ill). Diagnosis: on laboratory examination of feces, blood, urine, and other body fluids (see paracentesis abdominis and occipital puncture). Treatment: antibiotic drug in maximum doses, though should be one effective against particular organism. Pathology varies with infecting bacteria. Actinobacillus equuli (which causes sleepy foal disease) produces abscesses in kidney, adrenal glands, lungs and brain. E. coli causes pneumonia and inflamed alimentary tract. Streptococci cause pleurisy.

septicemic Of septicemia.

septum (L.; pl. septa) Any dividing wall, eg that between nostrils (**s. nasi**).

sequestrum Detached piece of bone which degenerates because blood no longer supplies it. Result of injury or infection. Should be surgically removed. See osteosis.

serology Study of antigen/antibody (qv) reaction in laboratory, eg for identifying influenza virus.

serum (pl. sera) Clear liquid which separates from red blood clot, ie whole blood minus cells and fibrinogen. See blood. **s. glutamic oxaloacetic transaminase** (SGOT) Enzyme of muscles and liver. Normal blood level approx. 150 units/100ml. of **s.** Increases in setfast, muscle damage and liver disease. **s. glutamic pyruvic transaminase** (SGPT) Enzyme present in blood, produced by kidney. Normal level: 8/100ml. of **s.** Increases in acute liver disease but levels in horse remain too low to be reliable guide. **s. gonadotrophin** (trade names: Antostab, Gestyl, PMS) Dry, sterile preparation of follicle stimulating hormone obtained from **s.** of pregnant mares. Stimulates growth of follicles in many species, but results in mares are disappointing. Cf pregnant mare's **s. gonadotrophin. s. hepatitis** See hepatitis.

sesamoid bones Small bones inserted into tendons where pressure occurs. **proximal s.b.'s** Two small bones behind fetlock joint attached to cannon bone and pastern bone by ligaments. Each is shaped like three-sided pyramid and forms back of fetlock joint, beneath deep flexor tendon. **distal s.** (syn. navicular bone) Flat, elongated bone behind joint formed by 2nd and 3rd phalanges (corono-pedal joint). **s.b.'s, fracture of** Caused by trauma; results in lameness. Diagnosis: on X-ray examination. See sclerosing agent.

sesamoiditis Inflamed sesamoid bones (suspensory ligament and distal sesamoidean ligaments may also be affected). Caused by strain, nutritional disturbance and trauma. Symptoms: pains and swelling around back of fetlock joint and, in severe cases, lameness. Diagnosis: on X-ray examination. Disproportion of one sesamoid bone best seen from point several paces behind horse, first on one side, then other.

setfast (syns. azoturia, Monday morning disease, paralytic myoglobin-uria, tying up) Painful condition of large muscle masses with degeneration of fibres. Occurs in horses on highly nutritious diets, eg race-horses and brood mares. Onset follows exercise especially after period of rest, as at weekends. Cause: thought to be rapid use of glycogen laid down by liver during idleness. When horse works production of lactic acid exceeds removal and destroys muscle fibres. The pigment myoglobin is liberated, colouring urine red. Some individuals seem particularly susceptible. Symptoms: profuse sweating, stiffness, reluctance to move, hard and painful muscles, particularly in back and hindquarters, restlessness, rapid respiration and pulse, raised temperature and sometimes difficult passing of port-coloured urine. Symptoms develop several hours, or immediately, after exercise. Most horses recover in matter of hours if rested but some lie down, cannot get up and die. Diagnosis: on characteristic symptoms, confirmed by urine colour and rise in SGOT and CPK enzymes in blood (see blood tests). Treatment: do not exercise horse, give anti-inflammatory drugs, corticosteroids and pain reliever. When recovered, reduce grain ration, give regular exercise and if attacks recur, give salicylates. Pathology: kidney damage, extensive pale discoloration of large muscle masses, giving cooked appearance. See anti-inflammatory, carbohydrate, corticosteroid, metabolism, muscle.

seton (Fr. seton, L. seta, bristle) Strip of silk or linen drawn through wound to help drainage, as in infection of frontal sinus. See sinusitis. Cf tape suture.

sex (L. sexus) Distinction between male and female based on genitalia, qv. See chromosome, intersex. **female s. hormones** Oestrogens: oestradiol, oestrone, oestriol, equilin, equilenin. Progestogens: progesterone, ethinyltestosterone. Responsible for female **s.** characters, oestrous cycle and maintenance of pregnancy. **male s. hormones** Androgens: testosterone, androstenediol, androsterone, androstenedione found in testes (and ovaries), adrenal cortex and in placenta of mare. Responsible for male **s.** characters and libido. **other s. hormones** Follicle stimulating hormone (FSH), luteinising hormone (LH), pregnant mare serum gonadotrophin (PMSG).

SGOT See serum glutamic oxaloacetic transaminase.

SGPT See serum glutamic pyruvic transaminase.

shaft Main part of long bone. See bone.

sheath Structure enclosing and protecting another. **artificial s.** See condom. **s. of penis** Colloq. for prepuce. Double fold of skin covering free part of penis when not erect. Consists of outer and inner folds and an opening or ring (orifice). Glands of lining produce fatty, evilsmelling secretion (smegma). See masturbation. **synovial s.** One secreting synovial fluid which lubricates contained part (eg tendon), reducing friction. Main **s.s.'s** are those of deep and superficial digital flexor tendons of front and hind legs; and tendons of common digital extensor, extensors carpi radialis and obliquus, lateral and long digital extensors, tibialis anterior and ulnaris lateralis.

Shetland pony Probably strongest member of Equidae in relation to its size. (Limited by stud book rules to 10.3 hands, but averages less.) May have originated in S. Isles of Scotland, where now bred. Good child's pony, usually long-lived. Seems to have some immunity to grass sickness. Most colours including piebald and skewbald. Assn: S. Pony Soc., c/o D. M. Patterson, 8 Whinfield Road, Montrose, Angus, Scotland (Montrose 683).

shigellosis See sleepy foal disease.

shin Front of cannon bones. See bucked s., periostitis.

Shire Largest English draught horse, usually over 17 hands. Takes name from the shires, eg Lincolnshire, Huntingdonshire, Cambridgeshire, where usually bred. Bays and browns most common and all colours have white around legs. Assn: S. Horse Soc., c/o R. W. Bird, The Showground, Alwalton, Peterborough PE2 0XE, Northamptonshire (Peterborough 64451).

shivering Involuntary quivering of muscles of hindlegs and tail; forelegs occasionally affected. Cause unknown, but may be damaged nerves supplying hindleg. Best seen on flexing hindleg and pulling it to side; as leg returns to ground it will shake and tail is elevated and quivers. Should not be confused with s. of shoulders and forelegs due to nervousness, eg before race. Foals normally shiver during first 2 hours of life to maintain body temperature.

shock Condition of failure in blood circulation characterised by pale mucous membranes, clammy skin, decreased blood pressure, feeble, rapid pulse, slow breathing and eventual unconsciousness. Caused by surgery, severe injury, reaction to injected drugs (anaphylaxis), hemorrhage, acute allergy or infection. Treatment: give large amounts of intravenous fluid initially, then more slowly over next few hours (normal saline, antibiotics, corticosteroids); ensure adequate ventilation (possibly oxygen direct into windpipe or through mask); treat underlying cause of s. and use good general nursing.

shoe Piece of iron or aluminium fitted to circumference of foot to protect it. Used on most ridden horses (should be removed from hindfeet if horse is turned out with others). S. consists of toe, quarter and heel, usually with groove (fullering) in surface which meets ground. Groove contains about 3 or 4 nail holes on either side (branch). **bar s.** One with full or half bar across heels to increase pressure on frog. **half rim s.** One which raises side of foot worn down when horse puts too much weight on it. **tip s.** One which covers only toe, throwing weight on heels and frog. **surgical s.** One which reduces injury through faulty action, eg roller toe s. which, fitted on hindfoot, tempers bruising if horse over-reaches (catches heel on forefoot). Cf plate. See plate 43.

shoeing (syn. farriery) Art of applying horseshoes. Good s. can lessen faults, eg contracted heels, tendency to develop corns.

shoulder blade (scapula) Flat bone on side of chest with muscles of shoulder and forearm attached; forms joint with humerus bone. See skeleton.

sidebones False bones caused by hardening of cartilages of pedal bone. See quittor.

side-effect Unintended happening or result of giving drug, eg tranquilliser may cause **s.-e.** of inco-ordination. See donkey.

siderocyte Red blood cell containing non-hemoglobin iron. Presence of large numbers suggests swamp fever, qv.

sign (L. signum) Evidence of abnormality/disease seen by person tending horse, rather than reported to him second hand (a symptom).

Silbeverm Trade name. See piperazine salts.

silver (L. argentum) Soft white metal. **s. nitrate** Colourless bitter-tasting odourless crystals. Used in weak solution as astringent or antiseptic; in eye lotion to treat ulcers; in concentrated form on warts or proud flesh to reduce bleeding. **s. n. poisoning** Occurs in overdose. Symptoms: abdominal pain, diarrhoea and possibly convulsions, paralysis and death from shock. **s. weed** (Potentilla anserina) Common roadside weed with high tannin content. May cause death if large amount is eaten.

sinew Tendon of a muscle.

sinus (L. a hollow) Body space containing blood or air. **s. arrhythmia** See arrhythmia. **s. of head** Cavity connected directly or indirectly to nasal cavity. 4 pairs; maxillary, frontal, sphenopalatine and ethmoidal. Functions: to lighten head (which if solid would be too heavy for horse to carry), to provide space for roots of teeth. Sometimes site of infection (see sinusitis).

sinusitis Infected air sinuses of head, causing pain, thick discharge (usually from only 1 nostril) and swollen lymph node between angles of lower jaw. Discharge may be evil-smelling if bone of skull is diseased. Cause: bacterial infection (most common), trauma causing broken bone, or growth (rare). Treatment: antibiotics and/or surgery (opening sinus from outside, flushing and causing free drainage into nasal passage).

351

Siwalik Pony originally from S. (Himalayan foothills) but now all over India. Up to about 13.2 hands, narrow and poor looking but hardy.

skeleton (from Gr., dried mummy, body) Body's framework of bones, all cartilage in embryo, gradually hardening throughout life until brittle in old age. Contains average of 210 bones: 37 in skull, including 3 small bones (auditory ossicles) in each ear, 2 branches of lower jaw, 54 vertebrae (7 cervical, 18 thoracic, 6 lumbar, 5 sacral, 15–21 coccygeal (tail)), 36 ribs (some breeds, eg. Arab, sometimes have 37 or 38), 1 sternum, 40 forelimb, 40 hindlimb (including pelvis). See bone, cartilage and individual bones.

skewbald See coat colouring.

skin (syn. cutis) Outer covering of body. Consists of epidermis (4 layers) and dermis (2 layers) containing hair follicles, sweat glands and sebaceous glands. It is 3.8mm. thick on average and 6.2mm thick, where mane and tail emerge. **s., diseases of** Dermatitis, ringworm, external parasites (louse, tick, harvest mite), acne, baldness (alopecia), cracked heels, mud fever, warble fly, photosensitisation, sores, eg from poorly-fitting saddlery, Queensland itch.

skull Bones of head—37 in all including 3 in each ear (auditory ossicles). Divided into cranium (which surrounds brain) and face. Those of cranium (10): occipital, sphenoid, ethmoid and intraparietal (single bones) and parietals, frontals and temporals (paired). Bones of face (21): vomar, mandible and hyoid (single) and maxilla, incisive, palatine, pterygoid, nasal, lacrymal, zygomatic (or malar) upper and lower turbinated (paired) bones. Lower jaw is formed by mandible which has 2 branches (rami).

slab fracture Break in third carpal bone (in knee joint) in which bone is split so that a slab becomes detached in front of joint. Treat by surgical removal or screwing together. See also carpal bones, fracture of.

sleep See behaviour.

sleepy foal disease (syn. shigellosis) Fatal disease of newborn foal caused by Actinobacillus equuli (shigella equirulis). Infection may start in utero or may enter through mouth or navel after birth. Symptoms include fever, sleepiness, rapid breathing and loss of strength to get up

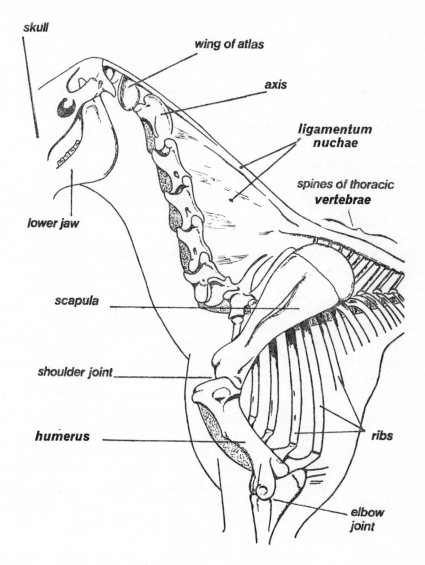

skull

wing of atlas

axis

ligamentum
nuchae

spines of thoracic
vertebrae

lower jaw

scapula

shoulder joint

humerus

ribs

elbow
joint

32 Part of skeleton

and suck. Death may occur within 24 hours, but some foals live several days. At post-mortem kidneys, adrenal glands, brain and possibly joints contain abscesses. See also septicemia of the newborn.

smegma (Gr. smegma, soap) Thick, cheesy, evil-smelling secretion in sheath of penis.

smooth muscle (syn. involuntary muscle) One of 3 types of muscle; that not under voluntary control and found in walls of such organs as bladder, uterus and alimentary tract. Cf striped muscle, heart muscle.

Smudish See Estonian.

snake bite Unlikely to kill horse. Usually occurs on head or legs, causing swelling around site, pain and possibly nosebleed. Treatment: cut open fang wounds, draw off venom and give antibiotics to prevent secondary infection. **s. venom** Used in some anti-blood clotting agents (anticoagulants).

sneeze Sudden expulsion of air through nostrils (horse cannot normally breathe through mouth). May be due to excessive dust, inflamed mucous membranes infected with influenza virus, cerebral irritation through tumour, infection or hemorrhage. See neonatal maladjustment syndrome.

snotty nose (syns. equine viral rhinopneumonitis, cold, catarrh, stable cough) Mild disease of upper respiratory tract caused by equine herpesvirus I (syns. EHVI, rhinopneumonitis), rhinovirus, adenovirus. Some sub-types of EHVI cause abortion but more usually a cold with nasal discharge, at first watery, then pus-like. May also cause coughing, fever and enlarged lymph nodes of throat. Common in foals and yearlings, lasting weeks or months, but rare in adults. Cf influenza.

soap (L. sapo) Compound of one or more fatty acids with an alkali. Used to clean skin before operation and as enema: 1 part to 20 parts warm water.

Society for the Study of Animal Breeding (SSAB) c/o R. Clarke, Somerset Cattle Breeding Centre, Ilminster, Somerset (Ilminster 2258).

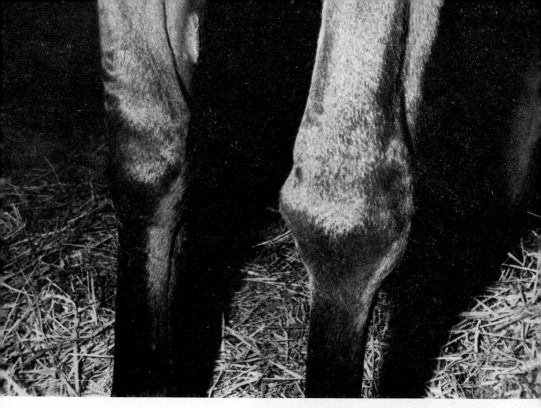

40 Near-fore with a popped knee. See *carpitis*. Note chestnut, qv, above inside of offfore knee

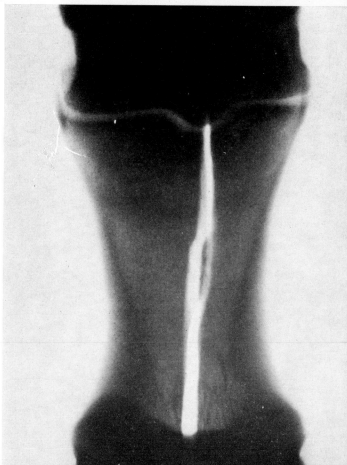

41 X-ray photograph of a split pastern. See *pastern*

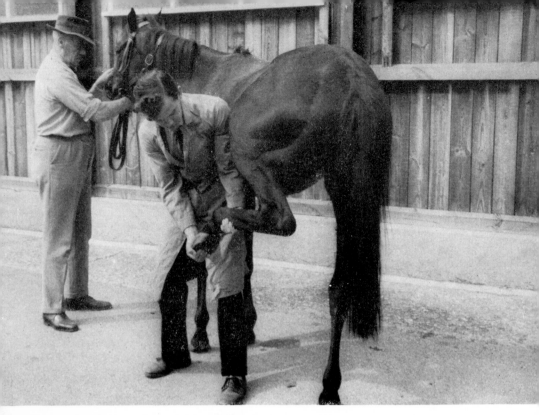

42 Flexing the hock for signs of lameness. See *spavin*

43 Types of special shoe; l to r: full-bar, T-bar, three-quarter-bar. See *shoe*

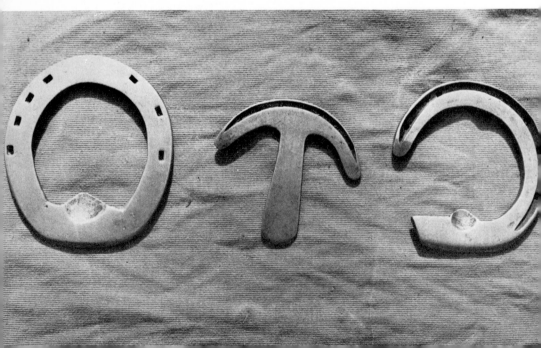

soda lime Hard granules, white or coloured with indicator to show when their capacity for absorbing carbon dioxide is exhausted. Used in anaesthetic breathing circuits to absorb carbon dioxide. See anaesthesia.

sodium acid citrate White odourless salty-tasting powder. Used to prevent clotting of blood intended for transfusion. 1.7–2% with 2.5% dextrose in 120ml. water will prevent clotting of about 420ml. blood. See anticoagulant. **s. a. phosphate** Colourless crystals or white crystalline powder with acid, saline taste. Used to treat low phosphate conditions, 30gms. followed by 15gms. daily, by mouth.

sodium bicarbonate White opaque odourless crystals, with saline taste. Given by mouth to treat excess staling; intravenously in 5% solution, to foals suffering from convulsions or diarrhoea. Dose: by mouth (adult) 15–60gms.; IV: 200–500ml. See polyuria, neonatal maladjustment syndrome. **s. calcium edetate** (trade names: Calcium Disodium Versenate, Edathamil Calcium Disodium) White tasteless powder with slight odour. Used to treat poisoning by lead and other heavy metals, eg mercury. Given intravenously: 75ml./kg. body wt. **s. chloride** (1) Common salt of the body. Imbalance will show as pale, livid red or purple mucous membranes of gums, cheeks and eyes. (2) Colourless odourless crystals with salty taste. Used to treat colic (30–90gms.) or as purgative (125–500gms.). **s. citrate** White odourless crystals or powder. Used in solution as anticoagulant. Solution 2.5–3.8% prevents clotting of blood for laboratory study. **s. glycarsamate** (trade name: Astryl) Odourless tasteless creamy-white crystalline powder. Given to treat redworm infestation (best after soft food, eg bran mash). Should not be given if intestines are inflamed. Dose, adults: 8–24gms., foals: 4–8gms. **s. morrhuate** Salt of morrhuic acid. See sclerosing agent. **s. oleate** See sclerosing agent. **s. salicylate** (syn. aspirin) Colourless odourless salty-tasting crystals or powder. Reduces temperature by depressing heat-regulating centre of brain. See also acetylsalicylic acid. Dose: 15–120gms. **s. sulphate** (syn. glauber's salt) Colourless to light-brown odourless bitter-tasting crystals. Acts as laxative. Dose: 30–60gms.; purgative dose: 240–360gms. Should be given by stomach tube with large volume of water. **s. thiosulphate** Colourless odourless crystals with salty taste. Given to reduce flatulence and fermentation in stomach/intestines, also to treat poisoning by arsenic, bismuth, mercury, and some other metals. Dose: 8–10gms. as 10–30% solution IV.

soft palate Membrane of muscles which separates mouth from pharynx except when swallowing. Continuation of hard palate (mouth) with upper surface forming end of nasal cavities. Undersurface forms back of throat (seen in man as uvula). Sides of **s.p.** merge with walls of pharynx and contain tonsils, which are not compact, as in man, but consist of a series of lymphoid tissue and mucous glands. Average length of **s.p.** is 15cm. (6ins.) and its shape probably explains why horses cannot normally breathe through the mouth. Muscles of **s.p.** are the palatinus, levator palati and tensor palati. Their action is to shorten, tense and raise the **s.p.** during swallowing. Nerves supplying palate are from the trigeminus, vagus and glosso-pharyngeal cranial nerves. Symptoms of **s.p.** condition (when **s.p.** interferes with breathing) include gurgling, roaring or whistling at exercise (see wind). Treatments include injection of sclerosing agent (qv), cautery, reducing size of **s.p.** by surgery. All measures have limited value. Cause unknown but may be virus infection affecting nerve supply to **s.p.** muscles.

sole (L. solea, plata) Undersurface of foot (hoof). Usually concave and non-weight-bearing. **dropped/flat s.** One which has lost its concavity and is susceptible to bruising.

Solupen Trade name. See benzylpenicillin.

soma (Gr. soma, body) Body tissue (as distinguished from germ cells).

soporific (L. soporificus) Drug or substance which induces sleep.

sore Colloq. (1) for any lesion on skin or mucous membrane; (2) for feeling of stiffness. **s. shin** See bucked shin. **summer s.** See stomach worm.

Sorraia Native pony of Spain, usually dun-coloured with dorsal stripe. Similar to Przewalski and Tarpan.

sound (L. sonus) Energy waves of frequency between 20 and 20,000 cycles per second. Normal or abnormal noise heard in body, eg murmur, râle, borborygmus, roaring. See equine sounds, percussion, stethoscope, wind.

soundness State of health or fitness to carry out particular function, eg sound for racing, breeding, etc (recent move to avoid use of word 'sound'). **s. examination** Methods used by veterinarian to ascertain state of horse at a given time, eg before it changes hands or is insured. Misrepresentation Act (1967) and Trade Descriptions Act (1968), which give remedy through civil courts if buyer has been influenced by incorrect statement, resulted in Royal College of Veterinary Surgeons and British Veterinary Association making recommendations on the examining of horses for a buyer:

Stage 1   preliminary examination
      2   trotting up
      3   strenuous exercise
      4   a period of rest
      5   second trot and foot examination

Stage 1—preliminary examination. This is best conducted in stable . . . note animal's general appearance and condition. Veterinarian should develop habit of examining horse methodically part by part, so there is no chance of inadvertently overlooking any part. Teeth should be examined, age assessed . . . resting heart should be auscultated for comparison with its action after exercise. Eyes should be examined with an ophthalmoscope. Veterinarian should run hand over animal's body and legs to ensure he has not missed abnormalities or lesions. Horse should be turned right around in stable and each foot picked up and examined and leg joints flexed to detect pain or limitation of movement. Horse should then be brought outside and inspected from all sides in daylight.

Stage 2—trotting up. Animal should be walked and trotted on hard, level ground. . . . Horse should be walked 20 yards away from veterinarian, turned and walked back. Horse should then be trotted away for 30 or 40 yards and trotted back. . . . If animal is not fit to be exerted . . . or if it is lame when trotted examination should not be continued. . . .

Stage 3—strenuous exercise. . . . age, condition and fitness should be considered. Animal should be given sufficient exercise (1) to make it breathe deeply and rapidly so that any unusual breathing sounds may be heard; (2) to increase action of heart so abnormalities may be more easily detected; (3) to tire animal so that strains or injuries may be revealed by stiffness or lameness after period of rest. Riding horse should be ridden at canter 5–10 minutes and pass close to veterinarian so that he can hear horse's breathing. Speed should then be increased to controlled gallop, again passing close to veterinarian until he indicates it should be pulled up. He can then auscultate heart and observe rate and depth of breathing. More exercise can then be given if necessary. Untrained animals and those too young or too small to be ridden can be lunged, which should be stated on certificate. [Racehorses are normally galloped past vet. for about 6 furlongs, then pulled up and immediately trotted back to him.] Horse is then returned to stable.

Stage 4—a period of rest. Horse should be allowed to stand quietly in stable for at least half an hour. . . . attention by groom defeats object of rest period. During this time vet. should observe breathing and check heart beat as it settles. He should write down name, colour, breed, sex, age and markings needed for animal's identification and also any conditions of disease or injury observed so far.

Stage 5—second trot and foot examination. Horse should be brought out and walked and trotted as before. It is then turned round sharply, first one way then the other and made to step back a few paces. If there is doubt about condition of feet, animal's shoes must be removed. Owner's permission should be obtained and it should be agreed his farrier replaces shoes.

Presenting facts and opinion in form of a certificate

A client . . . is entitled to clear opinion that horse is or is not a fit subject. . . . Certificate should be brief as possible but should indicate clearly on what grounds vet.'s decision has been based.

Certificates available from the British Veterinary Assn (see Veterinary Record) take following form:

Vet's name: .... Qualifications ....
Address ....
Description of horse:

name	colour	breed	sex	age	approx. height

(Certificates include diagram here)

Markings

Head ....

Body ....

Forelegs { left side ....
{ right side ....

Hindlegs { left side ....

{ right side ....

Acquired marks ....

This is to certify that at the request of (name and address) ....

....

I have examined the horse described above, the property of (name and address) ....

at (place of examination) ....

and I find no clinical signs of disease, injury or physical abnormality other than those here recorded.

Signs of disease and injury observed:

Opinion:

This clinical examination was carried out in accordance with the standard procedure recommended by the Royal College of Veterinary Surgeons and the British Veterinary Association (joint memorandum on the examination of horses, 1973).

* No radiological or other specialised techniques were included.

Time and date of examination ....

Signed ....

* Amend as required.

All injury and disease . . . should be recorded on certificate. If some are not included vet. may later be accused of having carelessly failed to see them. If none, certificate should conclude under the heading 'opinion':

'On this examination I find no physical abnormality likely to affect the animal's usefulness as a .... or its suitability for purchase for this purpose.'

If clinical signs of disease, injury or abnormality have been seen and listed on certificate, but animal meets requirements of buyer, certificate should conclude:

'In my opinion, on this examination, the conditions set out above do not affect the animal's usefulness as a .... or its suitability for purchase for this purpose.'

If clinical signs of disease, injury or abnormality have been seen and . . . animal is considered unsuitable for purchase, a certificate will normally not be issued. . . . if a certificate is specially requested, it should conclude:

'In my opinion, on this examination, this animal is not suitable for purchase as a ....'

Inclusion of phrase 'in my opinion' is an admission that there may be other interpretations of facts but it in no way reduces vet's responsibilities of careful observation. . . .

Vices . . . are objectionable habits and normally concern the vet. in his examination only if he notes that they have affected, or could affect. . . the animal's physical condition. If vices, or evidence of vices, are seen during examination, they should be recorded on certificate and taken into account in concluding opinion. [See vice.]

Height For the purposes of this examination, the exact height of a horse or pony is not the concern of the examining vet. Approximate height is included on certificate only to assist identification of animal.

Warranty If a buyer wants a warranty covering . . . exact height, freedom from vices, non-administration of drugs prior to examination, or the animal's existing performance as a hunter, showjumper, riding pony, eventer, etc he should be advised to seek it in writing from the seller, as these are matters between them and not responsibility of the vet.

The memorandum on examinations issued by the Royal College and the BVA points out that recommendations do not include taking blood sample.

This matter was most carefully considered in the hope of being able to provide further protection for purchasers and their veterinarians—with particular reference to the possibility that a vendor might have sought to mask lameness . . . by the use of anti-inflammatory medicaments. Unfortunately in the present state of scientific knowledge it is not possible to store and analyse blood samples in a manner . . . acceptable in terms of practicality and cost, yet . . . provide sufficient certainty that the analysis would lead to the detection of any anti-inflammatory medicaments present in the horse at the time of examination. A blood sample may, of course, be taken if the purchaser so requests and the vendor agrees. . . .

Special examinations, besides blood samples, include: X-ray, ECG (electrocardiogram) recordings, rectal palpatation (if examining mare for stud), palpation of external genital organs of colt (examination for stallion duties, then possibly collecting and examining semen—see artificial vagina).

South German Cold Blood (syn. Noric) Heavy harness breed, probably with Haflinger blood. Originally concentrated around Salzburg, Austria, now also common in S Germany.

Spaerophorus Bacteria which live only in absence of air (anaerobic); rod-shaped but also grow long filaments. **S. necrophorus** Cause of thrush, qv.

Spanish Andalusian See Andalusian.

Spanish Jennet Horse of middle ages developed from heavy Spanish horse, Barb, Arab, Persian and Turkish. Docile with showy action, including ambling gait. Extinct in pure form. Ancestor of Kladruber and others.

Sparine Trade name. See promazine hydrochloride.

spasm (L. spasmus, Gr. spasmos) Violent, involuntary contraction of muscle or group of muscles giving pain. **s. of alimentary canal** See colic. **tetanic s.** See lockjaw.

Spasmodin Trade name. See benzyl benzoate.

spavin Condition of hock joint or surrounding area. **bone s.** Inflamed bone or lining (periostitis or ostitis) affecting inner, upper end of cannon and inside of third and central small bones of hock joint, associated with arthritis. **jack s.** Bone s. of large proportions. **bog s.** Enlarged joint capsule of hock, see bog **s. occult s.** Typical hock lameness, without any visible X-ray or clinical changes. Cause—trauma, conformation (sickle and cow hocks), dietary deficiency or imbalance. Symptoms of hock lameness: shortened stride, excessive wear on toe. Exercise usually improves condition but may worsen severe cases. Diagnosis: on X-ray, nerve block (of posterior tibial and deep peroneal nerves). **s. test** Flex hock for minute or two, then trot. Increased lameness, especially in first few steps, indicates faulty hock. Treatment: corticosteroids, short-wave therapy and for bone s. surgical removal of part of cunean tendon. See plate 42.

species Division of animals or plants subordinate to a genus. **S.** of domestic horse is Equus caballus, qv.

specimen Sample of blood, urine, feces or tissue. Usually collected for laboratory examination. See blood tests, dope test.

speculum (L., mirror) Hollow metal tube for internal examinations, usually of vagina and cervix. See plate 31.

speedy cutting See interfering.

sperm Abbr. spermatozoa, spermatazoon.

spermatic cord Cord containing structures carried by testicle in its descent from abdominal cavity to scrotum, ie spermatic artery and veins, lymphatics, nerve, vas deferens, internal cremaster muscle and fold of peritoneum (tunica vaginalis).

spermatocyte Immature spermatozoon.

spermatozoa Pl. of spermatozoon, qv.

spermatozoon (spermato + Gr. zoon, animal; syns. sperm, seed) Male cell (gamete) consisting of head, mid-piece and tail. Contains hereditary material of stallion. Mature **s.** contains half number (haploid) of chromosomes of body cell. See semen.

sphincter (L., Gr. sphigkter, that which binds tight). Ring-like band of muscle fibres that constricts or closes natural opening, eg anus.

spinal (L. spinalis) Of spine. **s. column** See vertebral column. **s. cord** See cord.

Spiti Native pony of India named after mountainous **S.** area, where it thrives on little food in low temperatures. Most often grey and about 12.2 hands.

splint Slender bone, 1 either side of cannon bone. They represent second and fourth metacarpal and metatarsal bones, remnants from animal which had 3 toes on each forefoot (see evolution). Each **s.** consists of shaft, large upper end or head and small lower end or button. Shaft and head are closely bound to cannon bone by ligaments, the button sticks out and can be felt beneath skin. **S.** also colloq. for condition of the bone, usually the one on inside of cannon bone of foreleg; 3 types of **s.**: (1) fractured shaft causing a callus; (2) inflamed binding ligament; (3) inflamed lining of cannon bone (periostitis). Cause: a knock as when one foreleg strikes the other; faulty nutrition,

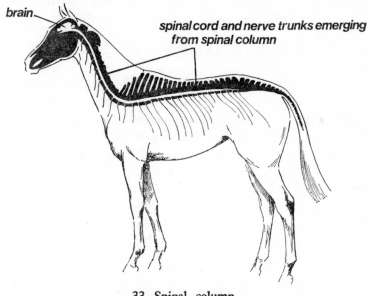

brain

spinal cord and nerve trunks emerging
from spinal column

33 Spinal column

eg deficiency of calcium, vitamin A or D; faulty conformation. Symptoms: lameness and heat, firm swelling over area. Diagnosis: on symptoms and X-ray. Treatment: rest, surgical removal of the bone, corticosteroid injections, irradiation.

split pastern See pastern.

spondylitis Inflamed vertebrae.

spot Small area, maybe with central core, on skin or mucous membrane. See acne, ringworm.

spotted horse See Appaloosa, Knabstrup.

spp. Abbr. species (pl.).

sprain (syn. strain) Abnormal stretching of a part causing torn fibres of ligaments, tendons, muscle, joint capsule, tendon sheaths and membrane lining outer surface of bones (periostium). Results in bleeding and typical inflammatory reaction, with heat, swelling and pain. Heals with fibrous or scar tissue (see inflammation). Severity is directly related to number of fibres torn.

SSAB See Society for the Study of Animal Breeding.

stable fly (syn. Stomoxis calcitrans) Common insect belonging to phylum Arthropoda. Resembles housefly but distinguishable by long, stout sucking tube (proboscis). Adult about 7mm. (approx ¼in.) long and darker coloured than housefly. **S.f.** usually lays eggs in horse manure mixed with straw and bites horses to suck blood. Larva develops, followed by a pupa stage lasting 6–20 days, though whole life cycle can be completed in 14 days. **S.f.** can transmit trypanasomes, encephalomyelitis and swamp fever. Cf tabanid fly.

staggers Colloq. for inco-ordination. See cerebellar degeneration, grass sickness, meningitis, wobbler syndrome.

stale Colloq. to urinate, micturate. See behaviour, urine sample.

stallion An entire (not castrated) male. Term usually reserved for horse used for breeding. Young s., up to 4–5, termed 'colt.' After that age, if not used for breeding, he is called 'an entire' or simply 'horse'. Cf gelding. See plates 3–5.

Standardbred Official type used for harness racing, either trotter (diagonally-gaited) or pacer (laterally-gaited). **S.** is large, long-legged and extremely tough. It dates from 1870s and traces through English Thoroughbred foundation sire, Messenger. Assn: United States Trotting Assn. See gait, whorlbone lameness.

stapes (L., stirrup) One of small bones of ear, qv.

staphylo-/staphyl- Combining form meaning resemblance to bunch of grapes, eg Staphylococcus. See bacteria.

Staphylococcal dermatitis See acne.

stasis (Gr. stasis, a standing still) Stoppage in flow of blood or other fluid.

Stat Trade name. See alum.

stay apparatus System of ligaments in all legs. Helps support horse while standing, reduces concussion in action and prevents over-extension of fetlock, pastern and corono-pedal joints. **s.a. of foreleg** Top-to-bottom: (1) serratus ventralis muscle, from ribs to shoulder blade (scapula); (2) biceps brachii tendon, from tuber scapulii to radius and tendon of extensor carpi radialis muscle—this muscle originates on front of humerus bone and inserts on to front upper part of cannon bone (metacarpal tuberosity); (3) long head of triceps muscle, from back of shoulder blade to point of elbow (olecranon); (4) superior

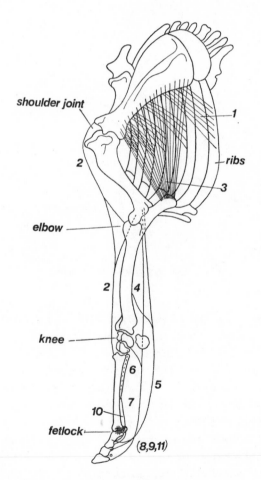

34   Stay apparatus of foreleg (for explanation of numbers, see text)

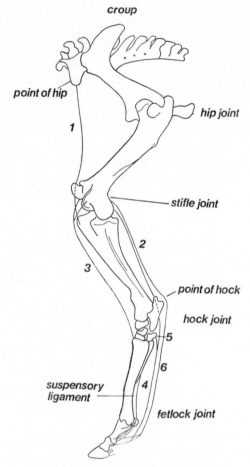

35 Stay apparatus of hindleg

check ligament, from back of radius and fuses with tendon of superficial digital flexor muscle, above knee joint; (5) superficial flexor tendon (muscle originates behind humerus and radius and inserts through its tendon on to back of first and second phalanges); (6) inferior check ligament, from back ligament of knee joint to deep flexor tendon (joint in middle third of cannon bone); (7) deep digital flexor muscle, from back of humerus and inner surface of elbow to third phalanx (pedal bone); (8) intersesamoidean ligament, binds 2 sesamoid bones of fetlock, forming groove for flexor tendons; (9) collateral sesamoidean ligaments, bind sesamoid bones to cannon and first phalanx (pastern bone); (10) suspensory (or interosseous) ligament, from back of cannon bone and lower row of knee (carpal) bones; lies on back of cannon bone and divides into 2 branches: 1 attaches to sesamoid bones on either side of fetlock joint, the other runs downward and forward to front of first phalanx; both join tendon of a common digital extensor muscle; (11) distal sesamoidean ligaments, join sesamoid bones of fetlock to first and second phalanges. **s.a. of hindleg** System similar to foreleg, except without superior check ligament: (1) tensor fascia lata, from point of hip to patella (knee cap) and outside of stifle joint; (2) gastrocnemius muscle, from femur bone to bone forming hock (tuber calcis); (3) peroneus tertius muscle, from lower end of femur to upper end of cannon bone and front of hock joint; (4) deep digital flexor, from back and upper part of tibia to pedal bone; (5) tarsal check ligament, from ligaments behind hock to tendon of deep digital flexor muscle, just below hock joint; (6) superficial digital flexor muscles, from back of femur to hock and upper end of second phalanx and lower end of first phalanx. Cf suspensory apparatus.

stem Stalk, eg brain **s.**

stenosis (Gr. stenosis) Narowing or stricture of duct or opening, eg **aortic s.** Narrowing of opening into aorta from heart due to thickened valves.

sterile (L. sterilis) (1) Infertile; barren. (2) Free from micro-organisms. See infertility.

sterilisation Destruction of micro-organisms by heat, eg steam under pressure, at 120°C., (248°F.) for 15 minutes; dry heat at 360°–380°C. (680°–684°F.) for 3 hours; chemical compounds.

sternum See breast bone.

steroids Important biological substances of body; based on system of 4 carbon rings joined in characteristic way; include oestrogens, progestins, androgens, adrenal cortex hormones (corticoids and corticosteroids), cholesterol, vitamin D, bile acids.

stethoscope (stetho- + Gr. skopein, to examine) Instrument for listening to heart, lung and gut sounds. See heart sounds. Cf percussion.

stick tight flea. See flea.

stifle Joint in upper hindleg, corresponds to human knee. Formed by lower end of femur and upper end of tibia with knee cap (patella) attached to front. Ligaments on front of joint: medial, middle and lateral patella. Cf knee. **s., inflammation of** (syn. gonitis) Arthritis of the joint due to infected or injured bones, cartilages or ligaments.

Stilboestrol. Trade name. See stilboestrol.

stilboestrol (syn. diethyl-**s.**) Colourless crystals or white crystalline odourless tasteless powder. A synthetic oestrogen used to induce heat, treat infections of uterus, dilate cervix at birth and expel afterbirth. Dose: 10–25mg. IM.

stilette (Fr.) (1) A thin instrument used to probe cavity. (2) Wire put through catheter (qv) or cannula (qv) to clear or stiffen it.

stillbirth Delivery of dead foal which has developed for more than 300 days. (Before this, term abortion should be used.) About 2% incidence in Thoroughbreds. Causes: infection, asphyxia.

stitch To unite edges of skin or other tissue with thread, catgut, wire or nylon threaded through needle. See wound, Caslick. Cf ligature, tape suture.

stomach (L. stomachus, Gr. stomakhos) Muscular bag inside rib cage. Digests food by secreting digestive (gastric) juices. Small in horse (see alimentary canal). **s. tube** Rubber or plastic tube used for passing fluid into stomach. Inserted up one nostril and, after horse swallows, end pushed gently down gullet to about chest, ie not into stomach. Varies in diameter according to horse (about 1cm.—approx. $\frac{1}{3}$in.—for foals, 3cm.—approx 1in.—for adults). Can be open-ended or blunt with opening on side. Used to feed foal (see neonatal maladjustment syndrome, food by **s.t.**) or to give liquid drugs. **s. worm** (1) Trichostrongylus axei, Nematode (roundworm) parasite of order Strongyloidea. Only roundworm not host-specific; found in **s.** of horse, donkey, pig, sheep and goat. Causes thickened, inflamed **s.** and possibly unthriftiness. Treatment: see thiabendazole, phenothiazine. (2) Habronema muscae, H. microstoma, H. megastoma, small Nematode (roundworm) parasites 8–20mm. (approx. $\frac{1}{3}$in.–$\frac{3}{4}$in.) long, of order Spiruroidea, found in **s.** Eggs pass out in feces and are eaten by fly maggot. This enters either wounds or horse's feed and finds its way to **s.** Larvae may cause itchy, fibrous walnut-sized nodules in skin. Nodules ulcerate and weep (condition known as summer sores, bursatti or habronemiasis and, in Australia, as swamp cancer). In **s.**, adult worm lays eggs, thus completing life-cycle. Habronema megastoma are found in tumours, eg in **s.** wall. Treatment: see carbon disulphide.

stomatitis (pl. stomatitides; syn. aphtha) Small white blister. See vesicular stomatitis.

stone (syn. calculus, pl. calculi) Accumulation of salts which form object the size of a grain to size of melon. May occur in kidney, bladder or urethra; more common in horses and geldings than in mares. Either rough, yellow to brown, composed mainly of calcium carbonate, or smooth and white, mainly phosphate.

strain See sprain.

strangles (L. strangulare) Infectious disease characterised by swollen throat. Occurs in all countries, especially in groups of horses, eg draught, Welsh Mountain ponies. Young horses particularly susceptible and about 2% of cases die. Cause: Streptococcus equi bacteria, specific to condition (should not be confused with Strep. pyogenes var. equi). Spread by eating or inhaling infected pasture droplets. Organism can live in empty stable for about 6 weeks. Symptoms (after 4–8 days incubation): fever, to 41°C. (106°F.), abscesses in lymph glands around throat which burst after about 10 days; watery nasal discharge becoming thick pus, inflamed eyes, lack of appetite, moist cough. Infection may spread to other organs (**bastard s.**), eg abscesses in lungs, brain, liver, muscles.

strawberry roan See coat colouring.

streptococcal Due to a streptococcus.

streptococci Gram-positive bacteria, shaped as minute beads and occurring in strings of varying length and sometimes in pairs (diplococci). See Streptococcus equi, Strep. pyogenes var equi.

Streptococcus equi Cause of strangles, qv; produces strong hemolytic toxin. In laboratory, grows as honey-like drop on blood agar medium, from pus or nasal discharge of infected case. **S. pyogenes var. equi** (syns. Strep. zooepidemicus, beta hemolytic streptococcus, BHS).

Ubiquitous germ which infects nasal passages, uterus, wound and any tissues damaged or made susceptible by virus infection, trauma or other cause of reduced resistance. May follow herpes infection of lungs and air passages or damage to uterus during foaling. (Does not cause epidemics as Strep. equi, therefore syn. zooepidemicus is a misnomer.)

streptomycin sulphate (trade name: Streptovex) White odourless slightly bitter-tasting powder from Streptomyces griseus. Antibiotic active against wide range of bacteria, often used to treat sleepy foal disease. Dose: 10mg./kg. body wt. (foals: 20mg./kg.).

Streptovex Trade name. See streptomycin sulphate.

stress fracture Minute break in bone, eg cannon, due to concussion. Less common in other bones. S.f.'s difficult to diagnose even on careful X-ray. They cause inflamed membrane around bone (periostitis). See bucked shin.

stridor Harsh, high-pitched respiratory sound, eg in spasm of voice box. May occur during removal of intratracheal tube at end of anaesthesia.

Strinacin Trade name. See sulphapyridine.

stringhalt Involuntary snatching up of hindleg and flexing of hock when walking. May affect both hindlegs. Cause unknown, but probably injured nerves. Considered an unsoundness and usually worsens, but some cases occur and disappear spontaneously. Treatment: remove tendon of lateral digital extensor muscle as it crosses outside of hock joint. See veterinary rules (Ministry of Agriculture).

striped horse See zebra. **s. muscle** One of 3 types of muscle; that concerned with voluntary actions, eg movement of legs, head, neck and back. Muscle fibres have irregular lines. Cf smooth muscle, heart muscle.

strongyle See redworm.

strychnine poisoning Often fatal condition caused by eating s. Symptoms: restlessness, muscular twitching, stiffness followed by convulsions, extended limbs and curved neck between periods of relaxation. (Diagnosis confirmed on recovery of s. from stomach.) Treatment: give potassium permanganate by stomach tube and anaesthetise.

styptic (Gr. styptikos) Drug or substance which stops bleeding by astringent action.

sub- Combining form meaning underneath.

sub-acute Between acute and chronic.

subchondral bone cyst Area of bone, less solid than normal, immediately below joint cartilage.

subcutaneous (abbr. sub. cut.) Situated or occurring beneath skin, eg s. injection of drug.

submandibular Below mandible.

Suffolk/S. Punch Draught horse, which takes name from English county of **S.** Always chestnut, usually docile and with feather-less legs. Dates back to 1500s. Assn: **S.** Horse Soc., 6 Church Street, Woodbridge, Suffolk (Woodbridge 2505).

sugar See carbohydrate. **s. beet poisoning** Caused by eating fresh, unwilted **s.b.** tops which contain oxalic acid. Horses particularly susceptible and suffer paralysis, restlessness, cold limbs, salivation and inability to swallow. Treatment: inject 0.2gm. of pilocarpine and feed artificially until swallowing power returns. See stomach tube, food by stomach tube.

sulphadimidine (trade name: Sulphamezathine) White odourless crystals or powder with bitter taste. Has actions similar to sulphanilamide, qv. Used to treat infections of upper respiratory tract, eg snotty nose in foals, sinusitis. Has advantage over many antibiotics of being well tolerated by adult horses, not causing side-effects such as diarrhoea. Dose: initially 0.2gm./kg. body wt. (IV or by mouth), then 0.1gm./kg. body wt. once daily.

Sulphamezathine Trade name. See sulphadimidine.

sulphanilamide Colourless odourless crystals or white crystalline powder with slightly bitter taste. Sulphonamide drug active against streptococci and, to lesser extent, against other micro-organisms. Used to treat septicemia, pneumonia and local infections caused by streptococci. Useful as wound powder, reducing production of excessive granulation (proud flesh). Dose: 0.15gm./kg. body wt.

sulphapyridine (trade name: Strinacin) Drug used to treat diarrhoea in foals.

sulphonamide Type of anti-infection drug, eg sulphadimidine. Overdosage may cause loss of appetite, weak pulse, debility, diarrhoea, jaundice, kidney dysfunction. Treatment: normal saline IV or through stomach tube.

sulphur poisoning May occur after exposure to the gas. Symptoms: diarrhoea, dullness, weak and rapid pulse, pale mucous membranes. Treatment: not effective once symptoms have developed.

summer sores (syn. habronemiasis) See stomach worm.

sunlight See photosensitisation.

supportive treatment Any measure which backs up specific therapy, eg giving warmth to scouring foal when main treatment is feeding anti-diarrhoea mixture. See newborn foal.

suppuration (L. sub, under + puris, pus) Forming and oozing of pus.

suprarenal (supra- + L. ren, kidney) Above kidney; of the s. gland.

suramin (trade names: Antrypol, Germanin, Moranyl, Naganol, Naphuride) White powder with no smell and slightly bitter taste. Used to treat trypanasome infections. Dose: 7–10mg. IV or, for prevention, 2gms. IV every 10 days.

surfactant Chemical substance (phospholipid) in lung. Reduces surface tension of air sac lining, enabling sac to remain expanded. If absent or destroyed, air sac deflates (atelectasis). See broken wind.

surgery (1) Colloq. for centre where surgical operations are performed or patients received for diagnosis and treatment (cf veterinary hospital). (2) Operation for repair, alteration, reconstruction or removal of part or parts. Performed by surgeon under sterile conditions and local or general anaesthesia.

orthopaedic s. Of bones, joints.

bowel s. Of gut, as in twists.

dental s. Of teeth.

opthalmic s. Of eye.

cosmetic s. Improves or alters appearance.

plastic s. Changes part by transplanting or moving skin or other tissue.

Common surgery of horse: Caslick
　　　　　　　　　　　　Hobday
　　　　　　　　　　　　castration
　　　　　　　　　　　　hernia
　　　　　　　　　　　　ruptured bladder of foal
　　　　　　　　　　　　knee chip, joint mice
　　　　　　　　　　　　fractured sesamoid
　　　　　　　　　　　　sinus infection
　　　　　　　　　　　　stringhalt
　　　　　　　　　　　　contracted tendons
　　　　　　　　　　　　dislocated patella
　　　　　　　　　　　　aberrant growth of tooth
　　　　　　　　　　　　internal fixing of fracture (by screws, plates)
　　　　　　　　　　　　growth (warts) removal
　　　　　　　　　　　　twisted gut
　　　　　　　　　　　　caesarian section

See also anaesthesia.

surra (in Algeria: mal de zousfana) Disease of horses and dogs in India and Africa, especially the Sudan. Caused by Trypanosoma evansi, spread by stable fly and tabanid (horse) fly.

suspensory apparatus Part of the stay apparatus (qv) that supports fetlock and prevents it touching ground. Includes: (1) suspensory ligament, (2) sesamoid bones of fetlock joint, (3) intersesamoidean ligament, (4) distal sesamoidean ligament (superficial, middle and deep), (5) short sesamoidean ligament, (6) superficial and deep flexor tendons (see stay apparatus). **s. ligament** (syns. interosseous tendon, superior sesamoidean ligament) Broad, elasticised band of fibrous tissue behind, and attached to, cannon bone. Runs between lower row of carpal bones (in hindlimb: tarsal bones) and sesamoid bones of fetlock. A branch continues across pastern bone to join extensor tendon inserted into front of pedal bone (see stay and suspensory apparatus). **s. ligament, sprain** Most common at insertion into sesamoid bones and at lower end of ligament. Symptoms: swelling, oedema, pain and sometimes lameness. Treatment: rest, corticosteroid injections, irradiation.

suture (L., a seam) (1) Type of fibrous joint. (2) Surgical stitch or series of stitches. See stitch, wound. Cf tape suture.

suxamethonium bromide/s. chloride (trade names: Brevidil, Scoline) White crystalline odourless saline-tasting powder. Given intravenously to relax muscle and may cause respiratory paralysis. Used in anaesthesia. Dose: 0.125–0.20mg./kg. body wt.

swab Wire or stick with end covered by tuft of sterilised cotton. Used to collect material for study in laboratory. **cervical s.** That put through speculum to cervix to aid diagnosis of uterine infection. See uterus, infection of.

swamp Marshland; natural habitat of some breeds, eg Camargue. **s. cancer** See stomach worm. **s. fever** (syn. infectious equine anemia) Contagious disease caused by virus, characterised by chronic illness alternating with acute attacks of fever, anemia and debilitation. Occurs in USA, Canada, Europe, but not reported in British Isles up to 1972. Affects only horses; most in an outbreak area will be affected, with death rate about 50%. Full recovery rare but convalescent animals remain carriers, greatly increasing danger of spread. All breeds and ages susceptible. Virus destroyed by sunlight but persists several months in urine, feces, dried blood and serum. Infection spread by biting flies, contaminated needles, etc. Virus present in body for many years prevents re-infection but is source of infection to other horses through secretions and excretions. Causes damage to walls of small blood vessels and inflammatory changes in most organs, particularly liver; also massive destruction of red blood cells. Symptoms (after 2–4 weeks' incubation): depression, weakness, inco-ordination, marked loss of body condition, fever rising to 41°C. (106°F.), jaundice, oedema of abdomen, hemorrhages in mucosa of mouth, tongue and eye, increased heart rate. After acute phase, there is temporary recovery, then relapses coincide with periods of stress. Diagnosis: on identifying virus in laboratory, but this is difficult. For many years transmission experiments have been only reliable method, but recently serological tests (Coggins test, qv) on blood have given promising results. There may be small hemorrhages on tongue associated with clinical symptoms and increase in sedimentation rate of blood. Treatment: none available. Control: euthanase carriers, eliminate biting insects (helped by draining marshy areas), sterilise surgical instruments.

sweat Salty fluid secreted by **s.** glands in skin on stimulation of sympathetic nerves or release of adrenaline. Evaporation of **s.** from skin causes cooling of body. Increased in exercise, hot surroundings, excitement, painful conditions, eg colic. **lack of s.** (syn. anhidrosis) See dry coat.

Swedish Strong, compact horse for agricultural work or riding. Developed from various breeds including Anglo-Norman and Hanoverian. **S. Ardennes** See Ardennes. **North S.** Cross between **S.** and Gudbrandsdal or Oldenburg. Breeding association formed about 1900.

sweeny Colloq. for wasting (atrophy) of shoulder muscles (supraspinatus and infraspinatus) due to damaged nerve supply (suprascapular nerve). See paralysis.

sweet itch Old name for eczema, qv.

swimming See physiotherapy.

symbol Written sign, usually used to save space. **S.**'s used by veterinarians include:

⌒	about
=	equals
♀	female
<5	less than 5
♂	male
>5	more than 5
±	plus or minus, eg $10 \pm 3 = 7\text{--}13$

sympathetic nervous system Part of autonomic nervous system, qv. Nerves which originate from spinal cord and supply blood vessels, secretory glands, hairs and smooth muscle of intestines. They stimulate increased blood flow, glandular secretions, sweating and intestinal movement. (See parasympathetic nervous system.)

symptom Reported state of horse. Cf sign.

symptomatic (Gr. symptomatikos) Of nature of a symptom.

synapse (Gr. synapsis, a conjunction, connection) Place of contact between 2 nerve cells, where nervous impulse is transmitted from cell to cell. See nerve cell.

syndrome (Gr. syndrome, concurrence) Set of symptoms which characterise particular disease, eg neonatal maladjustment **s.**

synovia (L., Gr. syn, with + oon, egg) Transparent, sticky fluid secreted by part of joint (synovial membrane). Present in bursa and helps lubricate joint.

synovitis Inflamed synovial membrane. See arthritis.

syringe (L. syrinxe, Gr. syrinx) Glass or plastic instrument for injecting liquid drug or other fluid into cavity.

system (Gr. systema, a complex or organised whole) Set of parts which function together, eg nervous system. See parasympathetic nervous system.

systole (Gr. systole, a drawing together) Contraction of heart chambers when blood is pumped into aorta and pulmonary artery. **extra s.** A beat which does not originate from usual point. See electrocardiogram.

systolic Occurring during contraction of heart chambers. **s. murmur** See heart sounds.

T

tabanid fly Large fly belonging to family Tabanidae of phylum Arthropoda; commonest British species: Chrysozona pluvialis (cloak or horse fly). Erroneously called gad fly (because it annoys animals causing them to gad about) but name is reserved for warble fly, qv. Other genera of **t.f.** found in different regions, eg Chrysozona caecutiens widespread in England, C. quadrata common in New Forest and South of England, Tabanus montanus common in hilly areas and T. suditicus (females of which may be 1in. long and emit a deep hum when flying) chiefly in Scotland. **T.f.** has powerful wings and large, irridescent, multicoloured eyes. It lays eggs on leaves of aquatic plants, on stones near water or on damp ground; larvae hatch, drop into water and feed on small aquatic animals; larval stage lasts 2–3 months, then larvae leave water and pupate on dry ground. Adults emerge during July or August for a brief period of activity and mating. **T.f.** bites host after host, so spreads trypanasomes (qv) and viruses of VEE and swamp fever (infectious anemia).

tachycardia (tachy- + Gr. kardia, heart) Excessively fast heart beat, qv.

tail (L. cauda, Gr. oura) End of spinal column from back of croup. Covered in short, furry hair in foal, develops into fall of hair to hocks in most adults (see American Saddle horse, Camargue, donkey). **t. rubbing** May be symptom of eczema or seatworms. **t. swishing** Common after defecation/urination (see behaviour), also considered sign of ill temper (eg in race). **t. (coccygeal) vertebrae** Vary in number, averaging 18.

Tanderil Trade name. See oxyphenbutazone.

tape suture Stitch made of linen, used for tying umbilical cord if this bleeds profusely after birth, but not recommended as routine procedure. Sometimes used to tie skin together after abdominal operation.

tapeworm Internal parasite belonging to class Cestoda with elongated, flat body without cavities or alimentary canal. The two genera of **t.** affecting horses (Anoplocephala and Paranoplocephala) belong to order Cyclophyllidea, family Anoplocephalidae. They are distinguished from other orders by having neither a protrudable part (rostellum) nor hooks on head (scolex). Anoplocephala magna—up to 80cm. long and 2cm. wide, lives in small intestine. A. perfoliata—up to 8cm. long and 3–4mm. wide with small head. Infests small and large intestines. Paranoplocephala mamillana—6–60mm. long and 4–6mm. wide, lives in small intestine. Each type has a number of segments containing male and female reproductive organs. Eggs are self-fertilised or cross-fertilised by male gametes from other segments and stored in uterus of segment, which breaks off and passes out in feces. An intermediate host, eg oribatid mite, feeds on eggs which develop into cysticercoids (bladderworms). These have an outer cuticle, inner germinal layer and central cavity filled with fluid, with head turned inwards. When mite and cysticercus is swallowed by a horse, cysticercus ruptures, releasing head, so t. has gone full cycle. Light infestations do not produce symptoms but cause ulcers in intestine. Large numbers cause digestive disturbances, shaggy coat and anemia and have been known to rupture the caecum. Diagnosis: on finding t. eggs in feces (by microscopic examination). Treatment (if considered necessary): turpentine, male fern extract or linseed oil, qv. See plate 26.

Tarbenian Breed centred on town of Tarbes in Pyrenees. Originally descended from local horses but after Arab and English Thoroughbred influence it is virtually Anglo-Arab. Has good action and conformation, most often chestnut or brown and around 15 hands.

Tarpan Wild horse, became extinct about 100 years ago; descended from horse of prehistoric times and influenced breeds including Spanish Sorraia and ponies on Greek island of Skyros. Was usually grey or dun with dorsal stripe and stripes on upper forelegs; coat colour sometimes changed to white in winter; mane had bushy hogged look; ears and nostrils large. Efforts now being made to re-establish type of wild **T.** in Poland, where similar semi-wild ponies live in forests.

tarsal (L. tarsalis) Of bones of tarsus. **t. bones** Small bones of hock joint (usually 6, occasionally 7). Arranged in 2 rows (proximal and distal). Proximal row: tibial bone, with 2 oblique ridges (trochlea) which articulate with tibia; fibular t. bone, largest bone of hock, forms tuber calcis (point of hock); central t. bone between tibial t. and third t. bone. Distal row: first and second t. bones, articulate with metatarsal bones (cannon and splints); third t. bone, between central t. and metatarsal bone (cannon); fourth t. bone articulates with fibular t. and other t. bones.

tarsus (Gr. tarsos, wickerwork frame) (1) Hock or spavin area. (2) Framework of eyelid.

tartar (L. tartarum, Gr. tartaron) Build-up of scaly deposit on teeth. Can be filed off during routine dental examination.

taste (L. gustus) (1) Sensation transmitted to brain via taste buds, mainly in tip of tongue. Horse who continually licks human hand may **t.** salty dried sweat and may be suffering from salt deficiency. (2) Colloq. for action of stallion or teaser when he nudges/licks mare's vulva.

TB Abbr. Thoroughbred, qv.

Tb Abbr. tuberculosis, qv.

t.d.s. Abbr. ter di'e sumen'dum. 3 times per day. Used on prescriptions.

tears (L. lacrimae, Gr. dakrya) Watery, slightly saline, alkaline secretion of lacrimal glands which moistens conjunctiva. See eye.

teaser Entire horse (see vasectomy) used to find out if mare will accept stallion. **T.** encouraged to nibble mare across trying (teasing) board. If she is in oestrus she will lean towards him and wink vulva, if not she will be hostile and may kick (board should prevent injury to **t.**). **T.** common in breeding of Thoroughbred, less so in other breeds. See plate 1.

teat Nipple of mammary gland.

teeth (pl. of tooth) Structures in upper and lower jaws for grasping and chewing food. Normally 40 in adults—12 front (incisor), 24 cheek (molar) and 4 tusks (canine). May also be up to 4 rudimentary wolf **t.** **T.** consist of a crown above gum, a neck embraced by gum, a root embedded in bony cavity (alveolus) of jaws. Each tooth has 5 surfaces: an upper chewing, an outer, presenting to lips or cheek, an inner presenting to tongue, plus two sides next to adjacent **t.** All except old **t.** contain a cavity open at top of root and containing pulp which nourishes hard structures of **t.** (dentine, enamel and cement). **t., growth of** Process of extending deeper and gradually outwards. Limit of jaw reached at about 7 years, when roots are formed and movement is outwards only. Rate of growth and outward movement parallels rate of surface wear. Entire tooth length lasts about 34 years, then horse would suffer malnutrition. **front (incisor) t.** 2 central **f.t.** in upper and lower jaws at birth; joined by 2 more (lateral **f.t.**) at 4–6 weeks; and a further 2 (corner **f.t.**) at 10 months. Centrals replaced by permanent **f.t.** at 2½ years, laterals at 3½ years, corners at 4½ years. **cheek (molar) t.** (syn. grinders) First 3 (temporary or milk **t.**) present at birth, on each side, upper and lower jaws. 1st and 2nd shed at 2½ years, 3rd at 3½

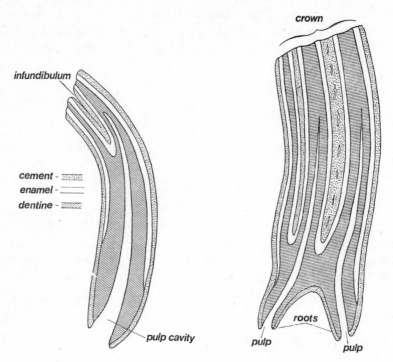

36 Section through front tooth   37 Section through back (molar) tooth

TABLE OF TEETH

Approx. age through gums	Front teeth				Cheek teeth					
	1	2	3		1	2	3	4	5	6
Birth	○									
4 weeks	○	○			○	○	○			
9 months	○	○	○		○	○	○	●		
1½ years	○	○	○		○	○	○	●	●	
2½ years	●	○	○		●	●	○	●	●	
3½ years	●	●	○		●	●	●	●	●	
4½ years	●	●	●		●	●	●	●	●	●

○ =a temporary, first or milk tooth
● =a permanent or 2nd tooth

years. They are pushed up and replaced by permanent t. and remain for short time as caps. Second 3 c.t. develop without milk t. (premolars). 4th cheek tooth in use by 12 months, 5th by 2 years, 6th by $4\frac{1}{2}$ years. **tusk (canine)** 1 on each side of upper and lower jaw by 4 years old in male (absent in female).

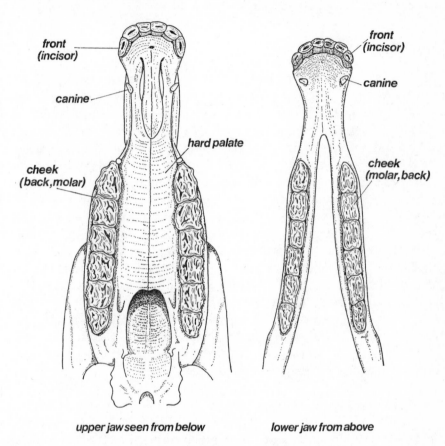

front (incisor)

canine

cheek (back, molar)

hard palate

front (incisor)

canine

cheek (molar, back)

upper jaw seen from below   *lower jaw from above*

38 Teeth in full mouth, ie 6 years or over

Horse's age can be estimated by noting which t. have erupted, which are in wear and amount of wear at grinding surfaces (see bishop; plates 27–9).

telemetry (from Gr. metron, measure) Transference of signals by radio, so that they can be recorded at distance, eg horse can be fitted with transmitter (usually strapped to back) and let loose or ridden so that electrocardiogram (qv) can be recorded at a distance.

383

teleological Serving an ultimate purpose in development, eg fact that foals are usually born at night gives them chance to establish contact with dams before joining herd. This helped ancestors of present-day breeds to survive in wild state. See behaviour.

Telmin Trade name. See mebendazole.

temperament See behaviour.

temperature Measurement of heat. **T.** of healthy horse: 38°C. (100.4°F.), usually taken per rectum (rectal **t.**) which is slightly lower than core **t.** in conditions of diarrhoeic or dry feces (when rectum is ballooned with air). **body or core t.** True **t.** of body, ie in centre. Measured only under experimental conditions by placing thermometer in oesophagus. **skin t.** Raised in any condition, local or general, when horse is afraid, in pain or body needs to lose heat, eg colic, 1st stage labour, inflammation, such as sprained tendon. Body has 4 ways of losing heat: convection (air blowing over skin), conduction (skin in contact with saddle, straw etc), evaporation (involving fluid, eg sweat on skin) and radiation. Skin is main route of heat loss, though urine, feces and lungs (evaporation) play small part. **raised t.** (hyperthermia) Occurs in infectious disease, after exercise, in some poisoning and in painful conditions, eg colic. Grave prognosis if **t.** reaches 41°C. (105.8°F.). See antipyretic. **sub-normal t.** (hypothermia) Common in foals (see neonatal maladjustment syndrome), also occurs in coma, chronic wasting and some poisoning. **T.** can be raised by reducing heat loss, eg with clothing or heated stable (see plate 32).

tendinitis/tendonitis Inflamed tendon. See sprain, bowed tendons.

tendon (L. tendo, Gr. tenon) (1) Fibrous cord which attaches muscle to bone (prominent below carpus and hock where horse has no muscles). See contracted tendons. (2) Colloq. for injured deep and/or superficial flexor **t.** of forelimb. See bowed **t.**, contracted **t.**

Tennessee/T. Walking horse (syn. Plantation Walking horse) Good, all-purpose breed, originally developed to carry farmers of S States over plantations at comfortable running walk (see gaits). Foundation sire was Black Allan, a Standardbred trotter, foaled in 1880s and taken to Tennessee. Usually has long mane and tail and may adopt dog-like stance, ie forelegs together, hindlegs together and behind (instead of underneath) quarters. Assn: **T.W.** Horse Breeders' Assn of America, c/o PO Box 87, Lewisburg, Tennessee (Zip no: 37091).

tenosynovitis/tenovaginitis Inflamed tendon sheath, usually after fibres of tendon have ruptured.

tension (L. tensio, Gr. tonos) (1) Stretching or being stretched. (2) Pressure of gas measured in millimetres of mercury. See pO_2, pCO_2, Boyle's law.

Terramycin Trade name. See oxytetracycline hydrochloride.

testes Pl. of testis.

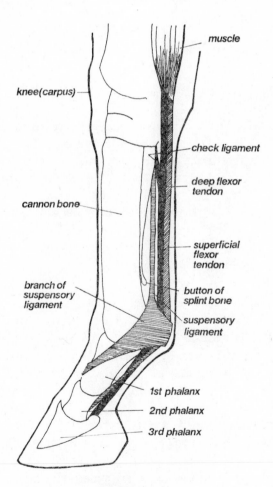

39 Tendons of foreleg

testis (syn. testicle) One of 2 reproductive glands of male; produces spermatozoa and male sex hormone testosterone. Each **t.** in adult stallion is about 5ins. long, 2ins. wide and weighs 300gms. (10oz.). The left is usually larger than right to 21 months, then right becomes larger. Size is related to sperm output so large testes desirable in stallion. Epididymis (qv) attached to upper border. See castration, descent of testes.

testosterone Sex hormone secreted by testes and responsible for male sex characters, libido and descent of testes. Also isolated or synthetic **t.**, white crystalline odourless powder, given by injection or subcutaneous implant to promote libido of stallion or teaser. Dose: 0.5–1gm. Cf castration.

tests (L. testum, crucible) See blood **t.**, laboratory **t.**, pregnancy **t.**

tetanus See lockjaw.

tetanus toxoid Vaccine for immunising against lockjaw (tetanus). Given in 2 injections at least 4 weeks apart followed by 3rd a year later and thereafter at 5-yearly intervals. Pregnant mares should have booster dose in 11th month to produce high level of protective substances (antibodies) in colostrum, qv. Foal will be protected against lockjaw for about 6 weeks. Can be vaccinated at 3 months. Dose: 2–5ml. by deep IM. Cf **Prevac T.**

tetany Muscle twitching.

tetrachloromethane See carbon tetrachloride.

tetracycline/t. hydrochloride (trade name: Achromycin) Yellow crystalline odourless powder with bitter taste. Antibiotic effective against gram-positive and gram-negative bacteria, eg streptococci, staphylococci, Corynebacterium equi. Given as pessary in uterus, by intravenous injection or in ointments. Used to treat strangles, sinusitis, infected wounds, frog thrush, joint ill, pneumonia. Dose: 60mg./kg. body wt. by mouth; 12mg./kg. body wt. IV. See septicemia.

thalamus (pl. thalami; L., Gr. thalamos, inner chamber) Part of brain, **qv.**

thallium poisoning Caused by rat poisons. Symptoms: excessive salivation, difficult swallowing, depression. Diagnosis: on symptoms, or at post-mortem: on hemorrhagic gastroenteritis, fatty degeneration of liver, congested organs, presence of t. in stomach and intestines. Treatment: intravenous glucose, saline, gastric sedatives, atropine.

Theocardin Trade name. Drug used to stimulate heart and lungs.

thermometer (thermo- + Gr. metron, measure) Instrument for measuring temperature. **clinical t.** In centigrade or fahrenheit. See temperature.

thiabendazole (trade name: Equizole) White to creamy-white odourless tasteless powder. Given in feed or by stomach tube, 50mg. (to treat redworm), 100mg. (whiteworm), per kg. body wt. Free of side-effects, including in pregnant mares. Little danger in overdose.

thiamine hydrochloride See aneurine hydrochloride.

thigh Part of hindleg between hip and stifle. **second t.** See gaskin.

thin sole Abnormally delicate sole of hoof; bruises easily. Can be covered with pad of leather or metal kept in place with a shoe.

thiopentone sodium (trade names: Intraval sodium; Pentothal) Yellowish-white powder with characteristic odour and bitter taste. Has tendency to absorb moisture if exposed to air. Used in anaesthesia as knock-down dose to induce sufficient unconsciousness to insert tube (intratracheal) into windpipe (see anaesthesia). Used alone, may cause inco-ordination during recovery. Dose: 10–15mg./kg. body wt. IV.

thirst (L. sitis, Gr. dipsa) The craving for a drink. Increases in hot weather, when in hard work and if salt intake is high. Excessive **t.** symptom of diarrhoea (especially in foals), kidney disease involving excess of urine and diabetes insipidus. (Colic case may swill water through mouth without drinking.)

thoracic vertebra One of vertebrae of withers region. Usually 18, sometimes 19. Articulates with rib and has well-developed spinous process (upper tip) which may fracture if horse falls over backwards.

thorax (Gr., pl. thoraces) Body between withers/shoulder and diaphragm (internal organ approx. beneath last rib).

Thorazine Hydrochloride Trade name. See chlorpromazine hydrochloride.

Thoroughbred (Arabic kelihan, pure all through; sometimes abbreviated TB) Breed most countries use for Flat and jump racing. Has been developed over more than 250 years; its athletic form is exploited and it commands far higher prices than other breeds. Every **T.** traces to one of 3 Oriental sires: the Byerley Turk (imported in 1860s), Darley Arabian (about 1700) and Godolphin Arabian/Barb (about 1730), but their close descendants, Herod, Eclipse and Matchem respectively, are better known. Though most **T.**'s have lost obvious Arab characteristics (eg dished profile) breed has inherited and improved Arab speed. As racing puts great stress on body structures and **T.** is raced before it has finished growing, breed has reputation for unsoundness. Paradoxically it is one of few breeds in which sires do not have to be licensed, to prevent defects being passed on (cf veterinary rules). **T.** more likely than other breeds to conceive twins and a fit **T.** stores more of its red blood cells in spleen than other breeds. Average height at week old: 41 inches, average girth: 35 inches (see also growth). Adult **T.** usually 15.1-16.3 hands. In N hemisphere official birthdate of all **T.**'s is 1 Jan. (in S hemisphere, 1 Aug.). Arbitrary date outside Flat racing season was chosen for easy administration (see veterinary rules), but imposes unnatural breeding season—generally accepted as 15 February to 15 July (see fertility rate). Assn: **T.** Breeders' Assn, 42 Portman Square, London W1H 0EN (01 486 4921); Jockey Club (controls Flat racing in Britain), Newmarket, Suffolk (Newmarket 4151); California **T.** Breeders' Assn, 201 Colorado Place, PO Box 750, Arcadia, California 91006 (213 447 7445); **T.** Breeders of Kentucky, PO Box 4158, Lexington, Kentucky 40501; Weatherbys (British Jockey Club secretaries), Sanders Road, Wellingborough, Northamptonshire NN8 4BX (Wellingborough 6241/4387). See plate 33.

thoroughpin Inflamed tendon sheath which encloses deep digital flexor tendon as it passes behind hock. Soft swelling appears approx. level with point of hock and extends from one side to the other beneath the tendons (gastrocnemius and superficial flexor) that cross over point of hock. Treat by draining fluid through needle and injecting corticosteroids. Often recurs, but seldom causes lameness. See plate 21.

thrill Tremor or vibration felt on body above (usually abnormal) condition, eg friction of air in mucus-filled air passage or badly damaged heart valve causing turbulence in blood flow.

throat (syn. pharynx) Area at back of tongue. Contains soft palate, glottis, epiglottis, openings to larynx (voice box), eustachian tubes and nasal cavities. See wind.

thrombotic Of a blood clot.

thrombus (Gr.) Blood clot in artery or vein. Acts as plug, restricting blood flow. Usually due to rough vessel lining, caused by bacterial infection, trauma, or migrating redworm larvae. Most common sites: mesenteric artery where it leaves aorta to the gut; aorta where it divides into iliac arteries, which pass to hindlegs. See iliac thrombosis.

thrush (syn. canker) Degenerative condition of frog characterised by black, evil-smelling material. In severe cases infection may erode most of frog, reaching sensitive laminae below. Caused by standing in soiled bedding and lack of attention to foot. Micro-organism usually involved is Sphaerophus necrophorus. Symptoms include lameness and contracted heels. Treatment: ensure bedding is kept clean, cut away rotting frog and apply chloramphenicol and gentian violet.

thymus Gland in chest. Source of blood lymphocytes. Particularly large and active in foal and concerned with immunity.

thyroid Ductless (endocrine) gland either side of voice box (larynx). Made up of vesicles (small balloon-like sacs) filled with colloid (sticky protein material which, in **t.** gland contains the iodine-containing protein thyroglobulin, part of which is thyroxine, qv). Lack of thyroxine causes hypothyrodism (goitre and cretinism) and is common in yearlings eating food with anti-thyroxine effect, eg kale. **T.** gland over-reacts, becomes fibrous and vesicles fill with colloid which is difficult to convert into thyroglobulin. Gland swells and can be felt by placing thumb and forefinger either side of larynx. See iodine. **t. extract** Cream-coloured powder with faint meat-like odour and taste, obtained from **t.** gland. Given by mouth, but slow to take effect. Maximum activity from single dose may take 10 days to develop and effects persist more than 14 days, therefore danger of overdosage by accumulation. Used to promote libido. Dose 1–2 mg./kg. body wt. **t. stimulat-**

ing hormone (syns. TSH, thyrotrophic hormone) Produced by front (anterior) lobe of pituitary gland. Acts on t. gland, causing it to produce colloid. See hyperthyroidism.

thyroxine Hormone produced by thyroid gland. Circulates in blood and when at certain level pituitary gland reduces its production of thyrotrophic hormone. Has many important effects: raises basal metabolic rate (BMR), helps liver to change glycogen into glucose, promotes absorption of glucose from the gut, accelerates heart rate and rate of calcium removal from bones.

Tibetan Pony descended from Mongolian and Chinese breeds, often dun.

tibia Long bone between stifle joint (above) and hock joint (below). Forms second thigh (gaskin).

tick Arthropod insect belonging to class Arachnida, order Acarina. Important in human and veterinary medicine because many types are parasitic and transmit disease. They live on skin and suck blood and, in large numbers, cause anemia and loss of condition. Can transmit infectious diseases including spirochaetosis (Spirochaeta theileri), biliary fever (Babesia equi and B. cabelli), the virus of equine encephalomyelitis (Western and Venezuelan types), swamp fever. Those affecting horses belong to family Ixodidae, the hard t. Male has chitinous shield over back; female's shield covers only small portion. Female lays small, round, dark brown eggs in one batch under stone or in sheltered spot, then dies. Larvae hatch and crawl on to grass or shrubs from which they fasten on to host. After feeding, larva moults and becomes nymph; nymph becomes an imago; male and female imagos copulate and, after feeding, female drops off host to lay eggs; males may stay on host for many months. T. classed as 1-, 2-, or 3-host depending on number of hosts it needs during life cycle. It is sensitive to change in temperature or moisture; some survive only in warm regions, others most active in cold, dry climates and not usually host-specific.

Important members of family:

Ixodus	**I. ricinus:** castor bean tick
	I. canisuya: British dog tick
Boophilus	**B. annulatus:** North American tick

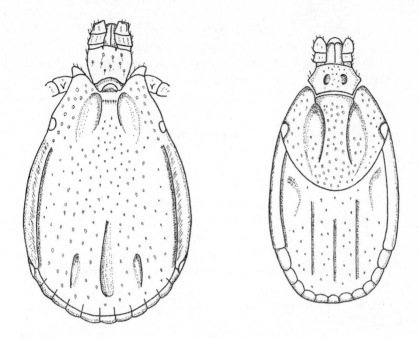

40 Male (*left*) and female tick—Rhipicephalus appendiculatus—from above

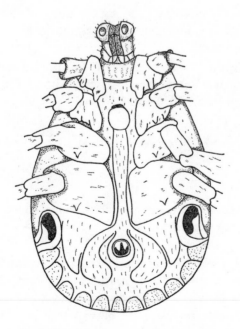

41 Male tick (genus Dermacentor)

B. decoloratus: blue tick in South Africa, transmits spirochaetosis of horses

Margaropus **M. winthemi:** Argentine tick, also in South Africa

Hyalomma **H. aegyptium:** bont-leg tick, in Africa, Asia and S Europe

Rhipicephalus **R. appendiculatus:** brown tick, in South Africa

R. evertsi: red tick, common in south Africa

R. bursa: common in South Africa, transmits equine piroplasmosis

Dermacentor **D. reticulatus:** in Asia and S Europe, transmits biliary fever

D. andersoni: transmits encephalomyelitis and Rocky Mountain spotted fever

Treatment: see benzene hexachloride, dicophane, gamma benzene hexachloride.

t.i.d. Abbr. L. ter in di'e, 3 times per day. Used on prescriptions.

Timor Hard-working harness or saddle pony of New Zealand and Australia. All colours, including mixtures similar to Appaloosa, qv.

tincture (L. tingere, to wet, to moisten) Solution of drug in alcohol, eg **t.** of chloroform and morphine (syn. chlorodyne), used to treat colic, especially of newborn foal. Dose 15–30ml.

tip (1) Pointed body part, eg **t.** of tongue. (2) Small metal plate used to shoe foal with slightly contracted tendons or deformed, upright feet. Cf plate, shoe.

tipped vulva Poor conformation in which vulval lips form concave line beneath anus. See Caslick.

tissue (Fr. tissu) Collection of specialised cells, eg fat (adipose) **t.**, connective **t.**, fibrous **t.** (see separate headings). **t. culture** Cells from kidney or other organs grown in laboratory specially for cultivation of virus. **t. fluid** Water, salts and dissolved gases which pass through capillary walls to bathe body cells (see oedema).

tocopheryl acetate (trade names: Davitamon-E, Ephynal, Germinol, Phytoferol) Pale-yellow odourless liquid. (Alpha-tocopheral is one form of vitamin E.) Essential to cell metabolism. Found in green foods and germ of cereals. Appears to be interchangeable to some extent with selenium, qv.

toe Colloq. end of limb, ie front of hoof. See base-wide, evolution.

Tolseran Trade name. See mephenesin.

tongue (L. lingua, Fr. glossa) Muscular, moveable pad of flesh on floor of mouth. Used extensively when grazing, to help teeth gather food. May be injured by rough edges on teeth or by bit of bridle (which should be on, not underneath, t.). **t. swallowing** Colloq. for abnormal gurgling noise made at fast paces. Some claim strapping down of t. stops gurgling and eases breathing, though this is doubtful. Cf wind.

tonic (Gr. tonikos) Colloq. for medicine believed to restore health and vigour, eg beer, stout or manufactured t. mixed in feed may put on weight and improve coat condition.

topical (Gr. topikos) Local, as in use of ointment.

tourniquet Rope, rubber band, or other device to compress blood vessels, control bleeding, eg after injury, during surgery. Must be placed at a point between heart and site of bleeding. Should not be applied longer than 30 minutes unless circumstances exceptional. Cf Esmarch bandage, twitch.

toxemia (toxin + Gr. haima, blood + -ia) Body's absorption of bacterial product, ie toxin, from focus of infection.

toxin (L. toxibum, poison) Poison or substance produced by bacteria, eg Clostridium tetani, cause of lockjaw, qv.

tracheotomy (tracheo- + Gr. tome, a cutting) Opening into windpipe so that tube can be inserted. See tube.

Trackehnen/Trakehner Popular German breed developed with Arab and Thoroughbred blood for about 200 years before Poles took over majority of horses after World War II. (Now bred as Masuren, qv.)

Those **T.** not commandeered formed basis of lighter type which excels as saddle horse, though some claim it is particularly susceptible to unsoundness.

tract (L. tractus) Passageway, eg urinary **t.**, alimentary **t.** or canal.

tragacanth mucilage Suspending agent for medicines and a base for drugs in tablets and pills.

tranquilliser (L. tranquillus, calm) Drug which allays fear and anxiety. Should be given only in minimum dose to donkeys as may cause inco-ordination. See dope test.

transference See immunity, passive.

transfuse To give liquid, eg blood into vein. See hemolytic jaundice.

transplant To take organ or part and use it in another horse (only in experiments) or in another part of donor, eg part of extensor tendon can be used to strengthen bowed tendon of foreleg. Cf skin graft.

transudate (trans- + L. sudare, to sweat) Fluid which passes through membrane as result of inflammation.

trauma Wound, injury or severe shock (adjective: traumatic). **birth t.** Injury to foal, usually chest, as it emerges through mare's pelvis. See birth.

trephine (L. trephina) Instrument for boring hole in sinus. See sinusitis.

triamcinolone (trade names: Vetalog, Ledercort veterinary) White odourless powder; synthetic cortisone with actions and uses similar to cortisone acetate, qv. Dose: 30mg. IM; 6–30mg. into joints.

Tribrissen Trade name. See trimethoprim.

Trichlorphon Trade name. See metriphonate.

tricuspid valve (syn. atrio-ventricular valve) Set of valves with 3 cusps guarding opening between first and second chambers on right side of heart. Cusps are attached to fibrous ring which forms atrio-ventricular (AV) opening. Free edges of cusps contain fibrous cords (chordae tendineae) the other ends of which are attached to wall of second chamber. Valve prevents blood regurgitating from second chamber to first. Valve may be infected with bacteria or redworm larvae, causing incompetence and back flow of blood during heart contraction (leaking valve). See endocarditis, mitral valve.

trimeprazine tartrate (trade name: Vallergan) White odourless bitter-tasting powder. Derivative of phenothiazine. Usd to sedate in pre-operative medication and as anti-histamine in allergy cases. Given by mouth, or by subcutaneous, intramuscular or intravenous injection. Dose: 1–4mg./kg. body wt.

trimethoprim (trade names: Tribrissen, Trivetrin) Drug used with sulphadiazine or sulfadoxine to treat bacterial diarrhoea in foals and infections of adult horses. Dose: 0.25gms./kg. body wt. twice daily.

Trivetrin Trade name. See trimethoprim.

trocar (Fr. trois quarts, three quarters) Pointed instrument used with cannula (hollow tube) which fits around a stilette. Used for paracentesis, qv.

trochanter (Gr.) Bony projection, eg parts of femur: major, minor and third t.'s.

trochanteric bursitis See whorlbone lameness.

trot See gait.

Trypanosoma (Gr. trypanon, borer + soma, body) Genus of parasite in blood of man and animals, including horse. Most live part of life cycle in insects, eg tabanid fly. **T. equinum** Species in mal de caderas, qv.

trypanosome Organism of genus Trypanosoma.

trypsin (Gr. tryein, to rub + pepsin) Enzyme secreted by pancreas.

TSH Abbr. thyroid stimulating hormone, qv.

tube (L. tubus) (1) Round, hollow pipe, eg air t. (any air passage). (2) Pipe of rubber or similar, used in treatment, eg stomach t. (qv). Cf

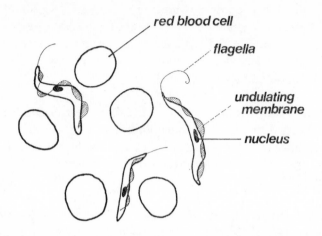

42 Trypanosoma evansi in blood. See *surra*

speculum. **intratracheal (or endotracheal)** t. One into windpipe (trachea). (3) Colloq. to operate on windpipe, inserting small t. (tracheotomy). Seen from outside as 1in. hole in neck beneath throat, covered with metal mesh to prevent objects being drawn in with air. Performed to counteract obstructed wind, ie when horse cannot get sufficient air into lungs at fast paces, via nostrils and throat (pharynx). Horse will drown if tubed part of neck is submerged.

tuber Pointed part, eg **t. coxae.** See pelvis.

tuberculin Liquid containing extracts from tubercle bacillus (from birds or mammals). **t. test** The liquid is injected into skin (intradermal injection) to test reaction 48 hours afterwards. See tuberculosis.

tuberculosis (Tb) Disease rare in horses due to limited exposure to infection and apparent resistance; caused by Mycobacterium tuberculosis or M. bovis. Most likely to cause fusion of neck (cervical) vertebrae, causing stiff neck and inability to get head down to graze. Pneumonia may develop, destroying air spaces and increasing breathing rate, with wasting and fluctuating temperature. **t. pneumonia** See pneumonia.

tumour See growth.

Turk Fast, light breed virtually extinct in original form even in Turkey, but known in England around 1700 when several were imported. White and Yellow **T.** both raced in England. According to some authorities, Byerley **T.** was an Arab. See Thoroughbred.

Turkoman (syn. Pouseki) Slender horse developed from Mongolian and Arab. Now bred almost exclusively by Kirghis tribesmen in Northern Persia (Iran). Ridden long distances in desert, often with little drinking water. Sometimes ewe-necked (qv). Many kept in racehorse-like trim with felt rugs which counteract heat in summer and cold in winter.

tush/tusk Colloq. for canine tooth. See teeth.

twin One of two foals of same pregnancy, usually developed from 2 fertilised ova. (The splitting of 1 ovum, producing identical **t.**'s, rare in horses.) About 1.7% of Thoroughbred pregnancies are **t.**; incidence much less in other breeds. Birth-weight one- to two-thirds less than single foal. See plate 33. **t. abortion** See abortion.

twist (syn. volvulus) Colloq. for torsion of part of alimentary tract, usually small intestine. May be complete, with tube tied in knot, or partial, involving membrane (mesentery) suspending gut. Results in strangulated blood supply and acute gut damage. Symptoms: as colic (qv) and unless treated surgically, death. Cause unknown, but sometimes follows damage done by redworm larvae.

twitch (1) Reflex action, particularly flashing of third eyelid (nictitating membrane) and muscle tremor, both symptoms of lockjaw (tetanus). (2) Length of cord or similar, looped at top of rod, usually about 12ins. long. Used to restrain horse by gathering flesh, usually upper lip, into loop and twisting rod until skin is pinched. May increase blood pressure so should be used with caution on pregnant, or recently foaled, mare.

tying-up syndrome Mild form of setfast, qv. May also be result of pulled muscle (myositis), ie tearing of fibres causing inflammation and pain. Diagnosis: on faradic stimulation causing muscle to contract and elicit pain, blood tests for raised enzyme (SGOT and CPK) levels. Treatment: corticosteroids, injected locally, salicylates, faradism (see physiotherapy).

tympany (Gr. tympanis) (1) Colloq. for cavity or sac distended with gas or air (tympanites), eg abdomen, guttural pouch. (2) A bell-like sound. Cf percussion.

tympanitic Of tympany. See colic.

U

udder See mammary glands, plate 35.

ulcer (L. ulcus) Inflamed area on mucous membrane with eroded surface cells. Sometimes found on gums, lining of gut. See mouth, injuries of; coital exanthema.

ulcerative enteritis Enteritis (qv) caused by ulcers in lining of alimentary tract due to redworm larvae. Cf aneurysm. **u. lymphangitis** Rare, occasionally fatal contagious disease characterised by swollen lower legs; caused by Corynebacterium pseudo-tuberculosis. Infection enters leg wounds and spreads to lymphatic vessels where abscesses develop. Symptoms: swelling and pain around pastern with nodules beneath skin. These rupture, discharging creamy-green pus and leaving ulcers with ragged edges. They heal in 1–2 weeks but fresh crops occur. (Should not be confused with glanders.) Diagnosis: on laboratory examination of pus. Treatment: antibiotics, especially penicillin. Control: good stable hygiene. See also lymphangitis.

ulna Smaller of 2 bones of forearm, upper part of which forms point of elbow (olecranon). Cf radius.

ultrasonic (ultra- + L. sonus, sound) Radiant energy with frequency beyond upper limit of human hearing, ie above 20,000 cycles per second. See physiotherapy, pregnancy tests.

ultraviolet Beyond violet end of spectrum; wave lengths between 1,800 and 3,900 angstroms. See filter, radiation.

umbilical (L. umbilicalis) Of the umbilicus. **u. abscess** Focus of pus at navel (umbilicus), usually in remnant of vein, which in fetal life carried blood from placenta to liver. May become infected when **u.** cord breaks after birth. Swelling is much harder than a hernia (qv) or may not show externally. Can harbour germ causing lockjaw, qv.

umbilicus (syn. navel) Point of attachment in fetus. At birth cord breaks about 3cm. from abdominal wall, forming stump which shrivels. Abdominal opening (umbilical ring) through which urachus and blood vessels passed in fetal life, closes during first week. Failure to close allows abdominal contents to push through ring. See hernia, plates 13 and 14.

ungulate (L. ungula, hoof) Mammal with digits protected by hoof, eg horse, pig. See evolution.

urachus (Gr. ourachos) Tube connecting fetal bladder with allantois (placenta). Cf pervious **u.**

uremia Abnormal increase in urea content of blood (above 40mg./ 100ml.). Occurs in kidney disease or after kidney damage by toxins or bacteria, eg sleepy foal disease. See septicemia.

ureter See kidney.

urethra, male Long tube from urinary bladder to glans penis. Passes backward on floor of pelvis, turns round brim of pelvis and comes forward as part of penis. Therefore divided into pelvic and extra-pelvic parts. See stone. **u., female** Duct which conveys urine from bladder to outside. About 7cm. (3ins.) long and 2.5cm. (1in.) wide, though capable of dilation.

urethritis Inflamed urethra.

urinary Of urine.

urinate (syns. micturate, stale) To void urinary bladder. See behaviour cystitis.

urine Fluid of water and soluble substances formed by kidneys and excreted after collecting in bladder. Adult horse may pass 2–10 litres per day, depending on water intake, amount of sweating and fluid content of feces. Colour depends on substances known as urochromes. High volume of **u.** dilutes them, so that fluid is pale; conversely, dark **u.** is due to concentration. Equine **u.** normally pale to brown, but red or black in setfast and red after phenothiazine intake. Cloudy **u.** is due to calcium carbonate crystals. Odour comes from volatile acids and breakdown of urea, producing ammonia. Specific gravity depends on volume, average 1.050. **U.** is usually alkaline (pH 7–9) but changes if left to stand and varies with diet (high-concentrate rations may cause slightly acidic **u.**). It normally has high mucin content. Abnormal substances in **u**: protein, sugar, red and white blood cells, hemoglobin, myoglobin, bilirubin. **u. sample** Small amount of **u.** collected (1) to aid diagnosis of conditions such as cystitis, (2) to discover any drug content, eg after race stewards can order course vet. to take **u.s.** from any runner. Horse may not urinate for an hour or more, but can be encouraged to do so if attendant whistles or shakes up straw bedding. **U.s.** must be collected in sterile container if analysis is to be accurate. See cystitis, dope test, phenylbutazone, veterinary rules.

urochrome (uro- + Gr. chroma, colour) Pigment in urine, qv.

urolith (uro- + Gr. lithos, stone) Urinary calculus. See stone.

urticaria See nettle rash.

uterine (L. uterinus) Of the uterus. **u. inertia** See uterus.

uterus Muscular, Y-shaped organ with 2 horns and body; horns are about 25cm. (10ins.) long, body 20cm. (8ins.) long. Horns are connected to fallopian tubes and body is separated from vagina by neck (cervix). Body and horns are suspended from abdominal wall by membrane, the broad ligament of **u.** Uterine wall has 3 layers: outer serous coat of peritoneum, middle, muscular coat and the inner mucous membrane (endometrium) containing glands. **u., inertia of** Weak uterine contractions during 2nd stage labour, causing delay in delivery. Cause: not established, possibly an imbalance of hormones, ie oxytocin, oestrogen and progesterone. Treatment: oxytocin and/or oestrogen. See birth. **u., infection of** Colloq. for any non-specific infection. Commonly caused by streptococci, E. coli, Pseudomonas pyocyanea and Klebsiella. Symptoms: thick discharge from cervix. May result in permanent infertility if not cleared. Diagnosis: on laboratory examination of discharge and, possibly, uterine biopsy (see biopsy). Cervical or uterine swab should be taken from mare before covering, to ensure she is free of infection. See metritis, endometritis. **u., involution of** Return of **u.** to non-pregnant size after foaling. See after-birth, retention of; birth. **u., prolapse of** Protrusion of **u.** through vagina. Inner lining is exposed as organ hangs from between vulval lips. Occurs in mares of all ages after foaling or, more rarely, abortion. Cause: unknown, but presumably result of slack ligaments retaining **u**. Treatment: mare should be kept standing and organ supported in clean sheet wetted with saline solution (teaspoonful of salt per pint of water). Replace **u**. by massaging at edge and squeezing gently towards vulva; when partially returned, complete process by working arm and clenched fist into vagina. Replacement helped by injecting muscle relaxant to abolish straining, and oxytocin to contract **u**. Tape sutures (qv) can be inserted across lips of vulva. Give antitenanus serum. If **u**. is not badly damaged and is replaced within about an hour, mare will breed normally after recovery. Complications include rupture of **u**. and prolapse of intestines, hemorrhage from uterine artery, infection of **u**. and laminitis. **u., rupture of** Tear in **u**. wall. May occur during 2nd stage labour or as result of prolapse. Signs include mare's reluctance to proceed with 2nd stage. Treatment: surgical repair under general anaesthesia.

V

vaccinate To inject vaccine to stimulate immunity.

vaccine (L. vaccinus) Solution containing live, altered (attenuated) or killed micro-organisms. May or may not have carrying agent (adjuvant). Injected to stimulate immunity to particular micro-organism. **V**.'s used on horses:

dead	Brucella abortus
	Clostridium tetani
	influenza (contains several strains)
live	African horse sickness (contains several strains)
	encephalomyelitis (Western, Eastern and Venezuelan types)
	herpesvirus I (rhinopneumonitis)

vagina Passage from neck of uterus (cervix) to vulva and about 20cm. (8ins.) long. Walls normally touch, but at mating, or if speculum is inserted, air can be sucked in to distend organ into large cavity. Cf artificial **v**.

vaginal Of the vagina. **v. bruising** May occur during birth, causing type of blood blister (hematoma) which can be seen just inside vulval lips. Swelling may burst, releasing blood. Cf birth hemorrhage.

vaginitis Inflamed vagina. May be caused by infection introduced at coitus, foaling or when mare takes air into vagina due to poor conformation. See Caslick.

vagus See nerves, table of.

Vallergan Trade name. See trimeprazine tartrate.

valve (from L. valvae, folding doors) Fold of membrane which regulates flow of a body fluid, eg heart **v.** See heart, plate 36.

valvular endocarditis Inflamed heart valves, ie tricuspid, mitral, or pulmonary and aortic semilunar valves. Caused by infection with bacteria, eg Streptococcus equi or Strep. pyogenes var. equi, resulting from damage by redworm larvae. May accompany inflamed heart lining (endocardium). Thickenings and cauliflower-like growths appear on edges of valves, causing incompetence (failure to close properly, allowing back flow of blood and reduced pumping capacity of heart). Symptoms depend on heart's ability to contract more strongly to overcome defect; if it compensates there are no symptoms; if not, there is decreased stamina, distress after exercise, filling of legs and/or sheath. Diagnosis: on signs, anemia, increased white blood cell count (see blood tests) and hearing a heart murmur, qv.

vas (pl. vasa) Tube for carrying fluid, eg **v.** deferens.

vascular Full of vessels.

vas deferens (pl. vas deferentia; syn. ductus deferens) Duct which carries spermatozoa from each testis to urethra. Together ducts form ejaculatory duct of penis.

vasectomy (vas + Gr. ektome, excision) Severence of vas deferens. Sometimes performed on colt used as teaser to allow him to mount mares without risk of conception.

vasoconstriction Reduced calibre of blood vessels; lessens blood flow; caused by action of sympathetic nervous system or substance, eg adrenaline, which mimics nervous stimulation. May be local, as in skin during cold weather to reduce heat-loss, or general, as in reaction to exercise or excitement, resulting in raised blood pressure.

vasoconstrictor Drug or substance that causes constriction of blood vessels.

vasodilation Dilated blood vessels, causing increased blood flow to part. See inflammation.

vasopressin (syn. pitressin) Antidiuretic hormone secreted by back (posterior) lobe of pituitary. Name is misnomer because it has little effect on vascular system. Decreases amount of water excreted by kidney.

Vecortenol Trade name. See prednisolone.

vector (L., one who carries, from vehere, to carry) Carrier, usually an Arthropod, which transfers infective agents from one host to another, eg tick carries organisms causing biliary fever, mosquito transmits encephalomyelitis.

VEE See encephalomyelitis.

vein (L. vena) Part of blood circulatory system. Carries de-oxygenated blood from capillaries of organs and muscles to heart. V.'s are thin-walled, non-muscular, relatively large-calibre tubes containing valves which help prevent back flow. In general, arranged like arteries (see arteries, table of). Largest v. known as vena cava. **jugular v.'s** One on either side of neck in jugular furrow, receive blood from head and convey it to anterior vena cava. **anterior vena cava** (syns. AVC, superior vena cava, SVC) Returns blood from head, neck, forelegs and chest to heart. **posterior vena cava** (syns. PVC, inferior vena cava, IVC) Returns blood from abdomen, pelvis, hindlegs and hindquarters to right, 1st chamber of heart. Lies close to aorta in roof of abdomen and passes through diaphragm. **portal v.** Collects blood from gut, pancreas and spleen, returning it to liver where it is distributed among cells and then carried by **hepatic v.** to posterior vena cava. **pulmonary v.'s** 7 or 8 v.'s which return blood from lungs to left side of heart. **cardiac v.'s** Collect blood from heart muscle and open into coronary sinus (a v.) which discharges into right atrium (first chamber) of heart.

velum palati Part of soft palate, qv.

vena cava See vein.

Venagmin Trade name. See oxallic acid.

venereal (L. venereus) Any infection passed on via coitus, eg Klebsiella.

Venezuelan equine encephalomyelitis (VEE) See encephalomyelitis.

venous (L. venosus) Of a vein, eg **v.** blood.

ventral (L. ventralis) Position which is below, ie towards belly or undersurface.

ventricle Small cavity, eg one of lower heart chambers. See heart. **v. stripping** Removal of membrane lining larynx, so that vocal cords stick to walls, preventing whistling, roaring etc. See Hobday, wind.

venula/venule A tiny blood vessel that joins capillary bed with vein.

vermicide (vermis + L. caedere, to kill) See anthelmintic.

vermifuge See anthelmintic.

Verocid Trade name. See piperazine salts.

vertebra One of 51–7 bones of spinal column.

vertebrae, lumbar 6 largest **v.** of column; with muscles of back attached. Tops of spinous processes can be felt in mid-line of back. May cause

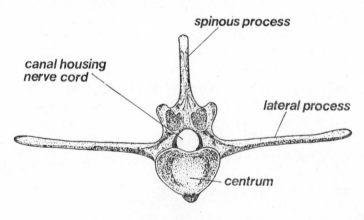

43 A back (lumbar) vertebra

pain and lameness if damaged (eg in jumping or falling) or if arthritis develops between **v.** Fused **v.** may cause horse to screw his jumps, ie jump to left or right.

vertebral column (syn. spinal column) Bones articulating in a line from head to tail and which house spinal cord. Numbers: 7 neck (cervical) vertebrae, 18 withers region (thoracic), 6 back (lumbar), 5 croup (sacral), 15–21 tail (coccygeal).

vesica (L., blister; pl. vesicae) Any sac or bladder for a secretion, eg urinary bladder.

vesicant A blistering agent. See blister.

vesicle (L. vesicula, dim. of vesica) Bladder or sac containing liquid, eg seminal **v.**, qv.

vesicular exanthema See coital exanthema. **v. stomatitis** Infectious disease caused by virus and characterised by blisters on mouth and feet. Indiana and New Jersey strains of virus have been isolated from horses, donkeys, cattle and pigs. Saliva and blister fluid are highly infective and biting flies probably spread disease which has occurred in USA and Mexico. Blisters appear on tongue, lips and lining of mouth; there is mild fever, salivation and loss of appetite. Similar to foot and mouth disease, which does not occur in horses. Recovery is spontaneous and no treatment required.

vessel Channel for carrying fluid, eg blood or lymph.

vestibule Anatomical term for space at entrance to an opening, eg part of vagina just inside vulva.

Vestland See Fjord.

Vetalog Trade name. See triamcinolone.

Veterinarians' Alliance New name for **V.** Union. See Veterinary Doctor.

veterinary (L. veterinarius) Of animals and their diseases. **v. anaesthetists** See Association of VA. **v. codex** See British **V.** Codex. **V. Doctor** (previously **V.** Digest) Journal published quarterly by Veterinarians' Alliance, 292 Southend Lane, London SE6 (0582 25892).

Distributed free to selected vets in general practice in Britain and those overseas listed in British register. **V. Drug** Monthly newspaper circulated to **v.** practices in UK. Published by Henderson Group One, 23a Craven Street, London WC2N 5NT (01 839 3707) for **V.** Drug Co (York). See manufacturers. **V. History Society** Asociated with Worshipful Society of Apathecaries of London, c/o S. A. Hall, **V.** Investigation Centre, Madingley Road, Cambridge CB3 0ER. **v. hospital** Treatment centre. From 1965 Royal College of **V.** Surgeons has allowed premises of sufficiently high standard to be described as **v.h.**; more than 55 in UK in 1973. See also British **V.** Hospital Association. **V. Journal** See British **V.** Journal. **V. Matters** Magazine, published 3–4 times a year by the Association of the British Pharmaceutical Industry. **V. Practice** Bi-monthly newspaper, published by A. E. Morgan Ltd, 172 Kingston Road, Ewell, Surrey (01 393 0941). Sent, free, to vets in private and hospital practice and to training centres. **v. radiologists** See British **V.** Radiological Association. **V. Record** Journal founded in 1888 by William Hunting, FRCVS, an Edinburgh graduate and President of the Royal College of **V.** Surgeons 1894–5. Published weekly by British **V.** Association, 7 Mansfield Street, London W1M 0AT (01 636 6541). **V. Review, The** Tri-annual magazine, free to the profession, published by May & Baker Ltd. See manufacturers. **v. rules** Can be divided into those of Jockey Club (which controls Thoroughbred racing in Britain); of various breed societies (see particular breed; of **v.** bodies, eg Royal College of **V.** Surgeons; of Ministry of Agriculture and (recommendations) of Thoroughbred Breeders' Assn, British **V.** Assn and British Equine **V.** Assn (see also soundness). Jockey Club rules of a **v.** nature include:

14 (vi) [The stewards of a meeting have full power] — At any time to order an examination by such person or persons as they think fit, of any horse entered for a race, or which has run in a race.

32 (i) Passports [qv] will be issued annually for named two-year-old horses in the care of licensed trainers and other horses as authorised by the stewards of the Jockey Club. They are returnable on demand and are issued subject to the instructions contained therein.

(ii) The stewards . . . may require such passports to be lodged with the clerk of the course for any race before the horses are declared under Rule 141 (i) so that the horse's identification may be verified by a **v.** surgeon before running.

(iii) The following fees are payable:

for initial use of a passport	£2
for replacement of a passport	£5
for endorsement to a passport for horse travelling abroad	£1

33 A horse which (a) was foaled outside or which has been outside Great Britain, Ireland or the Channel Islands (but not from one to the other), (b) is trained in Ireland or which has been in Ireland since Jan 1, 1972, may not be declared a runner . . . until either (i) a passport has been lodged with the clerk of the course for verification by a v. surgeon; or (ii) the following certificates have been lodged at Racing Calendar Office:

A certificate of pedigree stating name, pedigree, age, sex, colour and markings of the horse, issued by a recognised stud book authority or in the absence of a stud book authority, by the recognised Turf authority of the country in which the horse was foaled. A certificate of age and markings signed in Britain or Ireland or the Channel Islands by a v. surgeon who is neither owner nor trainer of the horse nor a person for whom the trainer of the horse holds a current identity card. The requirements of this rule shall not apply . . . after . . . the passport or papers are first lodged, provided the horse has remained in Britain during the intervening period.

34 A horse which is trained outside Britain or which has been out of Britain within the previous 6 months shall not be declared a runner . . . until there has been deposited with the clerk of the course either: (i) A passport with the vaccination section endorsed by a v. surgeon or by a recognised Turf authority to the effect that it has received 2 primary injections against equine influenza and thereafter a booster injection within each successive 14 months, or (ii) In cases where no passport has been issued, vaccination certificates signed by a v. surgeon stating that it has received the vaccination required under sub-rule (i) of this rule. The requirements of this rule shall not apply . . . after . . . the horse is first declared a runner in any race provided it has remained in Britain during the intervening period.

. . . When a passport is endorsed for a horse to go abroad and the horse does not travel for any reason, the trainer must return the passport to the Racing Calendar office within 48 hours of the original travelling date for the endorsement to be cancelled.

91 (ii) (a) Yearlings shall not run for any race.

(iii) . . . Two-year-olds shall not run—
  (a) more than 5 furlongs before June 1.
  (b) more than 6 furlongs before July 1.
  (c) more than 7 furlongs before September 1.

148 No horse shall run in shoes which have protrusions on the ground surface other than calkins on the hind, limited to $\frac{1}{4}$in. in length.

180 (ii) Where a horse has been the subject of an examination under Rule 14 (vi) and has been found to have received any substance (other than a normal nutrient) which could alter its racing performance at the time of racing, the horse shall be disqualified for the race in question and may, at the discretion of the stewards . . . be disqualified for such time and for such races as they shall determine.

The case of Rock Roi (disqualified after winning the 1971 Ascot Gold Cup because oxyphenbutazone was found in his urine) was followed by a Jockey Club statement on 21 October 1971. This said although it had been suggested phenylbutazone and other anti-inflammatory drugs should be permitted (as in some States in America) the Jockey Club did not intend to alter existing rule.

It also laid down proceedure if an official sample is reported positive—

(a) on a request from the trainer a portion of the sample will be sent direct from the forensic laboratory to an analyst nominated by the trainer, or (b) facilities will be provided at the laboratory for the trainer's analyst either to be present during examination of the specimen or to carry out tests in the presence of the director.

182 A horse is not qualified to start for any race—(iv) if he has been tubed on the day of the race.

Originally, this rule was to prevent horses racing with anaesthetic in blood. Such a case would now be covered by rule 180 (ii) and no present-day trainer is likely to want to race horse immediately after surgery. See tube.

The Royal College of Veterinary Surgeons issued, on 5 November 1971 (following the Rock Roi case, see Jockey Club rule 180 (ii)) a statement including:

If a veterinarian recommends the discontinuance of any such drug (anti-inflammatory) not less than 8 days before racing (even although such a period may be longer than is necessary in many instances) he should be able to feel sure that he has catered for all but the most exceptional case.

The College issues a 53-page guide to professional conduct which states:

> . . . it is still unprofessional for a veterinarian to advertise or describe himself to the public by titles such as consultant, specialist, canine surgeon or equine surgeon. To do so is to claim, by the use of a distinctive style, to be possessed of exceptional knowledge and skill and this would be the very essence of advertising. . . . This general rule does not, however, preclude the announcement by a veterinarian to fellow vets that he is available for consultation in any speciality.

Ministry of Agriculture rules include: **breeding** Stallions of most breeds other than Thoroughbred must have a licence (£11.55) or permit from the Ministry (Livestock Improvement Branch, Great Westminster House, London SW1).

> Horse Breeding Rules 9. The following diseases . . . shall render a stallion unsuitable for breeding . . . cataract, roaring, whistling, ringbone (high and low), side bone, bone spavin, navicular disease, shivering, stringhalt or defective genital organs.

> 11 . . . a licence shall not be revoked on the ground only of the stallion being affected in its wind if it has attained the age of 9 and a licence . . . has been in force for 2 years.

Export, transit and import (Diseases of Animals Act 1950)

> 37 (i) . . . Any horse over $14\frac{1}{2}$ hands . . . and a foal travelling with its dam if the dam is over that height, shipped from any port or aerodrome in Britain to any . . . outside the UK, Channel Islands and Isle of Man, to be examined by a **v.** inspector immediately before being shipped . . . except:
> a) any horse shipped to any port or aerodrome which is in the Republic of Ireland or which is not in Europe and any foal travelling with its dam. . . .
> b) any horse which the Minister is satisfied is intended for exhibition, breeding, racing, jumping, riding or polo, or

c) a foal travelling with its dam if the dam is any such horse as referred to in paragraph b)

... in every case in which paragraph b) or c) shall apply, a permit authorising the shipment of the horse shall be obtained. ...

39 If any horse . . . has a limb broken or is otherwise seriously injured . . . so as to be incapable of being disembarked without cruelty, the master of the vessel on which a horse is shipped shall carry a proper killing instrument. ...

Rules also require horses to be rested before shipment, except approx. those categories exempt from examination. Lighting, ventilation, stalls etc on ships/planes which carry horses are also subject to Ministry rules. All imports of equine animals are subject to licence and there is no statutory list of prohibited countries. This means applications to import from countries previously infected with disease but now clear, are considered on individual merits. Rules are covered by following sections of Diseases of Animals Act:

Export of Horses (Excepted Cases) Order 1969
Export of Horses (**V.** Examination) Order 1966
Export of Horses (Protection) Order 1969
Horses (Sea-transport) Order 1952 (Amendment 1958)
Transit of Horses Order 1951
Horses (Landing from N Ireland and Republic of Ireland) Order 1954
Equine Animals (Importation) Order 1973

All are available from HM Stationery Office, PO Box 569, London SE1 or 49 High Holborn, London WC1.

Notifiable diseases (ie those of which Ministry must be informed) affecting horses: epizootic lymphangitis (qv); anthrax (qv); glanders (qv, Glanders or Farcy Order 1938); parasitic (see mange, sarcoptic, Order 1938); rabies (qv. Order 1938). Ministry can also restrict movement of horses when diseases such as foot and mouth are evident (Foot And Mouth Disease, Infected Areas Restrictions Order 1938).

Pit ponies Rules governing use of horses (ponies, mules and donkeys) in mines and quarries include:

No horse to be taken below ground until it is 4 or more; if it is blind; unless it has been certified free of glanders; is examined by a vet at least once a year; and is fit.

Rules also govern stabling above and below ground, horse's general care and number of hours it is allowed to work.

Quarantine Regulations vary according to where horse began its journey, whether or not it has been vaccinated, eg against encephalomyelitis (not yet a notifiable disease in Britain) and the diseases with which it might have been in contact. The Thoroughbred Breeders' Association recommends quarantine measures to reduce risk of virus abortion by equine herpesvirus I (formerly rhinopneumonitis):

1 Wherever possible mares should be foaled at home and sent to stallion with healthy foal at foot. . . .

Disadvantages are: (1) Foal will not gain passive immunity—from dam's colostrum—against environment in which it will live. (2) Cost of supervising foaling (sitting up) at home is great. (3) Risk of virus abortion small compared with other causes of abortion.

2 Where this is not possible, the best solution would be that at least 1 month before a mare foals, she should be sent to stud where the stallion is standing and put into group isolation. . . .
3 Mares in late pregnancy which have come from a sale constitute a risk to the stud where the mare is sent. . . .
4 Most abortions result from infection from aborted fetus, although infection through respiratory tract cannot be ruled out.
5 Present evidence indicates no harm is done if mare is covered 1 month after she has had an abortion caused by rhinopneumonitis virus.

General.
(i) Foals or yearlings arriving on a stud from abroad should be isolated or at least kept apart from pregnant mares. They should be watched for any nasal discharge and not have contact with foaling mares for at least 6 weeks from time of arriving on stud or disappearance of any respiratory trouble.
(ii) It is essential that cleansing and disinfection of horse conveyances are carried out strictly in accordance with the regulations of the Ministry of Agriculture, Fisheries & Food and that an approved disinfectant is used.

(iii) Isolation facilities should be provided at all studs to prevent spread of rhinopneumonitis and other infections. The design and construction should be in consultation with a veterinary surgeon who should also be consulted about the precautions to be taken to prevent spread of infection by the attendant.

Action to be taken when abortion occurs.

(i) Action should be taken in the case of any abortion, or of a foal being born dead, or dying within 7 days of birth. The stud's veterinary surgeon must be notified immediately . . . and fetus or carcase sent to the Equine Research Station . . . or similar centre for post-mortem examination.

(ii) The mare should be put into strict isolation pending result of post-mortem, . . . all bedding and traces of foaling should be burnt, the mare washed down with disinfectant, such as Cetrimide BP and box thoroughly cleansed using water under pressure or steam and subsequently disinfected using a disinfectant approved for general purposes by the Ministry of Agriculture. . . . Before the box is used again for horses, it should be hosed down with clean water to remove residual disinfectant.

(iii) If rhinopneumonitis is diagnosed at a stud the Association (TBA) should be notified immediately. At the same time owners or their agents with mares at the stud or due to send mares should be informed. Those studs to which mares from the infected premises have been, or are to be, sent, should also be informed. . . .

(iv) Barren and maiden mares and those which have foaled at home, can be accepted on the stud at any time.

(v) These mares . . . can leave the stud at which abortion has occurred after 1 month from date of the last abortion provided they are isolated from in-foal mares at their home stud for 2 months.

(vi) The stud's own mares can visit other studs at any time after 1 month from the date of the last abortion provided they can be isolated for 2 months from in-foal mares at the stud they are visiting. . . .

(vii) Mares returned from studs where rhinopneumonitis virus abortion has occurred during the previous season should be foaled in isolation at home.

v. surgeon (syns. veterinarian, vet, probably from L. vetus, old or veterinae, old hack) Anyone whose name is on register of Royal College of Veterinary Surgeons. In Britain **v.s.** qualifies, usually after 5 years, at one of 7 universities: Bristol, Cambridge, Dublin, Edinburgh, Glasgow, Liverpool, London. He or she is entitled to initials MRCVS (Member of Royal College) and is now required to pass degree set by particular university, eg Bachelor of Veterinary Science (BVSc—Bristol, Liverpool); Bachelor of Veterinary Medicine (Vet MB—Cambridge); Bachelor of Veterinary Medicine and Surgery (BVMS—Edinburgh, Glasgow); Bachelor of Veterinary Medicine (BVetMed—London); Bachelor of Veterinary Medicine (MVB—Dublin). Higher qualifications are masters' degrees and doctorates, eg Master in Veterinary Medicine (MVM—Cambridge and Dublin); Master of Veterinary Science (MVSc—Liverpool); Master of Veterinary Surgery (MVS—Glasgow); Master of Philosophy (MPhil—London); Doctor of Veterinary Science (DVSc—Liverpool); Doctor of Veterinary Medicine (DVetMed—London); Doctor of Veterinary Medicine (DVM—Glasgow); Doctor of Veterinary Medicine and Surgery (DVM&S—Edinburgh); Doctor of Philosophy (PhD); Master of Science (MSc); Doctor of Science (DSc). (Initials of other higher degrees included in dictionary under BV, Dr, DV, FR, MB, MV, VetMB, VM.) Fellowship of the Royal College (FRCVS) is gained by thesis, additional exam, contribution to learning or by election. (Approx. 200 Fellows in 1973.) Vets work in general practice (about 3,900 in Britain at last census, 1970); in teaching or research; overseas; for Ministry of Agriculture or for Royal Army Veterinary Corps. Each racecourse appoints one or more **v.s.**'s to work at its meetings and the College approves vets to inspect riding schools. See also Royal College. **V. Times** Monthly newspaper published by Shape Newspapers, 308 Kew Road, Richmond, Surrey (01 836 3605).

Vetidrex Trade name. See hydrochlorothiazide.

VetMB Abbr. Bachelor of Veterinary Medicine.

vice Act of atypical, usually unpleasant, behaviour. Either declarable at most sales (eg weaving); aggressive towards humans (eg biting, kicking); or developed against restraint, eg bucking. **V.**'s usually declarable; crib-biting, weaving, wind-sucking, shivering. (Hobday or other wind operation or state of being a rig should be stated.) Any of these conditions can affect soundness, qv. Other habits considered a **v.** include rearing, bolting, jibbing or shying. These may have developed as a result of fear, faulty hearing or vision or may be sign of ill-temper or playfulness. See separate headings.

viral Of, or caused by, a virus. **v. arteritis** See equine **v.** arteritis. **v. abortion** See abortion.

viremia Presence of virus in blood.

virulence (L. virulentia, from virus, poison) Micro-organisms' ability to cause disease, especially acute or fatal one.

virus Extremely small living particles which infect and cause disease in man, animals and plants. Unlike bacteria, they are not visible with ordinary microscopes; they reproduce only in living cells and can pass

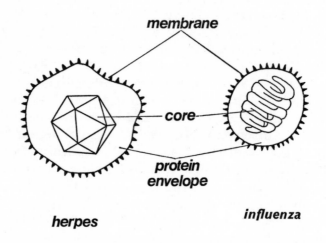

44 Herpesvirus and influenza virus, illustrating different shapes of nucleic acid core

through filters which trap bacteria. **v. abortion** See abortion. **v., classification of** Depends on size (measured in millimicrons—mμ), shape and chemical make-up. Group 1 contain ribonucleic acid (RNA); group 2 contain deoxyriboneucleic acid (DNA). Group 1: (a) myxovirus (80–120 mμ) A/equi 1 and A/equi 2—equine flu; (b) picornavirus (20–35 mμ) parainfluenza 3—acute upper respiratory infection; (c) reovirus (about 70 mμ)—diarrhoea, African horse sickness; (d) arborvirus (20–50mμ) Arthropod-borne virus—encephalomyelitis. Group 2: (a) equine herpesvirus (syns. EHV1, rhinopneumonitis, equine abortion virus—about 150mμ); at least 2 sub-types: Ky-D strain, isolated in Kentucky, USA 1952; army 183 strain and Japanese isolate H-45 strain—snotty nose, coital exanthema; (b) adenovirus (60–90 mμ)

—pneumonia; (c) papillomavirus (about 50 mμ)—**warts**. Unclassified: equine arteritis, equine infectious anemia (swamp fever). **v. diseases, diagnosis of** 2 methods: (1) By culture of v. in tissue. Sheets of cells grown in special media are innoculated with suspect material, such as nasal swabs from horses with influenza symptoms. The v. grows in cells, causing characteristic changes. (2) By blood examination. Serum is tested for presence of antibodies against a particular v. The concentration of antibodies is measured in terms of titre (qv). In a v. disease the concentration of antibodies rises from acute phase to convalescent stage, 2–4 weeks later. The increase of antibodies is diagnostic of disease because they are specific for the v. To test, it is necessary to have a captive v. (Influenza v. strains A/equi 1 and 2 are known and serum can be tested for them—it is impossible to test against an unknown strain.) See complement fixation test and hemagglutination test. **v.—immunity after infection** Recovery from most v. diseases is followed by strong immunity, though notable exceptions are equine herpesvirus 1 and, to a lesser extent, influenza. Immunity is based on production of antibodies which neutralise v. **v.—interference phenomenon** Animals innoculated with one v. may become resistant to innoculation with another. This interference is not fully understood but may be associated with production of interferon. This appears to be liberated by cells during a v. infection and to prevent further infection by that v. or any other which may enter cells. **v., laboratory study of** V. particles can be separated from bacteria or other matter with filters. (A relatively large v., influenza, is only a tenth of the size of a Staphylococcus bacterium.) An ordinary microscope can be used (1) to see changes in organs affected by v., (2) to detect inclusion bodies, qv, (3) to see changes in tissue culture, qv. An electron microscope (magnification: 1–200,000 diameters) is widely used to study v. V. can be cultivated in minced rabbit kidney and serum; on membranes of chick embryo and in its yolk sac; or in tissue culture, qv. V. cannot be isolated without suitable cells and the use of antibiotics to prevent growth of contaminating bacteria. **v., resistance of** Most v.'s are destroyed by heat and oxidising agents but are resistant to: dryness; low temperature; glycerin and weak concentrations of phenol (0.5%). They can be conserved for some time in glycerin at 0°C. **v., spread of** Similar to spread of bacteria, ie by direct contact, droplet or dust infection, ingestion or parasites.

viscera Organs, alimentary canal and other contents of abdomen, qv.

vision (L. visio, videre, to see) Act or sense of sight. See eye.

vitamin (from L. vita, life) Organic substance necessary for normal metabolism. **v.A** See concentrated **v.A** solution. **v.B₁** See aneurine hydrochloride. **v.B₁₂** (cyanocobalamin) Cobalt-containing substance produced in liver and gut. Dark red crystals essential for protein metabolism and therefore for growth and reproduction. Deficiencies can cause anemia but unlikely in horses. Dose: 2 micrograms/kg. body wt. **v.C** See ascorbic acid. **v.D** See concentrated **v.D** solution.

Vitavel K Trade name. See menaphthone sodium bisulphite.

vitreous (L. vitreus, glassy) Transparent. **v. humor** Fluid in back chamber of eye, qv.

viviparous (vivi + L. parere, to produce) That which produces offspring which has been nourished by a special organ (placenta), eg mare.

VMD Abbr. Doctor Veterinary Medicine (Stockholm and Pennsylvania Universities).

vocal cords Two string-like cords in voice box (larynx) which enable horse to whinny, neigh etc. See equine sounds, Hobday, wind.

voice box (syn. larynx) Short, connecting tube between throat and windpipe; regulates air intake, protects against inhaling dust and is site of voice. Composed of cartilages: 3 single (cricoid, thyroid and epiglottis) and 1 paired (arytenoid). See wind.

volemia Blood volume. **hyper-v.** Abnormally high volume of circulating blood. **hypo-v.** Abnormally low volume.

volume Measure of quantity. **blood v.** Total blood in body, approx. 1 tenth of total weight, eg foal: 3–4 litres; adult; 30–40 litres. **packed cell v.** See hematocrit, blood tests. **stroke v.** Amount of blood pumped by heart at each beat. **tidal v.** Amount of gas passing into or out of lungs during one breath.

volvulus (L. volvere, to twist round) Acute obstruction of alimentary canal. See twist.

vomit To regurgitate stomach contents. Rare in horses, indicating rupture of stomach, grass sickness (qv) and/or impending death.

Vonamycin Trade name. See neomycin sulphate.

vortex (L., whirl; pl. vortices) See whorl.

vulva End part or external opening of genital tract of mare. Opens into vagina and consists of 2 prominent, rounded lips (labiae) which protect clitoris. **V.** merges on either side with skin of perineum. **sloping v.** Poor conformation. See Caslick. **winking of v.** Action of in-season or urinating mare in which clitoris is exposed. See plate 1.

vulval Of vulva, eg **v.** lips.

W

Waler See Australian.

walk See gait.

walking disease Result of cirrhosis (hardening) of liver due to plant toxins such as Crotalaria and Senecio, which contain alkaloids. Symptoms: walking in circles, pressing head against objects. Diagnosis: on jaundiced state and liver function tests (lowered blood albumin and increased serum enzymes). **W horse** See Tennessee.

wall eye Lack of pigment in iris of eye, showing more white than usual around pupil. Said to be sign of ill-temper. See behaviour, marking. **w. of foot** See foot.

wanderer See neonatal maladjustment syndrome.

warble fly Two species significant in UK because their larvae, or warbles, occasionally live in horses (cattle are natural hosts). Hypoderma bovis and Hypoderma lineatum found all over Britain, except in Orkney and Shetland Isles. Also live in Europe, Canada and USA. They are large flies resembling bees. H. lineatum is black with yellow or orange bands; H. bovis, black and yellow. They lay eggs on horse's coat and these stick to base of hairs—H. lineatum eggs in rows, as many as 20 to each hair; H bovis eggs attached singly. 3–6 days later larvae about one fiftieth of an inch long emerge and develop into maggots. These crawl down hairs, burrow into skin and migrate through host's body. In cattle, H. lineatum spend autumn in tissues of leg, chest and belly, then find their way to gullet. In February they migrate to skin under back causing swelling with small hole through which maggot breathes.

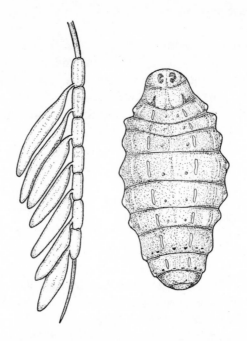

45 Warble fly eggs (H. lineatum) attached to hair
and larva (Hypoderma bovis)

Each maggot forms small abscess and 1–8 days later it moults to
become third and last larval stage. The translucent larvae feed on
inflammatory exudate and turn dark brown. After about 30 days they
leave back through holes in skin, fall on ground and pupate. Adult
flies emerge in May and life cycle is complete. As horse is an unnatural
host, larvae may act unusually, eg migrate to flank or form abscesses
and fail to break through skin. Larvae should never be squeezed; warm
poultices will encourage them to emerge. Tracts leading to swellings are
inflamed lymph channels and not, contrary to popular belief, tracts
made by the maggot. Treatment: see derris, metriphonate.

wart Fleshy or scaly growth on skin. See growth, milk wart, sarcoid.

wasting Loss of weight. Symptoms of red or whiteworm infestation,
tuberculosis, liver disease, chronic infection, ragwort poisoning,
diarrhoea, kidney disease or poor feeding. See metabolism.

water (chemical symbol: H_2O) Should always be available to horse, except in large quantities before hard work, eg race, or being anaesthetised. Washing **w.** through mouth without drinking usually symptom of colic. See fluid balance.

wax (L. cera) Colloq. for dry colostrum at end of teat just before foaling. See birth.

w.b.c. White blood cell (qv) or white blood (cell) count.

wean To separate mare and foal.

weaning Separation of mare and foal. Occurs gradually under natural conditions; feeding becomes less frequent and mare discourages foal by kicking, biting or hindering it. **W.** usually completed by 10–11 months, ie just before birth of next foal. Thoroughbred usually weaned at 5–6 months, by (1) taking group of foals from mares, confining foals to loose boxes for 2 or 3 days, until calling and anxiousness has died away (mares must be out of calling distance); (2) programme **w.**, kinder method in which group of mares and foals have one or two mares taken away at regular intervals of say, 2 days, until finally one mare is left with all the foals. Then she is removed. Mares usually taken away as group is let free in paddock and weaned foals are returned to own boxes at getting-in time. Method can be equally effective if mares and foals are out day and night. Group members should know one another and their paddock; mares with difficult temperaments should be taken first. **w., preparation for** Foal should be encouraged to eat away from its dam (with bars over small manger and creep feeding in paddock, ie rails foal can walk beneath, but mare cannot). After **w.**, protein in feed should be increased to compensate for loss of milk. (See food.) **w. problems** Mare's udder may become hot, swollen and tender, but it rarely needs treatment. Milking udder to relieve pressure stimulates formation of more milk and should be done only in exceptional circumstances. Liniments, ointments etc on outside of udder are unnecessary. If extensive swelling develops and mare is reluctant to move or goes off feed, suspect mastitis (qv). Quantity of food can be reduced, but not drastically, as sudden cutback may be harmful to pregnant mare. Water intake should not be restricted as it may cause stoppage. Exercise is helpful. Foals may fret and go off feed, especially if method (1) was used. They may weave, crib-bite and box-walk, but pairing foals is unsatisfactory because fretting will develop when pairs are split. Grids between boxes may settle restless foals.

weave To shift weight from one foreleg to the other and, usually swing neck and head from side to side. Considered bad nervous habit which takes off condition and may weaken tendons of forelegs. See vice.

WEE Abbr. Western equine encephalomyelitis. See encephalomyelitis.

weight Measure of heaviness. **birth w.** Measured to help determine maturity/immaturity. Thoroughbred: 50kg. (approx 110lb.), pony; 18–32kg. (approx. 40–70lb.). **w. loss** See wasting, metabolism.

weights and measures

MASS

metric

1 kilogram (kg.)	= 15,432 grains or 35.274 ounces or 2.2046 pounds
1 gram (G. or gm.)	= 15.432 grains
1 milligram (mg.)	= 0.015432 grains
(1,000 mg.=1 gm.)	

imperial

1 ton (2,240lb.)	= 1,016 kilograms
1 hundredweight (112lb.)	= 50.80 kilograms
1 stone (14lb.)	= 6.35 kilograms
1 pound (avoirdupois)	= 453.59 grams.
1 ounce (oz.)	= 28.35 grams
1 grain (gr.)	= 64.799 milligrams

CAPACITY

metric

1 litre (l.)	= 1.7598 pints
1 millilitre (ml.)	= 16.894 minims

imperial

1 gallon (gal.) (160fl.oz.)	= 4.546 litres
1 pint (pt.)	= 568.25 millilitres or 0.56825 litres
1 fluid ounce (fl.oz.)	= 28.412 millilitres
1 fluid drachm (fl.dr.)	= 3.5515 millilitres
1 minim (min.)	= 0.059192 millilitres

LENGTH

metric

1 kilometre (km.)	= 0.621 miles
1 metre (m.)	= 39.370 inches
1 decimetre (dm.)	= 3.9370 inches
1 centimetre (cm.)	= 0.39370 inch
1 millimetre (mm.)	= 0.039370 inch
1 micron (μ)	= 0.0039370 inch

imperial

1 mile	= 1.609 kilometres
1 yard	= 0.914 metres
1 foot	= 30.48 centimetres
1 inch	= 2.54 centimetres or 35.40 millimetres

TEMPERATURE
conversion tables

Centigrade	Fahrenheit	Centigrade	Fahrenheit
110°	230°	38°	100.4°
100	212	37.5	99.5
95	203	37	98.6
90	194	36.5	97.7
85	185	36	96.8
80	176	35.5	95.9
75	167	35	95
70	158	34	93.2
65	149	33	91.4
60	140	32	89.6
55	131	31	87.8
50	122	30	86
45	113	25	77
44	111.2	20	68
43	109.4	15	59
42	107.6	10	50
41	105.8	+5	41
40.5	104.9	0	32
40	104	−5	23
39.5	103.1	−10	14
39	102.2	−15	+5
38.5	101.3	−20	−4

To convert Fahrenheit into Centigrade: subtract 32, multiply remainder by 5 and divide result by 9.

To convert Centigrade to Fahrenheit: multiply by 9, divide by 5 and add 32.

Approx. equivalent doses in metric and imperial (apothecaries') systems *

grams (gms.)	grains (gr.)	grams (gms.)	grains (gr.)
10	150	2	30
8	120	1.6	25
6	90	1.2	20
5	75	1	15
4	60	0.8	12
3	45	0.6	10
2.5	40	0.5	8

Approx. equivalent doses in metric and imperial (apothecaries' systems)*

milligrams (mg.)	grains (gr.)	milligrams (mg.)	grains (gr.)
400	6	6	1/10
300	5	5	1/12
250	4	4	1/16
200	$3\frac{1}{2}$	3	1/20
150	$2\frac{1}{2}$	2.5	1/24
120	2	2	1/30
100	$1\frac{1}{2}$	1.5	1/40
80	$1\frac{1}{3}$	1.2	1/50
75	$1\frac{1}{4}$	1	1/60
60	1	0.8	1/80
50	$\frac{3}{4}$	0.6	1/100
40	$\frac{3}{5}$	0.5	1/120
30	$\frac{1}{2}$	0.4	1/160
25	$\frac{2}{5}$	0.3	1/200
20	$\frac{1}{3}$	0.25	1/240
15	$\frac{1}{4}$	0.2	1/300
12.5	$\frac{1}{5}$	0.15	1/400
10	$\frac{1}{6}$	0.12	1/500
8	$\frac{1}{8}$		

Approx. equivalent doses in metric and imperial
(apothecaries' system) *

millilitres (ml.)	minims (min.)	millilitres (ml.)	minims (min.)
10	150	0.8	12
8	120	0.6	10
6	90	0.5	8
5	75	0.4	6
4	60	0.3	5
3	45	0.25	4
2.5	40	0.2	3
2	30	0.15	$2\frac{1}{2}$
1.6	25	0.12	2
1.3	20	0.1	$1\frac{1}{2}$
1	15		

1 fluid ounce = approx. 30ml.
1 fluid drachm = approx. 4ml.
15 minims = approx. 1ml.

*Tables can be used for direct transference of doses from one system to the other; but multiples should not be used as approximation might raise figure significantly.

To convert grams per 100ml. into grains per ounce multiply by 4,375.
To convert grams into ounces, multiply by 10 and divide by 283.
To convert litres into pints, multiply by 88 and divide by 50.
To convert kilos into pounds, multiply by 1,000 and divide by 454.

Welsh Cob Good-natured breed developed from **W.** Mountain pony and with some of that breed's hardiness. Heavy type used in harness has high-stepping trot, but is now dying out, leaving riding type. Usually 14–15 hands, compact and can carry 14-stone rider. Most colours including dun, but piebald and skewbald not favoured. **W. Mountain** Breed often thought most beautiful of British mountain and moorland types. Origins are lost but looks indicate Arab blood. Strong, willing, up to 12 hands; makes good child's pony. Some authorities believe breed is more susceptible than most to cryptorchidism (see rig) and that condition is inherited from free-running rig ponies. Assn: **W.** Pony and Cob Soc., c/o T. E. Roberts, 32 North Parade, Aberystwyth, Cardiganshire (Aberystwyth 2924).

Westland See Fjord.

wheat (Triticum sativum) Cereal plant, husk of which (bran) fed to horses. The grain should not be given as likely to cause laminitis or eczema and, in amounts over 7lb., death.

whirlpool treatment See physiotherapy.

whistling Noise made by horse unsound in wind, qv.

white See albinism, coat colouring. **w. blood cells** (syns. w.b.c., leucocytes) Cells in blood stream, tissues and organs. 5 types: neutrophil (poly-morphonuclear leucocyte) which eats bacteria, dead cells and debris by amoeboid action; lymphocyte, which helps produce antibodies; eosinophil, which deals with allergic conditions and parasites; monocyte, which has similar function to neutrophil; basophil, which is part of inflammatory reaction (see also platelet, which helps clotting of blood). Normal **w.b.c.** count 5–10,000 per cu.mm. Any increase (leucocytosis) indicates bacterial and (lymphocytosis) viral infection; decrease (leucopenia) suggests arteritis or other virus infection. See blood tests. **w. bryony poisoning** Caused by eating **w.b.** plant Symptoms: sweating, severe purging, convulsions, stupor, sometimes death. No specific treatment available. **w. line** Junction of wall of foot with sole. Seen in upturned hoof as line inside circumference of wall.

whiteworm Nematode (roundworm parasite) of order Ascaroidea (see plate 26). Ascaris equi/equorum is largest roundworm in horses; male 15–30cm. (6–12ins.), female 12–24cm. (5–9½ins.). Life history is direct: adults live in small intestine, females lay eggs, which pass out in droppings; infective larvae develop and are swallowed, then burrow through intestinal wall. Blood stream carries them to liver, heart and lungs. From lungs they travel up windpipe to throat and are swallowed. Larvae pass through stomach to intestines, where they grow into adults, completing the cycle in about 12 weeks. A female can contain 27 million eggs and lay 200,000 a day. The eggs live many months, are resistant to many chemicals and are most dangerous to young horses. Can cause unthriftiness, lung damage and occasionally rupture of gut. Diagnosis: on finding eggs in dung. Treatment: see carbon disulphide, piperazine salts.

whorl (syn. vortex) Spiral twist, eg in muscles around heart; hairs in coat (usually about 1in. wide and on neck; see marking).

whorlbone lameness (syn. trochanteric bursitis) Lameness common in Standardbred (qv) after fall or strain in training. Caused by inflamed bursa beneath tendon of gluteus muscle where it passes over part of femur (great trochanter). Symptoms: pain on pressure over hip area, leg flexed at rest, weight put on outside of foot during action. Treatment: pain-killers and corticosteroid injections into bursa.

wild Untamed; animal whose ancestors have never been domesticated. The 5 w. species of living Equidae: Przewalski, Asiatic wild ass, common zebra, mountain zebra, Grevy's zebra. Cf feral.

wind (colloq. for breathing) Important part of soundness examination, qv. **gone in the w.** Any fault in respiration. **heaves/broken w.** (syn. emphysema) See broken w. **w. infirmities** roaring, whistling, gurgling. All sounds made by horse with partially blocked nasal passages, **w. pipe** (trachea) or voice box (larynx.) Obstruction may be wart or growth (rare), soft palate or vocal cords. If cartilage (arytenoid) and muscles of voice box are weak they will not pull aside cords when horse inhales; cords will stay in relaxed (exhaling) position, ie centre of voice box. (Cords are arranged like 2 half-cups facing upwards against sides of voice box. Air can easily escape, but cannot as easily enter, unless cups are pulled aside.) Diagnosis: on hearing noise as horse inhales at gallop—not to be confused with normal breathing-out sounds (cf soft palate, tongue swallowing). Viewing with larnygoscope (qv) can reveal lack of cord movement and deformed shape of voice box. Treatment: Hobday or similar operation. **w. pipe** (syn. trachea) Cartilaginous tube from voice box to lungs; extends down front of neck, then branches into 2 main bronchi. Lined with epithelial (qv) cells which have tiny hairs (cilia) attached. These wave in the air flow to trap any particles which can be coughed out.

windgall (syn. wind puff) Swelling of joint (articular **w.**, caused by arthritis) or of tendon sheath (tendinous **w.**), caused by sprain (tearing of fibres in tendon or tendon sheath). Swellings also appear in general ill-health, eg allergy, infection. See plate 22.

wind-sucking Gulping and swallowing of air. May be accompanied by crib-biting, qv. Nervous habit which impairs digestion and may increase foul-smelling flatus; considered a vice, qv.

wink Colloq. to contract lips of vulva, exposing clitoris. Seen in mare in oestrus and after urinating. See behaviour.

withers Top of shoulders, between neck and back; formed by 3rd–9th thoracic vertebrae (see vertebral column). Highest point of **w.** usually higher than back (cf donkey) and used in measuring horse's height. See hand, fistulous **w.**

wobbler syndrome (syns. ataxia, inco-ordination) Condition of poor co-ordination, especially of hindlegs and sometimes forelegs. May appear from 3 months to 3 years, although older horses can be affected. Onset may be gradual or sudden; there is dragging of toes of hindlegs and unsteadiness in pulling up, backing or turning. Horse may be able to cope with condition but some cannot get up and have to be destroyed. Mildly affected mares may be used for breeding, but in some cases it is unwise to allow stallion to mount. There is no known treatment and most insurance companies allow destruction on humane grounds and meet claims. Cause may be injury to spinal canal or cord, malformed or fractured cervical vertebrae, nutritional deficiency, abscesses. True **w.s.** may be inherited condition of malformed vertebrae. Cf neonatal maladjustment syndrome, cerebellar degeneration, segmental myelitis.

wolf tooth See teeth.

womb See uterus.

Wood's filter See filter.

wound Breach in continuity of skin made by kick, blow, sharp object, etc. **open w.** Cut. **lacerated w.** Tear, eg from barbed wire. **puncture w.** Small, penetrating hole produced by nail, pitchfork, etc. **W.** healing is by 1st intention (when edges of skin are stitched together and epithelium grows into direct union without scar tissue) or by 2nd intention (when proud flesh fills gap between edges of skin before epithelium grows). Treatment: wash with weak antiseptic and remove debris, stitch (suture) as soon as possible. Once granulation tissue starts to grow, ie after about 12 hours, 1st intention healing becomes more difficult. Lotion, eg of zinc sulphate, helps prevent proud flesh. Skin **w.** over bone heals better than over muscle, due to absence of swelling and oedema. All **w.'s** heal faster in presence of oxygen, therefore dressing should be permeable, eg polypropylene sheeting (filmy plastic-like material used especially on site of operation). Antitetanus serum should be given unless horse has previously been immunised.

wry neck Type of difficult birth (dystocia) in which head of fetus is bent backwards. Difficult to straighten manually as neck vertebrae usually damaged. Dismemberment of fetus (embryotomy) or caesarian section usually necessary.

X

X Female sex chromosome. See chromosome.

xerosis (Gr.) Abnormally dry, eg coat, eyes, in dehydrated state. See dehydration, dry-coat.

X-ray (syn. Rontgen ray) Energy wave of same type as light ray, but of much shorter wave-length (approx. 5×10^7cm.). See radiation, plate 41.

xylocaine hydrochloride Trade name. See lignocaine hydrochloride.

Y

Y Male sex chromosome. See chromosome.

yellow body (syn. corpus luteum) Structure in ovary formed after rupture of follicle and shedding of egg (ovulation); produces progesterone and lasts about 15–17 days. It is then destroyed—probably by hormone prostaglandin secreted in uterus. Follicle fills with blood clot; luteal cells grow into clot and organise themselves into **y.b.**, which controls dioestrus. **y.b. of pregnancy** One which lasts beyond usual span of 17 days (if a fertilised egg arrives in uterus during dioestrus). It is joined by accessory **y.b.**'s which maintain pregnancy to about day 150. After this fetus produces progesterone and ovaries become quiescent. **y. star thistle (centaurea soostitialis) poisoning** Causes chewing disease, with firming of muscles of face and muzzle, in N California.

yellows Colloq. for jaundice, qv.

yew poisoning Caused by eating y. (Taxus baccata), most poisonous tree native to Britain. Contains alkaloid taxine, which depresses heart action. Horse usually dies almost immediately. If death is delayed there may be intense inflammation of stomach. Diagnosis: on finding fragments of leaves in stomach and intestines. Treatment not usually possible.

yolk sac placenta Outgrowth of fetal gut, richly supplied with blood vessels. Nourishes fetus up to about 30 days' gestation and is then replaced by true placenta.

Yorkshire Coach horse Virtually extinct draught type developed from Cleveland Bay, qv.

Z

zebra (Amharic, striped) 3 types: common or Burchell's **z.** (Equus quagga burchelli, has 44 chromosomes); mountain **z.** (Equus zebra); and, largest and most horse-like, Grevy's **z.** (Equus grevyi, 46 chromosomes). Each lives in parts of Africa, may eat leaves and shoots instead of grass and has dark stripes and ass-like conformation, ie large ears, **thick neck, boxy hooves. Generally believed the more primitive a** species, the more striped or distinctly-marked it is. Different types of **z.** unlikely to become one breed because cross-breds are usually sterile. See chromosome, coat colouring.

Zeeland Heavy Dutch breed well known in middle ages but whose name is no longer officially recognised by Netherlands Ministry of Agriculture. More supple than its neighbour, Dutch Draught (qv) and has probably interbred with that massive type. Sometimes used as circus horse.

Zemaituka/s (from Zemaitifa, colloq. for W Lithuania; pl. Zemaitukai) Russian horse of great stamina, known in 13th century and probably developed from Przewalski (qv) and Arab. Up to about 15 hands and most often dun or mousey coloured with dorsal stripe.

Zephiran Trade name. See benzalkonium chloride solution.

zinc oxide White or yellowish-white soft odourless tasteless powder. Applied to skin in ointments, pastes and lotions as mild astringent and to protect. Heals saddle sores. **z. poisoning** Caused by taking in contaminated food or water (usually near brass foundry). More serious if lead is also ingested. Symptoms: constipation, gastroenteritis, arthritis, paralysed throat. **z. sulphate** Colourless crystals or white crystalline odourless powder with astrigent metallic taste. Solutions containing 10–25% used to treat proud flesh. See wound.

Zmudzin Type of Konik, qv.

Zolaphen Trade name. See phenylbutazone.

zygote (Gr. zygotos, yoked together) Fertilised egg. See embryology.

DRUG MANUFACTURERS

BRITISH AND IRISH

The following is a list of drug and veterinary equipment manufacturers. (If an entry ends with a group of figures in parentheses this is the telephone number, the exchange for which is the town in the address.)

Abbott Laboratories Ltd, Queenborough, Kent (079 56 3371)

Allen & Hanburys Ltd, Bethnal Green, London E2 6LR (01 739 4343)

Arnolds Veterinary Products Ltd, 1 Cremyl Road, Reading, Berkshire RG1 8HF (54064)

Astra Chemicals Ltd, Eastern Way, Bury St Edmunds, Suffolk (2041)

BDH Pharmaceuticals Ltd, Birkbeck Street, London E2 (01 739 3451)

Beecham Veterinary Products, Great West Road, Brentford, Middlesex (01 560 5151)

Berk Pharmaceuticals Ltd, Cattershall Lane, Godalming, Surrey (4191)

Bioglan Laboratories, Hertford, Hertfordshire (01 284 2137)

Boots Pure Drug Co, Nottingham NG2 3AA (56111)

Boileau & Boyd Ltd, Dublin, Ireland

Bristol Veterinary Products, Station Road, Langley, Buckinghamshire (Slough 44511)

British Cod Liver Oils, Hull, Yorkshire HU9 5NJ

British Drug Houses. See BDH Pharmaceuticals Ltd

Brookwick, Ward & Co, 8 Shepherds Bush Road, London W6 (01 743 1847)

Burroughs Wellcome & Co, Berkhamsted, Hertfordshire (3333)

Ciba-Geigy Agrochemicals Ltd, Whittlesford, Cambridge (Sawston 3621)

Constant Laboratories Ltd, Co Dublin, Ireland

Crookes Laboratories Ltd, Telford Road, Basingstoke, Hampshire (3212)

Crown Chemical Co, Lamberhurst, Kent (491)

Cynamid of GB Ltd, Fareham Road, Gosport, Hampshire, PO Box 13 OAS (Fareham 6131)

Dales Pharmaceuticals Ltd, Barrows Lane, Steeton, Yorkshire

Duphar Veterinary Ltd, Gater's Hill, West End, Southampton, Hampshire (West End 2281)

Elanco Products Ltd, Broadway House, London SW19 1RR (01 542 6600)

Enzypharm Biochemicals Ltd, 179 Heath Road, Twickenham, Middlesex (01 892 2028)

Epsom Veterinary Remedies Ltd, Hyde End Farm, Shinfield, Berkshire

FAIR Laboratories Ltd, 179 Heath Road, Twickenham, Middlesex (01 892 2028)

Gillman & Spencer Ltd, Bilton Road, Bletchley, Buckinghamshire (77271)

Glaxo Laboratories Ltd, Greenford, Middlesex TW4 6JH (01 422 3434)

Hoechst Pharmaceuticals Ltd, Salisbury Road, Hounslow, Middlesex (01 570 7712)

Imperial Chemical Industries Ltd, Alderley Park, Macclesfield, Cheshire (Alderley Edge 2828)

Intervet Laboratories Ltd, Viking Way, Bar Hill, Cambridge CB3 8EW (Crafts Hill 503)

Leo Laboratories Ltd, 27 Uxbridge Road, Hayes, Middlesex (01 573 6224)

Loveridge Ltd, 6 Millbrook Road, Southampton, Hampshire (28411)

May & Baker Ltd, Dagenham, Essex RM1 07X5 (01 592 3060)

Merck Sharp & Dohme Ltd, Hoddesdon, Hertfordshire (67123)

Parke, Davis & Co, Pontypool, Monmouthshire NP4 8YH (2468)

Pfizer Ltd, Sandwich, Kent (3511)

Pittaway Laboratories, 40 Hertford Place, Coventry, Warwickshire (25751)

Radiol Chemicals Ltd, Stepfield, Witham, Essex (Witham 2538)

Reckitt & Colman Ltd, Hull, Yorkshire (26151)

Reducine Co Ltd, 147 Upper Rathmines Road, Dublin 6, Ireland

Robinson & Sons Ltd, Wheatbridge Mills, Chesterfield, Derbyshire (76931)

Shaw's Veterinary Chemists Ltd, Aston Clinton, Aylesbury, Buckinghamshire

Smith Kline & French Laboratories Ltd, Welwyn Garden City, Hertfordshire (25111)

Spillers Ltd, Kentford, Newmarket, Suffolk (75503)

Squibb & Sons Ltd, Regal House, London Road, Twickenham, Middlesex (01 892 0164)

Stafford-Miller Ltd, 166 Great North Road, Hatfield, Hertfordshire

Stayne Veterinary Ltd, Greenfields Road, Bishop Auckland, Co Durham (5281)

Syntex Pharmaceuticals Ltd, St Ives Road, Maidenhead, Berkshire (28424)

Tad Pharmaceutical Products Ltd, 127 Broad Street, Chesham, Buckinghamshire (72653)

Tasman Vaccine Laboratory (UK) Ltd, 208–12 Burnt Oak Broadway, Edgware, Middlesex HA8 0AP (01 952 7494)

Upjohn Ltd, Fleming Way, Crawley, Sussex (31133)

Vestric Ltd, Stonefield Way, Ruislip, Middlesex (01 845 2323)

Veterinary Drug Co, 129–33 Lawrence St, York (58166) also London (01 445 3624), Crewe (55239), Bury St Edmunds (5821)

Volac Ltd, Crayden Old Farm, Royston, Hertfordshire (01 692 3985)

Webster Sales, Livestock Market, Hall Road, Norwich, Norfolk NOR 74C (55971)

Willington Medicals Ltd, Alpha Laboratories, Whitchurch Road, Shrewsbury, Shropshire (52665)

Willows Francis Ltd, 73 Shackwell Lane, London E8 (01 254 6361)

Winton Laboratories Ltd, 54–6 Cheam Common Road, Worcester Park, Surrey (01 337 0731)

Wyeth & Brother Ltd, Huntercombe Lane, South Taplow, Maidenhead, Berkshire (28311)

UNITED STATES

AAM Inc, 5209 S Kedzie Avenue, Chicago, Ill 60632

Albion Laboratories Inc, 101 N Main Street, Clearfield, Utah 84015

Armour Pharmaceutical, Box 3113, Omaha, Nebr 68103

Bickmore, Inc, 1900 Ridge Avenue, Evanston, Ill 60201

Bio Vet, 24201 Frampton Avenue, Harbor City, Calif 90710

Blue Bell Remedy Co, Blue Bell, Pa 19422

Cadco, Inc, 10100 Douglas Avenue, Des Moines, Iowa 50322

Colorado Serum Company, 4950 York Street, Denver, Colo 80216

Corona Manufacturing Company, Box 1214, 345 Glen Iris Drive, Atlanta, Ga 30301

Croyden-Browne Co Inc, Three Caesar Place, Moonachie, NJ 07074

Cut-Heal Inc, 214 Garvon, Garland, Texas 75040

Cutter Labs, Veterinary Division, 12707 W 63rd Street, Sawnee Mission, Kan 66201

Daniels, Dr A. C., Inc, Box 450, RFD, Webster, Mass 01570

Diagnostic Data, Inc, 518 Logue Avenue, Mountain View, Calif 94040

Diamond Shamrock Chemical Co, Fine Chemicals, 60 Park Place, Newark, NJ 07101

Elanco Products Co, Div of Eli Lilly & Co, PO Box 1968, Indianapolis, Ind 46206

Farnum Companies, Inc, PO 21447, East Magnolia, Phoenix, Ariz 85036

Fiebing Chemical Co, 516 S Second Street, Milwaukee, Wisc 53204

General's Pet Products, 238 N 29th Street, Elwood, Ind 46030

General Scientific Equipment Co, Linekiln Pike & Williams Avenue, Philadelphia, Pa 19150

Gilkey Remedy Co, 4035 Lake Cook Road, Northbrook, Ill 60062

Hawthorne Laboratories, 3003 White Way, Louisville, Ky 40205

Hess & Clark, Inc, Div or Rhodia Inc, Seventh & Orange Streets, Ashland, Ohio 44805

Highsmith Co Inc, Hwy 106, Ft Atkinson, Wisc 53538

I-Deal Ideas Inc, PO Box 14, Pablo, Montana 59855

Jack Frost Laboratories, 810 NW 9th Avenue, Ft Lauderdale, Fla 33311

Kendall, Dr B. J. Co, Div of J. H. Guild Co, 10 Main Street, Rupert, Vt 05768

Last, Alvin, Inc, 145 Palisades Street, Dobbs Ferry, NY 10522

Legear Laboratories, Inc, 1304 Ashby Road, PO Box 12650, St Louis, Mo 63132

Martin, C. J. Co, 606 W Main Street, PO Box 1089, Nacogdoches, Texas 75961

McTarnahan's Pharmaceuticals, 145 N Santa Anita Avenue, Arcadia, Calif 91006

Merck & Co Inc, Rahway, NJ 07065

Miller Harness Co, Inc, 131 Varick Street, New York, NY 10013

Myers Laboratories, Div of Zampa, Inc, 578 Nepperhan Avenue, Yonkers, NY 10701

Naylor, H. W., Co, Inc, Main Street, Morris, NY 13808

Old Hickory Medicine Co, Inc, 5813 Lee Hwy, Chattanooga, Tenn

Philips, Roxane, Inc, Div of Anchor Labs Inc, 7621 N Belt Hwy, St Joseph, Mo 64507

Plummer, Dr A. B., Products Co, Inc, Millersburg, Ky 40348

Ralston Pureena Checkerboard Square, 835 S 8th Street, St Louis, Mo 63188

Safety K Stirrup, PO Box 1157, El Cajon, Calif 90222

Shell Chemical Co, Agricultural Div Animal Health, 2401 Crow Canyon Road, San Ramon, Calif 94583

Solvit Chemical Co, Div of Dr A. C. Daniels, Inc., Box 450, Webster, Mass 10570

Southeastern Labs, Inc, PO Box 2023, Jacksonville, Fla 32203

Spohn Medical Co, 202 N Main Street, Goshen, Ind 46526

Square Laboratories, Inc, 100 Mill Street, Revere, Mass 02151

Staley, A. E., Mfg Co, Speciality Feed Dept, PO Box 151, Decatur, Ill 62525

Stockman Brand, Inc, Animal Health Products, 1721 Baltimore Avenue, Kansas City, Mo 64108

Thoroughbred Remedy Corp, 251 Hempstead Turnpike, Elmont, LI, NY 11003

3M Co, Medical Products Div, 3M Center, St Paul, Minn 55101

Troy Chemical Co, Inc, Corral Park, Mount Kisco, NY 10549

Turbulator Co, 28929 Manchester Road, Westland, Mich 48185

Turf Laboratories, PO Box 425, Tustin, Calif 92680

Veach Saddlery Co, 22nd & Princeton Road, Trenton, Mo 64683

Vineland Laboratories, Inc, 2285 E. Landis Avenue, Box 70, Vineland, NJ 08360

Wagner Veterinary Drug Co, 3035 S 4th Street, Louisville, Ky

Western Instrument, 4950 York Street, Denver, Colo 80216

Whitmer Company, PO Box 685, Bowling Green, Ky 42101

Whitmoyer Laboratories, Inc, 19 N Railroad Street, Myerstown, Pa 17067

Zirin Laboratories, 199 W 24th Street, Hialeah, Fla 33010

REFERENCES AND FURTHER READING

Adams, O. R. *Lameness in Horses* (Lee & Febiger, Philadelphia, 2nd ed 1966)

Blood, D. C. and Henderson, J. A. *Veterinary Medicine* (Bailliere, Tindall & Cassel, London, 3rd ed 1968)

Bryans, J. T. and Gerber, H. *Equine Infectious Diseases*, Vol. II (Karger, Basel; New York, 1970)

Campbell, Judith. *Horses and Ponies* (Hamlyn Publishing, Feltham, Middlesex, 1970)

Davidson, Joseph B. *Horsemen's Veterinary Adviser* (Area Publishing Company, Inc, New York)

Dorland's *Medical Dictionary* (W. B. Saunders Co, Philadelphia, 24th ed 1965)

Gaylord Simpson, George. *Horses* (Oxford University Press, New York, 1951)

Glyn, Sir Richard. *The World's Finest Horses and Ponies* (Harrap & Co, London, 1971)

Hayes, M. Horace (revised by J. F. Tutt). *Veterinary Notes for Horseowners* (Stanley Paul, London, 15th ed 1964; Arco Publishing Company, Inc, New York)

Lepage, G. *Veterinary Parasitology* (Oliver & Boyd, Edinburgh and London, 2nd ed 1968)

Mahaffey, Leo W. (ed). *Stud and Stable Veterinary Handbook* (Stud and Stable, London, 1969)

Miller, W. C. and West, G. P. *Black's Veterinary Dictionary* (Adam & Charles Black, London, 8th ed 1967)

Naviaux, James L. *Horses—in Health and Disease* (Arco Publishing Company, Inc, New York)

Pharmaceutical Society of Great Britain. *British Veterinary Codex* (Pharmaceutical Press, London, 1965)

Rossdale, P. D. *The Horse from Conception to Maturity* (California TB Breeders' Assn, Arcadia, Calif, USA (91006), 1972)

Siegmund, O. H. (ed). *Merck's Veterinary Manual* (Merck & Co, Rahway, NJ, USA, 3rd ed 1967)

Sisson, S. and Grossman, J. D. *The Anatomy of the Domestic Animal* (W. B. Saunders Co, Philadelphia, 4th ed 1955)

Smith, Dr R. N. *An Anatomy of the Horse* (Quartilles International, Welwyn Garden City, Hertfordshire, 1972)

Summerhays, R. S. *Observer's Book of Horses and Ponies* (Frederick Warne & Co, London and New York, 1973)